Injury & Trauma Sourcebook

Learning Disabilities Sourcebook, 2nd Edition

Dental Care & Oral Health
Sourcebook

Mental Health Disorders Sourcebook, 3rd
   Edition

Mental Retardation Sourcebook

Movement Disorders Sourcebook

Multiple Sclerosis Sourcebook

Muscular Dystrophy Sourcebook

Obesity Sourcebook

Osteoporosis Sourcebook

Pain Sourcebook, 3rd Edition

Pediatric Cancer Sourcebook

Physical & Mental Issues in Aging
   Sourcebook

Podiatry Sourcebook, 2nd Edition

Pregnancy & Birth Sourcebook, 2nd
   Edition

Prostate Cancer Sourcebook

Prostate & Urological Disorders Sourcebook

Reconstructive & Cosmetic Surgery
   Sourcebook

Rehabilitation Sourcebook

Respiratory Disorders Sourcebook, 2nd
   Edition

Sexually Transmitted Diseases Sourcebook,
   3rd Edition

Sleep Disorders Sourcebook, 2nd Edition

Smoking Concerns Sourcebook

Sports Injuries Sourcebook,

Stress-Related Disorders So
   Edition

Stroke Sourcebook, 2nd Edi

Surgery Sourcebook, 2nd E

Thyroid Disorders Sourcebo

Transplantation Sourcebook

Travele

Urinary
   Dis

Vegeta

Women's Health Concerns Sourcebook, 2nd
   Edition

Workplace Health & Safety Sourcebook

Worldwide Health Sourcebook

ON LINE

Teen Health Series

Abuse and Violence Information for
   Teens

Alcohol Information for Teens

Allergy Information for Teens

Asthma Information for Teens

Body Information for Teens

Cancer Information for Teens

Complementary & Alternative
   Medicine Information for Teens

Diabetes Information for Teens

Diet Information for Teens, 2nd Edition

Drug Information for Teens, 2nd Edition

Eating Disorders Information for Teens

Fitness Information for Teens, 2nd
   Edition

Learning Disabilities Information for
   Teens

Mental Health Information for Teens,
   2nd Edition

Pregnancy Information for Teens

Sexual Health Information for Teens,
   2nd Edition

Information for Teens

ation for Teens

s Information for Teens,
on

ation for Teens

mation for Teens

rmation for Teens

Dental Care
and Oral Health
SOURCEBOOK

Third Edition

Health Reference Series

Third Edition

Dental Care and Oral Health SOURCEBOOK

Basic Consumer Health Information about Dental Care and Oral Health Throughout the Lifespan, Including Facts about Cavities, Bad Breath, Cold and Canker Sores, Dry Mouth, Toothaches, Gum Disease, Malocclusion, Temporomandibular Joint and Muscle Disorders, Oral Cancers, and Dental Emergencies

Along with Information about Mouth Hygiene, Crowns, Bridges, Implants, and Fillings, Surgical, Orthodontic, and Cosmetic Dental Procedures, Pain Management, Health Conditions That Impact Oral Care, a Glossary of Related Terms, and a Directory of Additional Resources

Edited by
Amy L. Sutton

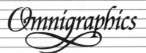
Omnigraphics

P.O. Box 31-1640, Detroit, MI 48231

Bibliographic Note

Because this page cannot legibly accommodate all the copyright notices, the Bibliographic Note portion of the Preface constitutes an extension of the copyright notice.

Edited by Amy L. Sutton

Health Reference Series

Karen Bellenir, *Managing Editor*
David A. Cooke, M.D., *Medical Consultant*
Elizabeth Collins, *Research and Permissions Coordinator*
Cherry Edwards, *Permissions Assistant*
EdIndex, Services for Publishers, *Indexers*

* * *

Omnigraphics, Inc.

Matthew P. Barbour, *Senior Vice President*
Kevin M. Hayes, *Operations Manager*

* * *

Peter E. Ruffner, *Publisher*

Copyright © 2008 Omnigraphics, Inc.

ISBN 978-0-7808-1032-7

Library of Congress Cataloging-in-Publication Data

Dental care and oral health sourcebook : basic consumer health information about dental care and oral health throughout the lifespan, including facts about cavities, bad breath, cold and canker sores, dry mouth, toothaches, gum disease, malocclusion, temporomandibular joint and muscle disorders, oral cancers, and dental emergencies : along with information about mouth hygiene, crowns, bridges, implants, and fillings, surgical, orthodontic, and cosmetic dental procedures, pain management, health conditions that impact oral care, a glossary of related terms, and a directory of additional resources / edited by Amy L. Sutton. -- 3rd ed.
    p. cm. -- (Health reference series)
   Summary: "Provides basic consumer health information about oral health concerns of children and adults, dental hygiene, and surgical, orthodontic, and cosmetic dental procedures. Includes index, glossary of related terms and directory of resources"--Provided by publisher.
   Includes bibliographical references and index.
   ISBN 978-0-7808-1032-7 (hardcover : alk. paper) 1. Dentistry--Popular works. 2. Mouth--Diseases--Popular works. 3. Mouth--Care and hygiene--Popular works. I. Sutton, Amy L.
   RK61.O66 2008
   617.6--dc22
                                                                                    2008038411

 ∞   0 1021 0239491 7

Table of Contents

Visit www.healthreferenceseries.com to view *A Contents Guide to the Health Reference Series*, a listing of more than 14,000 topics and the volumes in which they are covered.

Preface xv

Part I: Introduction to Dental Care and Oral Health

Chapter 1—The Structure of the Mouth and Teeth 3

Chapter 2—Why Are Dental Care and Oral Health So
Important? 9

Section 2.1—Dental Symptoms Can
Expose Health Issues 10

Section 2.2—The Relationship between
Poor Oral Health and Sys-
temic Disease 13

Chapter 3—Infant and Toddler Oral Health 19

Section 3.1—A Healthy Mouth for Your
Baby 20

Section 3.2—The Teething Process and
How to Ease It 22

Section 3.3—What Is Baby Bottle Tooth
Decay? 25

Section 3.4—Early Childhood Tooth Decay
in the United States 29

Section 3.5—Thumbsucking, Pacifier Use,
and Oral Health 33

Chapter 4—Oral Health in Children 35

    Section 4.1—Keeping Your Child's Teeth
                 Healthy...................................... 36

    Section 4.2—Your Child's Nutrition and
                 How It Affects Oral Health 40

Chapter 5—Oral Health in Adolescents 43

    Section 5.1—Oral Health Advice for Teens 44

    Section 5.2—Oral Piercings: What
                 Problems Can They Cause? 49

Chapter 6—Adult Oral Health 51

    Section 6.1—What Adults Can Do to
                 Maintain Good Oral Health 52

    Section 6.2—Dental Concerns in Women 54

    Section 6.3—Menstrual Cycle Affects
                 Periodontal Health 57

    Section 6.4—What Your Gums Can Expect
                 When You're Expecting 58

    Section 6.5—Why Is Dental Care Important
                 for Men?..................................... 60

Chapter 7—Oral Health Concerns in the Elderly 63

    Section 7.1—Overview of Oral Health
                 Concerns in Older Americans.... 64

    Section 7.2—Taking Care of Your Teeth
                 and Mouth as You Age 67

Chapter 8—Oral Care for People with Disabilities or
    Special Needs 71

    Section 8.1—Who Needs Special Dental
                 Care?.. 72

    Section 8.2—Helping Someone Care for
                 Their Teeth and Mouth: A
                 Caregiver's Guide 73

Chapter 9—Recent Research in Dental Care and Oral
    Health 79

    Section 9.1—Researchers Report Initial
                 Success in Promising Approach
                 to Prevent Tooth Decay 80

    Section 9.2—Salivary Diagnostic Device
                 Shows Promise 83

Section 9.3—New Vaccine May Decrease
        Risk of Oral Cancers 86

Section 9.4—The Phenomenon of Dental
        Tourism 88

Part II: Dental Hygiene at Home

Chapter 10—Toothbrushes, Toothpaste, and Other Home
Dental Care Products 95

Section 10.1—Choosing Dental Care
        Materials 96

Section 10.2—The Use and Handling of
        Toothbrushes 99

Section 10.3—Why Is Brushing with
        Toothpaste Important? 102

Section 10.4—Concerns over Imported
        Toothpastes 104

Section 10.5—Oral Irrigation Devices 107

Section 10.6—Mouth Rinses 113

Section 10.7—Denture Cleansers 115

Chapter 11—Cleaning Your Teeth and Gums 119

Chapter 12—Good Nutrition Linked to Healthy Mouths 125

Section 12.1—Vitamins and Minerals
        Needed for Oral Health 126

Section 12.2—Oral Health and Calcium 128

Section 12.3—Gum Chewers Have Reason
        to Smile 129

Section 12.4—Snack Smart for Healthy
        Teeth 132

Section 12.5—Soft Drinks and Oral Health 135

Chapter 13—Fluoride: Its Role in Cavity Prevention 137

Section 13.1—Fluoridated Water:
        Questions and Answers 138

Section 13.2—Your Child's Fluoride Needs 140

Section 13.3—Bottled Water Users: Are You
        Getting Enough Fluoride? 145

Section 13.4—Excess Fluoride Consumption:
        Enamel Fluorosis 152

Part III: At the Dentist's Office

Chapter 14—Finding and Choosing a Dentist 157

Section 14.1—What Are the Dental
Specialties? 158

Section 14.2—The Pediatric Dentist:
Teaching Kids and Teens
to Care for Their Teeth 161

Section 14.3—Choosing a Dentist 164

Section 14.4—Dental Insurance: What You
Need to Know 169

Chapter 15—Frequently Asked Questions about Teeth
Cleanings and Dental Visits 175

Chapter 16—Dealing with Dental Anxiety 179

Section 16.1—Calming the Anxious Child..... 180

Section 16.2—Tips on Easing Dental
Anxiety for Adults 181

Chapter 17—Holistic Dentistry: Considerations and
Cautions 183

Chapter 18—Avoiding Disease Transmission, Allergic
Reactions, and Dangerous Exposures at the
Dentist's Office 191

Section 18.1—Preventing Infectious
Disease Transmission............. 192

Section 18.2—Preventing Contact
Dermatitis and Latex Allergy
Reactions in Dental Settings ... 194

Section 18.3—Potential Risk for Lead
Exposure in Dental Offices 199

Chapter 19—X-Rays for Diagnosing Dental Problems 201

Section 19.1—How Do Dental X-Rays
Work? 202

Section 19.2—X-Ray Use and Safety in
Children 203

Chapter 20—Managing Pain at the Dentist's Office 205

Section 20.1—Conscious Sedation for
Adults 206

Section 20.2—Frequently Asked Questions
about Dental Anesthesia 209

Section 20.3—Air Abrasion: A Painless
Drilling Technique 211

Section 20.4—Minimally Invasive
Dentistry 213

Section 20.5—Lasers in Dentistry: How Do
They Work? 215

Part IV: Treating Common Dental Concerns

Chapter 21—Plaque and Tooth Decay 219

Section 21.1—Understanding Plaque 220

Section 21.2—What Is a Cavity? 221

Chapter 22—Sealants: Questions and Answers 225

Chapter 23—Dental Erosion and Tooth Sensitivity 229

Section 23.1—What Is Dental Erosion? 230

Section 23.2—What Are Sensitive Teeth? 231

Chapter 24—Tooth Pain 233

Section 24.1—Toothaches 234

Section 24.2—Abscessed Teeth 236

Chapter 25—Cracked Teeth 239

Chapter 26—Fillings 243

Section 26.1—Overview of Dental Filling
Options 244

Section 26.2—Tooth-Colored Fillings 254

Section 26.3—Questions and Answers on
Dental Amalgam 255

Section 26.4—Studies Evaluate Health
Effects of Dental Amalgam
Fillings in Children 257

Section 26.5—Mercury Exposure and
Dental Fillings 260

Chapter 27—Periodontal (Gum) Disease and Its Impact on
Health 265

Section 27.1—Facts and Fallacies about
Periodontal Disease 266

Section 27.2—Frequently Asked Questions
about Gum Disease and
General Health 269

Chapter 28—Causes, Symptoms, and Treatments for Gum
Disease 271

Section 28.1—Understanding Gum
Disease and Its Causes 272

Section 28.2—Fighting Gum Disease:
How to Keep Your Teeth 278

Section 28.3—Oral Rinse Fights Gum
Disease.................................... 287

Chapter 29—Tooth Injuries and Other Dental
Emergencies 289

Section 29.1—Tips on Dealing with Dental
Emergencies 290

Section 29.2—What to Do If a Tooth Is
Knocked Out 291

Section 29.3—Facial Trauma........................ 292

Section 29.4—Many Facial Sports Injuries
Are Preventable 295

Section 29.5—Mouth Guards Protect More
Than Teeth 298

Part V: Surgical, Orthodontic, and Cosmetic Dental Procedures

Chapter 30—Oral and Maxillofacial Surgery 303

Section 30.1—Types of Oral and
Maxillofacial Surgeries 304

Section 30.2—Home Care after Oral and
Maxillofacial Surgery 307

Chapter 31—Impacted Teeth 309

Section 31.1—Impacted Teeth and Their
Removal 310

Section 31.2—Removing Wisdom Teeth
during Adolescence Prevents
Problems 314

Chapter 32—Endodontic and Root Canal Treatment 317

Section 32.1—Root Canal Treatment............ 318

Section 32.2—Understanding Endodontic
          Surgery 321

Section 32.3—Endodontic Retreatment 324

Chapter 33—Prosthodontics: Extracting, Restoring, and
Replacing Teeth 327

Section 33.1—Overview of Prosthodontic
          Procedures 328

Section 33.2—Dental Implants:
          A Solution for Replacing
          Missing Teeth 331

Section 33.3—Dentures: Frequently Asked
          Questions 333

Section 33.4—What Are Crowns? 337

Section 33.5—Dental Bridges 339

Chapter 34—Orthodontics: Treating Bite Problems 341

Section 34.1—All about Orthodontia 342

Section 34.2—Overview of Braces and
          Appliances 347

Section 34.3—Straight Talk on Braces 349

Section 34.4—The Reality of Retainers 357

Chapter 35—Orthodontics for All Ages 361

Section 35.1—Space Maintenance in
          Young Children: Saving
          Room for Permanent Teeth..... 362

Section 35.2—Childhood Orthodontic
          Treatment 363

Section 35.3—Adolescent Orthodontic
          Treatment 371

Section 35.4—Can Adults Wear Braces? 376

Chapter 36—Cosmetic Dentistry: Improving Your Teeth's
Appearance 381

Section 36.1—How Can My Dentist
          Improve My Smile? 382

Section 36.2—What Should You Ask
          Your Dentist about Tooth
          Whitening Treatments? 384

Section 36.3—Veneers 386

Section 36.4—Enamel Microabrasion 387

Section 36.5—Decorative Dental Grills:
             Wearers Should Be Careful 389

Part VI: Jaw and Mouth Disorders

Chapter 37—Trigeminal Neuralgia: A Common Cause of
            Orofacial Pain 393

Chapter 38—Bruxism (Teeth Grinding and Clenching) 399

Chapter 39—Temporomandibular Joint and Muscle
            Disorders 403

Chapter 40—Oral Cancer 411

            Section 40.1—Oral Cancer Overview 412

            Section 40.2—The Oral Cancer Exam
                          Step-by-Step 414

            Section 40.3—Novel Device Shows
                          Potential in Better Detecting
                          Oral Cancer 415

Chapter 41—Lip and Oral Cavity Cancer 419

Chapter 42—Salivary Gland Cancer 427

Chapter 43—Dry Mouth and Burning Mouth Syndrome 435

            Section 43.1—Dry Mouth 436

            Section 43.2—Burning Mouth Syndrome 439

Chapter 44—Bad Breath (Halitosis) 443

Chapter 45—Canker Sores 447

Chapter 46—Infections That Affect the Lip and Mouth 451

            Section 46.1—Cold Sores
                          (Herpes Simplex Virus-1) 452

            Section 46.2—Oral Thrush (Oropharyngeal
                          Candidiasis) 455

Chapter 47—Taste and Smell Disorders 457

Part VII: Health Conditions That Impact Oral Care

Chapter 48—Autoimmune Diseases That Cause Oral
            Complications 467

            Section 48.1—Sjögren Syndrome 468

            Section 48.2—Pemphigus 476

Chapter 49—Oral Health and Bone Disease 483

    Section 49.1—Osteoporosis 484

    Section 49.2—Bisphosphonate-Associated
                  Osteonecrosis of the Jaw 486

Chapter 50—Oral Health and Cancer Treatment 489

    Section 50.1—Oral Complications of
                  Cancer Treatment.................... 490

    Section 50.2—Three Good Reasons to
                  See a Dentist before Cancer
                  Treatment 497

    Section 50.3—Head and Neck Radiation
                  Treatment and Your Mouth ... 499

    Section 50.4—Chemotherapy and Your
                  Mouth 504

Chapter 51—Oral Health and Diabetes 509

Chapter 52—Oral Complications in People with Eating
    Disorders 513

    Section 52.1—Oral Signs and Symptoms
                  of Eating Disorders.................. 514

    Section 52.2—Eating Disorders May
                  Be Detected at the Dental
                  Office 515

Chapter 53—Oral-Facial Clefts 517

    Section 53.1—All about Cleft Lip and
                  Palate..................................... 518

    Section 53.2—Scientists Discover How
                  Maternal Smoking Causes
                  Cleft Lip and Palate 524

Chapter 54—Oral Concerns in People with Heart
    Problems 529

    Section 54.1—New Antibiotic Recom-
                  mendations for People with
                  Valve Disease Undergoing
                  Dental Procedures 530

    Section 54.2—Patients with Drug-
                  Eluting Stents Should Not
                  Discontinue Antiplatelet
                  Therapy Prior to Dental
                  Procedures 534

Chapter 55—Mouth Problems and Human
            Immunodeficiency Virus (HIV) 537

Chapter 56—Neurological Disorders That Involve the
            Tongue and Mouth 541

    Section 56.1—Melkersson-Rosenthal
                  Syndrome 542

    Section 56.2—Parry-Romberg Syndrome 543

Chapter 57—Obstructive Sleep Apnea and Snoring:
            Oral Appliances May Help 545

Chapter 58—Tobacco and Drug Addiction and Oral
            Health 555

    Section 58.1—Oral Problems in Tobacco
                  Users 556

    Section 58.2—Spit Tobacco: A Quitting
                  Guide 559

    Section 58.3—Methamphetamine Use Can
                  Leave Users Toothless 568

Part VIII: Additional Help and Information

Chapter 59—Glossary of Terms Related to Dental and
            Oral Health 573

Chapter 60—Directory of Agencies That Provide
            Information about Dental and Oral Health 581

Chapter 61—Sources for Charitable and Accessible Dental
            Care 589

Index **595**

Preface

About This Book

According to federal government estimates, employed adults lose more than 164 million hours of work every year due to oral health problems and dental visits. Having unhealthy teeth and gums can leave patients feeling insecure or ashamed about missing, cracked, chipped, crooked, or stained smiles. Cosmetic dental concerns, however, are not the only issue. Recent research has uncovered surprising links between poor oral health and an increased risk of heart disease, diabetes, and other health complications. Fortunately, research also suggests that many dental problems can be prevented with daily hygiene and preventive care checkups.

Dental Care and Oral Health Sourcebook, Third Edition provides updated information about the structure of the mouth and teeth, age-related oral health concerns, and the link between poor oral health and systemic disease. It describes some of the most common dental concerns, such as plaque, cavities, tooth pain, cracked teeth, and gum disease, and it discusses oral and maxillofacial surgery, endodontic and root canal treatments, and orthodontic and cosmetic procedures. Jaw and mouth disorders and other health conditions that impact oral care are also addressed, and the book concludes with a glossary of related terms and a directory of additional resources.

How to Use This Book

This book is divided into parts and chapters. Parts focus on broad areas of interest. Chapters are devoted to single topics within a part.

Part I: Introduction to Dental Care and Oral Health provides general information about the structure of the mouth and teeth and examines the relationship between poor oral health and systemic disease. This part also offers specific facts about oral health in infants and toddlers, children, adolescents, adults, and seniors, and it highlights research advancements in the field of dental care.

Part II: Dental Hygiene at Home offers details about choosing and using home dental care products, including toothbrushes, toothpaste, oral irrigation devices, and mouth rinses. Step-by-step instructions on proper care of the teeth and gums with brushing and flossing and nutrition tips for optimal oral health are also included, along with facts about fluoride and its role in cavity prevention.

Part III: At the Dentist's Office suggests strategies for finding and choosing professional dental care, and it provides information to help readers understand the complexities of dental insurance benefits. It answers questions about teeth cleanings and dental visits, safety procedures, diagnostic tools, and pain management techniques, and it addresses the problem of dental anxiety in children and adults.

Part IV: Treating Common Dental Concerns provides facts and treatment options for a variety of common dental issues, including plaque and tooth decay, dental erosion and tooth sensitivity, tooth pain, cracked teeth, periodontal disease, and tooth injuries.

Part V: Surgical, Orthodontic, and Cosmetic Dental Procedures offers information on oral and maxillofacial, endodontic, and prosthodontic surgeries used to extract, restore, and replace teeth. Included in this part are details on braces, retainers, and other appliances used in orthodontics and tips for children, adolescents, and adults seeking orthodontic treatment to straighten teeth and correct malocclusion. The part concludes with information about dental procedures that can improve the appearance of teeth, such as tooth whitening, veneers, and enamel microabrasion.

Part VI: Jaw and Mouth Disorders discusses orofacial pain, teeth grinding (bruxism), oral cancer, dry mouth, bad breath, canker sores, taste and smell disorders, infections, and other disorders that cause pain and impede the function of the jaw and mouth.

Part VII: Health Conditions That Impact Oral Care highlights specific conditions that cause or result in oral complications, including bone disease, autoimmune disease, cancer treatment, diabetes, eating disorders, oral-facial clefting, heart problems, human immunodeficiency virus, sleep apnea and snoring, and tobacco and drug addiction.

Part VIII: Additional Help and Information includes a glossary of important terms, a directory of organizations for dental patients and their families, and a list of sources for charitable and accessible dental care.

Bibliographic Note

This volume contains documents and excerpts from publications issued by the following U.S. government agencies: Centers for Disease Control and Prevention (CDC); National Cancer Institute (NCI); National Guideline Clearinghouse; National Institute of Arthritis and Musculoskeletal and Skin Diseases (NIAMS); National Institute of Child Health and Human Development (NICHD); National Institute of Dental and Craniofacial Research (NIDCR); National Institute of Environmental Health Sciences National Toxicology Program; National Institute of Neurological Disorders and Stroke (NINDS); National Institute on Aging (NIA); National Institutes of Health (NIH); National Institutes of Health Clinical Center; U.S. Army Center for Health Promotion and Preventive Medicine; and the U.S. Food and Drug Administration (FDA).

In addition, this volume contains copyrighted documents from the following organizations: A.D.A.M., Inc.; Academy of General Dentistry; American Academy of Dental Sleep Medicine; American Academy of Pediatric Dentistry; American Academy of Periodontology; American Association of Endodontists; American Association of Orthodontists; American Board of Oral and Maxillofacial Surgery; American College of Prosthodontists; American Dental Association; American Dental Hygienists Association; American Dental Society of Anesthesiology; American Heart Association, Inc.; California Dental Association; Canadian Dental Association; Ceatus Media Group, L.L.C.; Cleveland Clinic Foundation; *Lake Mary Life Magazine;* Massachusetts Dental Society; Medical College of Wisconsin; Mississippi State Department of Health; National Eating Disorders Association; National Maternal and Child Oral Health Resource Center; Nemours Foundation; New York State Dental Association; Ontario Dental Association; Oral Cancer Foundation; Partnership for a Drug-Free America; PennWell Corporation; Quackwatch; Science News for Kids; State of Connecticut Department of Public Health; University of Pittsburgh Medical Center; and the Wisconsin Dental Association.

Full citation information is provided on the first page of each chapter or section. Every effort has been made to secure all necessary rights to reprint the copyrighted material. If any omissions have been made, please contact Omnigraphics to make corrections for future editions.

Acknowledgements

Thanks go to the many organizations, agencies, and individuals who have contributed materials for this *Sourcebook* and to medical consultant Dr. David Cooke and document engineer Bruce Bellenir. Special thanks go to managing editor Karen Bellenir and research and permissions coordinator Liz Collins for their help and support.

About the Health Reference Series

The *Health Reference Series* is designed to provide basic medical information for patients, families, caregivers, and the general public. Each volume takes a particular topic and provides comprehensive coverage. This is especially important for people who may be dealing with a newly diagnosed disease or a chronic disorder in themselves or in a family member. People looking for preventive guidance, information about disease warning signs, medical statistics, and risk factors for health problems will also find answers to their questions in the *Health Reference Series*. The *Series*, however, is not intended to serve as a tool for diagnosing illness, in prescribing treatments, or as a substitute for the physician/patient relationship. All people concerned about medical symptoms or the possibility of disease are encouraged to seek professional care from an appropriate health care provider.

A Note about Spelling and Style

Health Reference Series editors use *Stedman's Medical Dictionary* as an authority for questions related to the spelling of medical terms and the *Chicago Manual of Style* for questions related to grammatical structures, punctuation, and other editorial concerns. Consistent adherence is not always possible, however, because the individual volumes within the *Series* include many documents from a wide variety of different producers and copyright holders, and the editor's primary goal is to present material from each source as accurately as is possible following the terms specified by each document's producer. This sometimes means that information in different chapters or sections may follow other guidelines and alternate spelling authorities. For example, occasionally a copyright holder may require that eponymous terms be shown in possessive forms (Crohn's disease *vs.* Crohn disease) or that British spelling norms be retained (leukaemia *vs.* leukemia).

Locating Information within the Health Reference Series

The *Health Reference Series* contains a wealth of information about a wide variety of medical topics. Ensuring easy access to all the fact sheets, research reports, in-depth discussions, and other material contained within the individual books of the *Series* remains one of our highest priorities. As the *Series* continues to grow in size and scope, however, locating the precise information needed by a reader may become more challenging.

A Contents Guide to the Health Reference Series was developed to direct readers to the specific volumes that address their concerns. It presents an extensive list of diseases, treatments, and other topics of general interest compiled from the Tables of Contents and major index headings. To access *A Contents Guide to the Health Reference Series*, visit www.healthreferenceseries.com.

Medical Consultant

Medical consultation services are provided to the *Health Reference Series* editors by David A. Cooke, M.D. Dr. Cooke is a graduate of Brandeis University, and he received his M.D. degree from the University of Michigan. He completed residency training at the University of Wisconsin Hospital and Clinics. He is board-certified in Internal Medicine. Dr. Cooke currently works as part of the University of Michigan Health System and practices in Ann Arbor, MI. In his free time, he enjoys writing, science fiction, and spending time with his family.

Our Advisory Board

We would like to thank the following board members for providing guidance to the development of this *Series*:

- Dr. Lynda Baker,
  Associate Professor of Library and Information Science,
  Wayne State University, Detroit, MI

- Nancy Bulgarelli,
  William Beaumont Hospital Library, Royal Oak, MI

- Karen Imarisio,
  Bloomfield Township Public Library, Bloomfield Township, MI

- Karen Morgan,
  Mardigian Library, University of Michigan-Dearborn,
  Dearborn, MI

- Rosemary Orlando,
  St. Clair Shores Public Library, St. Clair Shores, MI

Health Reference Series *Update Policy*

The inaugural book in the *Health Reference Series* was the first edition of *Cancer Sourcebook* published in 1989. Since then, the *Series* has been enthusiastically received by librarians and in the medical community. In order to maintain the standard of providing high-quality health information for the layperson the editorial staff at Omnigraphics felt it was necessary to implement a policy of updating volumes when warranted.

Medical researchers have been making tremendous strides, and it is the purpose of the *Health Reference Series* to stay current with the most recent advances. Each decision to update a volume is made on an individual basis. Some of the considerations include how much new information is available and the feedback we receive from people who use the books. If there is a topic you would like to see added to the update list, or an area of medical concern you feel has not been adequately addressed, please write to:

Editor
Health Reference Series
Omnigraphics, Inc.
P.O. Box 31-1640
Detroit, MI 48231
E-mail: editorial@omnigraphics.com

Part One

Introduction to
Dental Care and Oral Health

Chapter 1

The Structure of the Mouth and Teeth

Your smile, formed by your mouth at your brain's command, is often the first thing people notice when they look at you. It's the facial expression that most engages others. With the help of the teeth—which provide structural support for the face muscles—your mouth also forms your frown and lots of other expressions that show on your face.

The mouth also plays a key role in the digestive system, but it does much more than get digestion started. The mouth—especially the teeth, lips, and tongue—is essential for speech. The tongue, which allows us to taste, also enables us to form words when we speak. The lips that line the outside of the mouth both help hold food in while we chew and pronounce words when we talk.

With the lips and tongue, teeth help form words by controlling air flow out of the mouth. The tongue strikes the teeth as certain sounds are made. The th sound, for example, is produced by the tongue being placed against the upper row of teeth. If your tongue touches your teeth when you say words with the s sound, you may have a lisp.

The hardest substances in the body, the teeth are also necessary for chewing (or mastication)—the process by which we tear, cut, and

"Mouth and Teeth," August 2006, reprinted with permission from www .kidshealth.org. Copyright © 2006 The Nemours Foundation. This information was provided by KidsHealth, one of the largest resources online for medically reviewed health information written for parents, kids, and teens. For more articles like this one, visit www.KidsHealth.org, or www.TeensHealth.org. Updated and reviewed by: Lisa A. Goss, R.D.H., B.S., and Garrett B. Lyons, Jr., D.D.S.

grind food in preparation for swallowing. Chewing allows enzymes and lubricants released in the mouth to further digest, or break down, food. Without our teeth we'd have to eat nothing but soft, mashed food. Eating would not be quite as enjoyable!

Read on to find out how each aspect of the mouth and teeth plays an important role in our daily lives.

Basic Anatomy of the Mouth and Teeth

The entrance to the digestive tract, the mouth is lined with mucous membranes. The membrane-covered roof of the mouth is called the palate. The front part consists of a bony portion called the hard palate, with a fleshy rear part called the soft palate. The hard palate divides the mouth and the nasal passages above. The soft palate forms a curtain between the mouth and the throat, or pharynx, to the rear. The soft palate contains the uvula, the dangling flesh at the back of the mouth. The tonsils are located on either side of the uvula and look like twin pillars holding up the opening to the pharynx.

A bundle of muscles extends from the floor of the mouth to form the tongue. The upper surface of the tongue is covered with tiny bumps called papillae. These contain tiny pores that are our taste buds. Four kinds of taste buds are grouped together on certain areas of the tongue—those that sense sweet, salty, sour, and bitter tastes. Three pairs of salivary glands secrete saliva, which contains a digestive enzyme called amylase that starts the breakdown of carbohydrates even before food enters the stomach.

The lips are covered with skin on the outside and with slippery mucous membranes on the inside of the mouth. The major lip muscle, called the orbicularis oris, allows for the lips' mobility. The reddish tint of the lips comes from underlying blood vessels. The inside portion of both lips is connected to the gums.

There are several types of teeth. Incisors are the squarish, sharp-edged teeth in the front of the mouth. There are four on the bottom and four on the top. On either side of the incisors are the sharp canines. The upper canines are sometimes called eyeteeth. Behind the canines are the premolars, or bicuspids. There are two sets, or four premolars, in each jaw.

The molars, situated behind the premolars, have points and grooves. There are 12 molars—three sets in each jaw called the first, second, and third molars. The third molars are the wisdom teeth, thought by some to have evolved thousands of years ago when human diets consisted of mostly raw foods that required extra chewing power.

But because they can crowd out the other teeth, sometimes a dentist will need to remove them.

Human teeth are made up of four different types of tissue: pulp, dentin, enamel, and cementum. The pulp is the innermost portion of the tooth and consists of connective tissue, nerves, and blood vessels, which nourish the tooth. The pulp has two parts—the pulp chamber, which lies in the crown, and the root canal, which is in the root of the tooth. Blood vessels and nerves enter the root through a small hole in its tip and extend through the canal into the pulp chamber.

Dentin surrounds the pulp. A hard yellow substance consisting mostly of mineral salts and water, it makes up most of the tooth and is as hard as bone. It's the dentin that gives teeth their yellowish tint. Enamel, the hardest tissue in the body, covers the dentin and forms the outermost layer of the crown. It enables the tooth to withstand the pressure of chewing and protects it from harmful bacteria and changes in temperature from hot and cold foods. Both the dentin and pulp extend into the root. A bony layer of cementum covers the outside of the root, under the gum line, and holds the tooth in place within the jawbone. Cementum is also as hard as bone.

Normal Development of the Mouth and Teeth

Humans are diphyodont, meaning that they develop two sets of teeth. The first set of 20 deciduous teeth are also called the milk, primary, temporary, falling-off, or baby teeth. They begin to develop before birth and begin to fall out when a child is around 6 years old. They're replaced by a set of 32 permanent teeth, which are also called secondary or adult teeth.

Around the 8th week after conception, oval-shaped tooth buds consisting of cells form in the embryo. These buds begin to harden about the 16th week. Although teeth aren't visible at birth, both the primary and permanent teeth are forming below the gums. The crown, or the hard enamel-covered part that's visible in the mouth, develops first. When the crown is fully grown, the root begins to develop.

Between the ages of 6 months and 1 year, the deciduous teeth begin to push through the gums. This process is called eruption or teething. At this point, the crown is complete and the root is almost fully formed. By the time a child is 3 years old, he or she has a set of 20 deciduous teeth, 10 in the lower and 10 in the upper jaw. Each jaw has four incisors, two canines, and four molars. The molars' purpose is to grind food, and the incisors and canine teeth are used to bite into and tear food.

The primary teeth help the permanent teeth erupt in their normal positions; most of the permanent teeth form close to the roots of the primary teeth. When a primary tooth is preparing to fall out, its root begins to dissolve. This root has completely dissolved by the time the permanent tooth below it is ready to erupt.

Children start to lose their primary teeth, or baby teeth, at about 6 years old. This begins a phase of permanent tooth development that lasts over the next 15 years, as the jaw steadily grows into its adult form. From ages 6 to 9, the incisors and first molars start to come in. Between ages 10 and 12, the first and second premolars, as well as the canines, erupt. From 12 to 13, the second molars come in. The wisdom teeth (third molars) erupt between the ages of 17 and 21. Sometimes there isn't room in a person's mouth for all the permanent teeth. If this happens, the wisdom teeth may not come through at all. Overcrowding of the teeth is one of the reasons people get braces during their teenage years.

What Do the Mouth and Teeth Do?

The first step of digestion involves the mouth and teeth. Food enters the mouth and is immediately broken down into smaller pieces by our teeth. Each type of tooth serves a different function in the chewing process. Incisors cut foods when you bite into them. The sharper and longer canines tear food. The premolars, which are flatter than the canines, grind and mash food. Molars, with their points and grooves, are responsible for the most vigorous chewing. All the while, the tongue helps to push the food up against our teeth.

As we chew, salivary glands in the walls and floor of the mouth secrete saliva, which moistens the food and helps break it down even more. Saliva makes it easier to chew and swallow foods (especially dry foods), and it contains enzymes that aid in the digestion of carbohydrates.

Once food has been converted into a soft, moist mass, it's pushed into the throat (or pharynx) at the back of the mouth and is swallowed. When we swallow, the soft palate closes off the nasal passages from the throat to prevent food from entering the nose.

Things That Can Go Wrong with the Mouth and Teeth

Proper dental care—including a good diet, frequent cleaning of the teeth after eating, and regular dental checkups—is essential to maintaining healthy teeth and avoiding tooth decay and gum disease. Some common mouth and dental diseases and conditions—some of which can be prevented, some of which cannot—are listed below.

Disorders of the Mouth

Aphthous stomatitis (canker sores). A common form of mouth ulcer, canker sores occur in women more often than in men. Although their cause isn't completely understood, mouth injuries, stress, dietary deficiencies, hormonal changes (such as the menstrual cycle), or food allergies can trigger them. They usually appear on the inner surface of the cheeks, lips, tongue, soft palate, or the base of the gums, and begin with a tingling or burning sensation followed by a painful sore called an ulcer. Pain subsides in 7 to 10 days, with complete healing in 1 to 3 weeks.

Cleft lip and cleft palate are birth defects in which the tissues of the mouth and/or lip don't form properly during fetal development. Children born with these disorders may have trouble feeding immediately after birth. Reconstructive surgery in infancy and sometimes later can repair the anatomical defects, and can prevent or lessen the severity of speech problems later on.

Enteroviral stomatitis is a common childhood infection caused by a family of viruses called the enteroviruses. An important member of this family is coxsackie virus, which causes hand, foot, and mouth disease. Enteroviral stomatitis is marked by small, painful ulcers in the mouth that may decrease a child's desire to eat and drink and put him or her at risk for dehydration.

Herpetic stomatitis (oral herpes). Children can get a mouth infection with the herpes simplex virus from an adult or another child who has it. The resulting painful, clustered vesicles, or blisters, can make it difficult to drink or eat, which can lead to dehydration, especially in a young child.

Periodontal disease. The gums and bones supporting the teeth are subject to disease. A common periodontal disease is gingivitis—inflammation of the gums characterized by redness, swelling, and sometimes bleeding. The accumulation of tartar (a hardened film of food particles and bacteria that builds up on teeth) usually causes this condition, and it's almost always the result of inadequate brushing and flossing. When gingivitis isn't treated, it can lead to periodontitis,

7

in which the gums loosen around the teeth and pockets of bacteria and pus form, sometimes damaging the supporting bone and causing tooth loss.

Disorders of the Teeth

Cavities and tooth decay. When bacteria and food particles stick to saliva on the teeth, plaque forms. The bacteria digest the carbohydrates in the food and produce acid, which dissolves the tooth's enamel and causes a cavity. If the cavity isn't treated, the decay process progresses to involve the dentin. The most common ways to treat cavities and more serious tooth decay problems are: filling the cavity with silver amalgam; performing root canal therapy, involving the removal of the pulp of a tooth; crowning a tooth with a cap that looks like a tooth made of metal, porcelain, or plastic; or removing or replacing the tooth. A common cause of tooth decay in toddlers is "milk bottle mouth," which occurs when a child goes to sleep with a milk or juice bottle in the mouth and the teeth are bathed in sugary liquid for an extended period of time. To avoid tooth decay and cavities, teach your child good dental habits—including proper tooth-brushing techniques—at an early age.

Impacted wisdom teeth. In many people, the wisdom teeth are unable to erupt normally so they either remain below the jawline or don't grow in properly. Dentists call these teeth impacted. Wisdom teeth usually become impacted because the jaw isn't large enough to accommodate all the teeth that are growing in and the mouth becomes overcrowded. Impacted teeth can damage other teeth or become painful and infected. Dentists can check if a person has impacted wisdom teeth by taking x-rays of the teeth. If, after looking at the x-rays, a dentist thinks there's a chance that impacted teeth may cause problems, he or she will usually recommend that the tooth or teeth be removed (extracted).

Malocclusion is the failure of the teeth in the upper and lower jaws to meet properly. Types of malocclusion include overbite, underbite, and crowding. Most conditions can be corrected with braces, which are metal or clear ceramic brackets bonded to the front of each tooth. The wires connecting braces are tightened periodically to force the teeth to move into the correct position.

Chapter 2

Why Are Dental Care and Oral Health So Important?

Chapter Contents

Section 2.1—Dental Symptoms Can Expose Health Issues 10
Section 2.2—The Relationship between Poor Oral Health
            and Systemic Disease 13

Section 2.1

Dental Symptoms Can Expose Health Issues

Without saying a word, your mouth can speak volumes about your general health. During an oral exam, dentists can find signs that point to everything from anemia to diabetes to heart or liver disease, diet deficiencies and eating disorders, gastrointestinal (GI) problems, arthritis, HIV [human immunodeficiency virus], osteoporosis, some autoimmune diseases, and even some pregnancy risks.

"Your mouth can reveal an awful lot," says Lee M. Radke, D.D.S., an Assistant Professor of Surgery at the Medical College of Wisconsin. "The correlation, or at least the association, between systemic health and a healthy mouth is becoming more and more evident."

In fact, in February 2006, the American Dental Association and the American Medical Association held a first-ever joint news conference in New York titled "Oral and Systemic Health: Exploring the Connection." As one of the speakers put it: "The fact that the mouth is connected to the rest of the body is often overlooked." Among the points discussed was the need for greater communication between dentists and physicians to reduce patients' risks for heart disease and stroke, worsening diabetic control, lung infections, and even premature births—risks that can manifest themselves in the patients' mouths.

Dr. Radke serves as the hospital dentist at the Oral and Maxillofacial Surgery Clinic, part of the Froedtert & The Medical College's Sargeant Health Center. The role of a hospital dentist can vary among institutions, he says. In Dr. Radke's case, he evaluates and treats a variety of patients, including some who are medically compromised because of suppressed immune systems, fragile health status, or behavioral problems.

Most Diseases Have Oral Symptoms

An unhealthy mouth, he says, can exhibit symptoms like dryness, gum swelling or infection, slow healing of sores, or rapidly advancing tooth decay and gum disease. It is estimated that 90% of all systemic diseases produce oral signs and symptoms.

"That's probably true," Dr. Radke says. "If the mouth is pale-colored, rather than the normal healthy pink color, it could indicate anemia. Unusual bleeding could indicate liver disease, medication overdoses, or coagulation disorders. A red, smooth tongue can indicate GI problems or diet deficiencies, especially a lack of vitamin B12 or folate. Erosion of tooth enamel can point to reflux or eating disorders. Erosions and patchy lesions could indicate cancers or immune diseases."

By contrast, a healthy mouth is free of infection, tooth decay, bad breath, or mouth sores. The patient's mouth and teeth look acceptable, and he or she can chew and speak without problems. Attaining a healthy mouth is simple, Dr. Radke says—practice good oral hygiene and smart lifestyle habits.

"That means daily brushing and flossing," he says, "although even today you have to convince people to do that. Diet is a major factor, but too many people make choices that aren't healthy. It's amazing the volume of soda and sugary snacks people consume. And then there's smoking and excessive alcohol use. So much is preventable and manageable."

Simply having a healthy mouth does not necessarily guarantee overall good health. But an unhealthy mouth can indicate problems elsewhere in the body. "If you do have a healthy mouth and still get infections or sores, it could indicate an underlying medical condition," Dr. Radke says.

Healthy Mouth Can Prevent Infection

"A healthy mouth is a great defense against bacteria, viruses, and fungi that can cause disease," he says. "If the mucosa—the pink stuff— is intact, it forms a good barrier that wards off infection."

During a dental exam, dentists look for decay and gum disease, and check for signs of cancer of the mouth or throat. They look under the tongue and in areas of the mouth that are difficult to see in a self-examination in front of a bathroom mirror, he says.

Approximately 500 different types of bacteria live in the mouth, and many of them have protective properties that help prevent over-growth of harmful microorganisms, Dr. Radke says. "There is a delicate balance between good and bad organisms in the mouth and throat, and maintaining this balance is what a healthy mouth is all about," he explains. "The saliva also contains antibodies and enzymes that protect against many bacteria and viruses."

"Oral bacteria can sometimes enter the bloodstream, especially after invasive dental procedures such as cleaning, extractions, and gum surgery," he notes. Patients with certain cardiac conditions, prosthetic joints, or immune compromises are often advised to take antibiotics before such procedures, he says.

Some researchers believe that in the future, saliva testing might replace blood testing as a means of diagnosing and monitoring diseases such as diabetes, Parkinson's disease, cirrhosis of the liver, and many infectious diseases. Right now, saliva testing is routinely used to measure illegal drugs, environmental toxins, hormones, and antibodies indicating hepatitis or HIV infection.

"Meantime," says Dr. Radke, "awareness of the association between oral infections and diseases like stroke, diabetes, and even preterm labor keeps increasing. It's quite a dynamic topic in the dental and medical literature. Cause and effect has not been proven yet, but the connection between oral infection and systemic disease is evolving rapidly. I think it's important to understand the relationship between oral health and overall health."

Section 2.2

The Relationship between Poor Oral Health and Systemic Disease

Excerpted from "Looking at the Periodontal-Systemic Disease Connection," from the National Institute of Dental and Craniofacial Research (NIDCR, www.nidcr.nih.gov), part of National Institutes of Health, July 2005.

Studies within the past 10 years have suggested an association between periodontal disease and the likelihood of delivering preterm, low-birthweight babies, developing cardiovascular disease, and having difficulty controlling blood sugar levels in people with diabetes. Some studies have also linked periodontal disease to respiratory infection in people with pulmonary problems.

Periodontal Disease and Preterm Birth

What led researchers to believe that women with periodontal disease may be at risk for delivering preterm and/or low-birthweight babies?

In the mid-1990s there were some studies by researchers at the University of North Carolina (UNC) that compared the birth outcomes of women with periodontal disease to those of women without periodontal disease. The studies showed that women who had periodontal disease were more likely to deliver preterm and/or low birthweight (PLBW) babies. These observational studies, so-called because they didn't involve treatment, were among the first to bring this association to light. Additionally, the UNC researchers did studies in hamsters where they found that maternal exposure to by-products of periodontal bacteria during pregnancy had harmful effects on the fetus.

There have also been a couple of clinical trials—particularly in South America. And those showed that treating periodontal disease resulted in fewer adverse birth outcomes in terms of PLBW. Those were the first intervention studies. A team of researchers in the United States also did a pilot interventional study. They found some trends that suggested periodontal disease therapy was associated with a

13

reduced incidence of preterm birth. However, these intervention studies were either relatively small or not designed to determine whether treating periodontal disease would reduce the risk of delivering preterm, low-birthweight babies.

There are also studies that have found no greater risk of pregnant women with periodontal disease delivering PLBW babies.

So we can't say that periodontal disease causes preterm birth or that treating periodontal disease will lower your risk of delivering a PLBW baby?

Right now, there's no proof that periodontal disease causes preterm birth or that preventing or treating periodontal disease will result in a lower incidence of delivering preterm or low-birthweight babies. We'll have to wait and see what these clinical trials tell us.

Periodontal Disease and Cardiovascular Disease (Heart Disease and Stroke)

What led researchers to believe there is an association between periodontal disease and cardiovascular disease?

Researchers looked at people with periodontal disease and found that they had a higher risk of heart disease. There were also some animal studies in which researchers injected periodontal bacteria into rabbits; they found the animals developed heartbeat irregularities and cardiac ischemia, or insufficient blood flow to the heart. But like the PLBW issue, there are conflicting data. There are some studies in humans that have shown an association between periodontal disease and cardiovascular disease and some that have not.

The evidence continues to mount with the observational studies, but the observational studies don't give a definite answer on whether the association is causal—that is, whether periodontal disease causes cardiovascular problems. Interventional studies, or clinical trials, are needed to clarify the relationship.

What are the challenges involved in studying the relationship between periodontal disease and cardiovascular disease?

First, a clinical trial of periodontal disease and its effect on cardiovascular health is a difficult study to do. If you randomly selected 40-year-olds with periodontal disease from the general population, you wouldn't have any idea how many, or if any, of them would ever have a heart attack or stroke. And it would not be ethical to do a clinical trial in which periodontal treatment was withheld for an indefinite period from half of the subjects.

So you probably need to do the trial with people who have already had a heart attack, because you're more likely to find the cause-and-effect relationship in that population. We know that, statistically, 3 to 7 percent of these people will have another cardiovascular event in the near future.

Conversely, in the preterm birth studies, 36–40 weeks after becoming pregnant there's definitely going to be an event for all the patients. Whether it's a birth, miscarriage etc., something is going to happen. With the heart disease study, you don't know whether people will ever have a cardiovascular event. Also, in the preterm birth studies you only have to delay treatment a few months in the delayed-treatment group—it isn't even nine months since they start the study in their second trimester. They're also being monitored, so that if anyone experiences progressive disease, they can be treated immediately.

Another challenge in studying the relationship between periodontal infections and cardiovascular disease is teasing out the effects of shared risk factors for both diseases, especially smoking. Smokers make up a large percentage of the participants in cardiovascular disease-periodontal disease observational studies. So how much of the observed association with heart attack might be due to periodontal infection as an independent risk factor and how much might result from smoking? That's something we still need to clarify.

Periodontal Disease and Diabetes

If you have diabetes are you more likely to get periodontal disease?

Yes. Diabetes does make you more susceptible to infection—any infection—including periodontal disease. And there is evidence that people with diabetes have more periodontal disease.

There also seems to be some evidence of the relationship going the other way—that if you control periodontal disease, it may help you control your blood sugar.

Having an infection, including periodontal disease, can impair the body's ability to process and/or use insulin. So the theory is that if you control the infection, it might be easier to control blood sugar.

We have one pilot study on this topic. Researchers are looking at people with diabetes who are having difficulty controlling their blood sugar and who also have periodontal disease. They are treating the periodontal disease to see if the treatment results in improved control of blood sugar levels. This study is finishing up and there are investigators who are going to propose similar studies.

What are the challenges in determining whether controlling periodontal disease will result in better blood sugar control?

The Diabetes Control and Complications Trial found that 'intensive' control of blood sugar reduced the risk for eye, kidney, and nerve disease compared to those using the 'standard' control. So if you are under intensive control, you wouldn't necessarily expect treating periodontal disease to bring down the blood sugar levels further. However, there are ongoing studies to see if it's feasible to do multi-center, interventional studies on this topic.

What led researchers to think there was any relationship between periodontal disease and diabetes?

For at least 50 years periodontists have felt that people with diabetes tended to have more severe periodontal disease and the bulk of the research does show an association between the two diseases. Several studies have shown that the more poorly controlled the diabetes, the more severe the periodontal disease is likely to be.

Periodontal Disease and Respiratory Infection

Isn't there some evidence that you can develop respiratory infection from inhaling periodontal pathogens?

Periodontal disease has been associated with pulmonary infections in people who are hospitalized or are in extended care facilities. Here again, there are no studies that have shown cause and effect. There are some studies in the pipeline looking at whether you can prevent respiratory problems by controlling dental plaque, particularly in patients who have existing breathing problems.

So to conclude, we can't tell people that periodontal disease causes preterm birth or heart disease, or results in difficulty controlling blood sugar levels or causes respiratory

infections. Nor can we say that preventing or treating periodontal disease will help you avoid these conditions?

That's right. At this time, we can't say whether or not periodontal disease causes any of these conditions or whether treating periodontal disease will prevent them. But we can tell people to treat periodontal disease for its own sake—to avoid tooth loss and to maintain oral comfort and function.

Chapter 3

Infant and Toddler Oral Health

Chapter Contents

Section 3.1—A Healthy Mouth for Your Baby 20

Section 3.2—The Teething Process and How to Ease It 22

Section 3.3—What Is Baby Bottle Tooth Decay? 25

Section 3.4—Early Childhood Tooth Decay in the United
States 29

Section 3.5—Thumbsucking, Pacifier Use, and Oral Health 33

Section 3.1

A Healthy Mouth for Your Baby

Excerpted from a brochure by the National Institute of
Dental and Craniofacial Research (NIDCR, www.nidcr.nih.gov),
part of the National Institutes of Health, April 2006.

Before Your Baby Is Born

What you eat when you are pregnant is important. Eating right
will help you and your growing baby stay healthy. Follow your doctor's
advice for eating the right foods and taking vitamins.

It's also time to think about how you'll feed your baby. Remember,
breastfeeding is best!

Protect Your Baby's Teeth with Fluoride

Fluoride protects teeth from tooth decay and helps heal early decay. Fluoride is in the drinking water of many towns and cities.

Ask your dentist or doctor if your water has fluoride in it. If it
doesn't, talk to your dentist or doctor about giving you a prescription
for fluoride drops for your baby.

Check and Clean Your Baby's Teeth

Check your baby's teeth. Healthy teeth should be all one color. If
you see spots or stains on the teeth, take your baby to your dentist.

Clean your baby's teeth as soon as they come in with a clean, soft
cloth or a baby's toothbrush. Clean the teeth at least once a day. It's
best to clean them right before bedtime.

At about age 2, most of your child's teeth will be in. Now you can
start brushing them with a small drop of fluoride toothpaste. Use a
drop of toothpaste.

Young children cannot get their teeth clean by themselves. Until
they are 7 or 8 years old, you will need to help them brush. Try brushing their teeth first and then letting them finish. And be sure that
you put the toothpaste on the brush—use only a pea-sized amount of
toothpaste.

Feed Your Baby Healthy Food

Choose foods that do not have a lot of sugar in them. Give your child fruits and vegetables instead of candy and cookies.

Prevent Baby Bottle Tooth Decay

Do not put your baby to bed with a bottle at night or at nap time. (If you put your baby to bed with a bottle, fill it only with water.)

Milk, formula, juices, and other sweet drinks such as soda all have sugar in them. Sucking on a bottle filled with liquids that have sugar in them can cause tooth decay. Decayed teeth can cause pain and can cost a lot to fill.

During the day, do not give your baby a bottle filled with sweet drinks to use like a pacifier.

If your baby uses a pacifier, do not dip it in anything sweet like sugar or honey.

Near his first birthday, you should teach your child to drink from a cup instead of a bottle.

Take Your Child to the Dentist

Ask your dentist when to bring your child in for his first visit. Usually, the dentist will want to see a child by his first birthday. At this first visit, your dentist can quickly check your child's teeth.

Section 3.2

The Teething Process and How to Ease It

"Teething Tots," June 2005, reprinted with permission from www.kidshealth .org. Copyright © 2005 The Nemours Foundation. This information was provided by KidsHealth, one of the largest resources online for medically reviewed health information written for parents, kids, and teens. For more articles like this one, visit www.KidsHealth.org, or www.TeensHealth.org. Updated and reviewed by: Garrett B. Lyons, D.D.S., and Lisa Goss, R.D.H., B.S.

Teething, the emergence of the first baby teeth through a baby's gums, can be a frustrating time for many babies—and their parents. It helps to know what to expect when your child is teething, and what you can do to make the process a little less painful for you and your child.

The Teething Process

Teething can begin as early as 3 months and continue until a child's third birthday.

Typically between the ages of 4 and 7 months, you will notice your child's first tooth pushing through the gum line. The first teeth to appear are usually the two bottom front teeth, also known as the central incisors. These are usually followed 4 to 8 weeks later by the four front upper teeth (central and lateral incisors). About 1 month later, the lower lateral incisors (the two teeth flanking the bottom front teeth) will appear. Next to break through the gum line are the first molars (the back teeth used for grinding food), then finally the eyeteeth (the pointy teeth in the upper jaw). Most children have all 20 of their primary teeth by their third birthday. (This is a general rule; if your child experiences significant delay, speak to your child's doctor.)

In some rare cases, children are born with one or two teeth or have a tooth emerge within the first few weeks of life. Unless the teeth interfere with feeding or are loose enough to pose a choking risk, this is usually not a cause for concern. If you have any questions it's a good idea to talk to your child's doctor.

Easing Teething

Whenever your child begins teething, you may notice that your child seems to drool more, and seems to want to chew on things. For some babies, teething is painless. Others may experience brief periods of irritability, and some may seem cranky for weeks, experiencing crying episodes and disrupted sleeping and eating patterns. Teething can be uncomfortable, but if your baby seems very irritable, contact your child's doctor.

Although tender and swollen gums could cause your baby's temperature to be a little higher than normal, teething, as a rule, does not cause high fever or diarrhea. If your baby does develop a fever during the teething phase, it is probably due to something else and your child's doctor should be contacted.

Here are some tips to keep in mind when your baby is teething:

* Wipe your baby's face often with a cloth to remove the drool and prevent rashes from developing.

* Give your baby something to chew on. Make sure it's big enough so that he or she can't swallow it and that it can't break into small pieces. A wet washcloth placed in the freezer for 30 minutes makes a handy teething aid—just be sure to wash it after each use. Rubber teething rings are also good, but avoid the ones with liquid inside because they may break. If you use a teething ring, be sure to take it out of the freezer before it becomes rock hard—you don't want to bruise those already swollen gums!

* Rub your baby's gums with a clean finger.

* Never tie a teething ring around a baby's neck, as it could get caught on something and strangle the baby.

* If your baby seems irritable, acetaminophen may help—but always consult your child's doctor first. Never place an aspirin against the tooth, and don't rub whiskey on your baby's gums.

Baby Teeth Hygiene

The care and cleaning of your baby's teeth is important for long-term dental health. Even though the first set of teeth will fall out, tooth decay can hasten this process and leave gaps before the permanent teeth are ready to come in. The remaining primary teeth may then crowd together to attempt to fill in the gaps, which may cause the permanent teeth to come in crooked and out of place.

Daily dental care should begin even before your baby's first tooth emerges. Wipe your baby's gums daily with a clean, damp washcloth or gauze, or brush them gently with a soft, infant-sized toothbrush and water (no toothpaste!). As soon as the first tooth appears, brush them with water.

Toothpaste is OK to use on your child's teeth once he or she gets old enough to spit it out—usually around age 3. Choose one with fluoride and use only a pea-sized amount or less in younger children. Don't let your child swallow the toothpaste or eat it out of the tube because an overdose of fluoride can be harmful for children.

By the time all your baby's teeth are in, it's a good idea to brush your child's teeth at least twice a day, and especially after meals. It's also important to get your child used to flossing early on. A good time to start flossing is when two teeth start to touch. Talk to your child's dentist for advice on flossing those tiny teeth. You can also get your toddler interested in the routine by letting him or her watch and imitate you as you brush and floss on a regular basis.

Another important tip for preventing tooth decay: don't let your baby fall asleep with a bottle. The milk or juice can pool in her mouth and cause tooth decay and plaque.

The American Dental Association recommends that children see a dentist by age 1, when six to eight teeth are in place, to spot any potential problems and advise parents about preventive care.

Section 3.3

What Is Baby Bottle Tooth Decay?

"Promoting Awareness, Preventing Pain: Facts on Early Childhood
Caries (ECC)" © 2004 National Maternal & Child Oral Health Resource
Center (www.mchoralhealth.org). Reprinted with permission.

Early childhood caries (ECC) is an infectious disease that can start as soon as an infant's teeth erupt. ECC can progress rapidly and may have a lasting detrimental impact on a child's health and well-being. ECC is a serious public health problem.

In a child age 71 months or younger, the presence of one or more decayed teeth, missing teeth (resulting from caries), or filled tooth surfaces in any primary tooth is known as ECC.[1]

Caries is a multifactorial disease process initiated by bacteria (primarily *Streptococcus mutans*).When food is consumed, bacteria are able to break down carbohydrates, producing acids that cause mineral loss from teeth. This mineral loss results in cavities when the attack is prolonged and exceeds an individual's resistance and ability to heal. Resistance and healing ability are determined partly by physiology and partly by health behaviors.

Because poor feeding and eating practices alone do not cause caries, terms such as "baby bottle tooth decay," "bottle mouth," and "nursing decay" are misleading. ECC is a term that better reflects the many factors involved in the disease process.[1]

ECC should be prevented to the extent possible and should be treated if it occurs.[2]

Who is at risk for ECC?

Among children in the United States, the number of teeth with treated or untreated caries has declined substantially since the 1970s.[2] However, ECC remains a significant problem for some children.

Among children from families with incomes at or below the federal poverty level, the amount of caries in the primary teeth remained unchanged from the early 1970s to the early 1990s.[2]

For children ages 2 to 5, 75 percent of caries is found in 8 percent of the population.[3] Children ages 2 to 5 who have not had a dental visit within the past 12 months are more likely to experience caries in primary teeth than children who have.[4]

Mexican-American children ages 2 to 5 are more likely than their non-Hispanic black and non-Hispanic white peers to experience caries in primary teeth.[4]

For children ages 2 to 5 from families with incomes above the federal poverty level, the likelihood of experiencing caries in primary teeth is significantly greater among those who do not eat breakfast daily or who eat fewer than five servings of fruit and vegetables per day than among those who do.[4]

What are the costs of ECC?

Children diagnosed with ECC may be highly susceptible to future caries development.[5] Manifestations of ECC may go beyond pain and infection. ECC has the potential to affect speech and communication, nutrition, productivity, and quality of life, even into adulthood. ECC has significant financial consequences. Many children with ECC require restorative treatment in an operating room under general anesthesia. State Medicaid expenditures for restorative dental care delivered under general anesthesia range from $1,500 to $2,000 per child per year.[6,7]

How can ECC risk be reduced?

The infectious nature of ECC, its early onset, and the potential of early interventions all point toward an emphasis on preventive oral health care.

Fluoride is safe and effective for preventing caries in children. Community water fluoridation is a major factor responsible for the decline in caries during the second half of the 20th century.[8] Fluoride toothpastes, varnishes, mouth rinses, gels, and dietary supplements can also help prevent caries.[9]

Preventing ECC requires good dietary and oral hygiene practices and access to preventive and restorative dental care.[10]

Programs directed toward families with young children, such as the Special Supplemental Nutrition Program for Women, Infants and Children (WIC), can contribute to the prevention of ECC.[11] Other programs such as Head Start can also help prevent ECC. Nutrition education and counseling for the purpose of preventing ECC aims to teach parents the importance of reducing their infant's or child's high-frequency exposures to foods containing sugar.[10]

The Early and Periodic Screening, Diagnosis and Treatment (EPSDT) component of the Medicaid program could be a powerful tool for identifying and treating ECC early. However, Healthy People 2010 baseline data indicate that only 20 percent of children eligible for dental services under Medicaid/EPSDT received a single preventive dental service.[12]

What can health professionals do?

As part of any routine health supervision visit, primary care health professionals should perform an oral health screening that includes the lips, tongue, teeth, gums, interior surface of the cheeks, and roof of the mouth.

Health professionals can help ensure that infants and young children receive the care they need by referring infants to a dentist for an oral examination within 6 months of the eruption of the first primary tooth, and no later than age 12 months, and by establishing the child's dental home.[1]

Health professionals can provide parents with anticipatory guidance on oral development, caries transmission, gum/tooth cleaning, feeding and eating practices, and fluoride. Since caries is an infectious disease that may be transmitted from the parent, especially the mother, to an infant or child,[13] anticipatory guidance on oral health should also be provided to pregnant women, new mothers, and other caregivers.

References

1. American Academy of Pediatric Dentistry, American Board of Pediatric Dentistry, College of Diplomates of the American Board of Pediatric Dentistry. 2003. Policy on early childhood caries (ECC): Unique challenges and treatment options. *Pediatric Dentistry* 24(7):27–28.

2. Brown LJ, Wall TP, Lazar V. 2000. Trends in total caries experience: Permanent and primary teeth. *Journal of the American Dental Association* 131(2): 223–231.

3. Macek MD, Heller KE, Selwitz RH, Manz MC. 2004. Is 75 percent of dental caries really found in 25 percent of the population? *Journal of Public Health Dentistry* 64(1):20–25.

4. Dye BA, Shenkin JD, Ogden CL, Marshall TA, Levy SM, Kanellis MJ. 2004. The relationship between healthful eating

practices and dental caries in children ages 2–5 years in the United States, 1988–1994. *Journal of the American Dental Association* 135(1):55–66.

5. Almeida AG, Roseman MM, Sheff M, Huntington N, Hughes CV. 2004. Future caries susceptibility in children with early childhood caries following treatment under general anesthesia. *Pediatric Dentistry* 22(4):302–306.

6. Griffin SO, Gooch, BF, Beltran E, Sutherland JN, Barsley R. 2000. Dental services, costs, and factors associated with hospitalization for Medicaid-eligible children, Louisiana 1996–97. *Journal of Public Health Dentistry* 60(1):21–27.

7. Kanellis MJ, Damiano PC, Momany ET. 2000. Medicaid costs associated with the hospitalization of young children for restorative dental treatment under general anesthesia. *Journal of Public Health Dentistry* 60(1):28–32.

8. Centers for Disease Control and Prevention. 1999. Achievements in public health, 1990–1999: Fluoridation of drinking water to prevent dental caries. *Morbidity and Mortality Weekly Report* 48(41):933–940.

9. U.S. Preventive Services Task Force. 2004. Prevention of dental caries in preschool children: Recommendations and rationale. Rockville, MD: Agency for Healthcare Research and Quality.

10. Tinanoff N, Palmer CA. 2000. Dietary determinants of dental caries and dietary recommendations for preschool children. *Journal of Public Health Dentistry* 60(3):197–206.

11. Nurko C, Skur P, Brown JP. 2003. Caries prevalence of children in an infant oral health educational program at a WIC clinic. *Journal of Dentistry for Children* 70(3):231–234.

12. U.S. Department of Health and Human Services. 2000. *Healthy People 2010: Volume II* (2nd ed.). Washington, DC: U.S. Department of Health and Human Services.

13. Li Y, Dasanayake AP, Caufield PW, Elliott RR, Butts JT, 3rd. 2003. Characterization of maternal mutans streptococci transmission in an African American population. *Dental Clinics of North America* 47(1):87–101.

Section 3.4

Early Childhood Tooth Decay in the United States

"Early Childhood Caries," reprinted with permission from the
State of Connecticut Department of Public Health, www.ct.gov/dph.
This document is undated.

What is early childhood caries (ECC)?

Early childhood caries (ECC) is the development of often severe
tooth decay in infants and young children.

Excessive use of a baby bottle or cup with juice, milk, formula, or
another drink containing sugars may cause sugary fluids to pool in
the mouth, and create an environment in the mouth that encourages
bacteria to multiply and produce the acids that eat away at tooth
enamel.

Most cases of ECC are preventable. Early detection is necessary
to prevent or stop the progression of this disease.

What does ECC look like?

ECC is not simply any dental decay appearing in early childhood.
The clinical appearance of ECC does not follow the typical pattern of
dental decay. Instead, it most often affects the pits and fissures of the
chewing surfaces of teeth. ECC presents with specific defining characteristics:

- ECC is a rapidly developing type of decay that characteristi-
  cally affects the 4 upper front teeth—although molars may also
  be affected.

- The upper front teeth come into the mouth between 6 and 9
  months of age. ECC is found, therefore, in very young children—
  between 6 months to 2 years of age.

- The decay typically (but not necessarily) starts as a dull white
  band on the smooth surface of the tooth at the gum line, followed

by yellow discoloration. Ideally, this is the time for the dentist to begin treatment intervention.

- As the condition advances, a soft brown or black collar surrounds the tooth, progressing slowly toward the chewing surface of the tooth until only a small amount of enamel-covered tooth remains.

- Eventually, the tooth breaks off, leaving only a decayed stump where a healthy tooth once was.

It is important to realize that the patterns described above may be the most typical, but different conditions may reveal different clinical patterns. In any case, decay in the teeth of very young children should raise a red flag.

Why was ECC once known as baby bottle tooth decay (BBTD)?

ECC has been linked to certain feeding habits such as overuse of a bottle by infants. In 1962, a Connecticut dentist, Dr. Elias Fass, first described a specific pattern of dental decay found in infants and young children. He termed this condition "nursing bottle mouth" based on the observation that children with this pattern of decay were often put to bed with a bottle. The specific pattern of decay has been labeled in many ways since then. The most common name is baby bottle tooth decay (BBTD).

Why is BBTD no longer an appropriate name for ECC?

In addition to frequent use of the bottle, experts now agree that the causes of ECC are more complex, including dietary practices, social, cultural and economic influences, genetic influences, and more. Changing feeding habits and use of the bottle, therefore, are not the only steps necessary to prevent dental decay in infants and young children. Defining this disease by only one cause minimizes the magnitude, complexity, and infectious nature of ECC.

How does severe ECC impact the child later in life?

The primary teeth (baby teeth) are very important and contribute to a child's overall development. Permanent (adult) teeth will eventually replace them, but this does not reduce the importance of primary teeth.

Dental decay in primary teeth is an infectious process that can be very painful, spread, and affect the development of the adult teeth.

Dental decay in primary teeth most often means there will be dental decay in the adult teeth.

Healthy primary teeth are important for:

- proper chewing, which helps assure the infant's proper nutrition;
- proper speech development;
- holding the space in the dental arch until the permanent teeth are ready to come into the mouth; and
- the development of the facial structure.

How widespread is ECC?

A 1997 survey of over 5,000 children found that active untreated dental decay was present in:

- 6 percent of 1 year olds;
- 22 percent of 2 year olds; and
- 35 percent of 3 year olds.

Connecticut surveys indicate that the prevalence of ECC may be as high as 25 percent in high-risk populations. As many as 65 percent of parents and caregivers in these populations use feeding practices that may put their infants at risk for ECC.

What role does diet and nutrition play in the development of ECC?

Food and drink containing carbohydrates are necessary ingredients in the development of ECC (and dental decay, in general). Carbohydrates are sugars and starches found in many foods and are not limited to soda, cookies, and cakes.

Milk, fruits, breads, cereals, grains, and some vegetables contain carbohydrates. These foods, however, contain many valuable and necessary nutrients, as well. Processed foods, on the other hand, like soda, candy, cakes and chips, have very high amounts of sugars added to them ("refined" sugars) and have limited or no nutritional value.

Unfortunately, bacteria do not distinguish between the sugars in nutritious versus non-nutritious foods. These bacteria metabolize either form to create the acid that eats away at the tooth.

31

What are the most common risk behaviors associated with ECC?

The most common risk behaviors associated with ECC are frequent snacking and the nighttime, naptime, or at-will use of a baby bottle or cup with juice, milk, formula or another drink containing sugars. The sugary fluids pool in the mouth after the baby falls asleep or all day long, in the case of at-will feeding, creating the environment in the mouth that encourages *S. mutans* to multiply and produce the acids that eat away at tooth enamel. It's not just what you eat but how often.

What can be done to help prevent ECC?

Don't use a bottle to calm or put an infant to bed. Instead of a bottle use:

- A favorite blanket or toy
- A clean pacifier
- Holding, patting, rocking
- Reading: It is never too soon to read to the baby
- Softly talking or singing: though they might not understand the words, a familiar voice will be comforting; or
- Let the baby cry. It is normal, in most situations, for a baby to cry when first put to bed. Generally, after the third night, the baby will drift off to peaceful sleep without crying.

The baby may have a sleep disturbance that should be discussed with the pediatrician.

Switch to a "sippy cup" or other small cup as soon as possible. A child should be encouraged to start using a cup as soon as he or she can sit up unassisted. Parents should be encouraged to transition their child from bottle to cup by 12 months of age. Similarly, the young child should be transitioned to the cup whenever the mother is ready to discontinue breast-feeding.

If a child must be pacified or put to sleep with a bottle, give a bottle filled with plain water. If a child does not adapt initially to the plain water, it may be necessary to fill the bottle with a mixture of juice and water, reducing the amount of juice slightly each night until it is filled with only water.

Section 3.5

Thumbsucking, Pacifier Use, and Oral Health

Why do children suck on fingers, pacifiers, or other objects?

This type of sucking is completely normal for babies and young children. It provides security. For young babies, it's a way to make contact with and learn about the world. In fact, babies begin to suck on their fingers or thumbs even before they are born.

Are these habits bad for the teeth and jaws?

Most children stop sucking on thumbs, pacifiers, or other objects on their own between two and four years of age. No harm is done to their teeth or jaws. However, some children repeatedly suck on a finger, pacifier, or other object over long periods of time. In these children, the upper front teeth may tip toward the lip or not come in properly.

When should I worry about a sucking habit?

Your pediatric dentist will carefully watch the way your child's teeth come in and jaws develop, keeping the sucking habit in mind at all times. For most children the American Academy of Pediatric Dentistry (AAPD) recommends encouraging these habits cease by age three.

What can I do to stop my child's habit?

Most children stop sucking habits on their own, but some children need the help of their parents and their pediatric dentist. When your child is old enough to understand the possible results of a sucking habit, your pediatric dentist can encourage your child to stop, as well as talk about what happens to the teeth if your child doesn't stop. This advice, coupled with support from parents, helps most children quit. If this approach doesn't work, your pediatric dentist may recommend a mouth appliance that blocks sucking habits.

Are pacifiers a safer habit for the teeth than thumbs or fingers?

Thumb, finger, and pacifier sucking all affect the teeth essentially the same way. However, a pacifier habit is often easier to break.

Chapter 4

Oral Health in Children

Chapter Contents

Section 4.1—Keeping Your Child's Teeth Healthy 36
Section 4.2—Your Child's Nutrition and How It Affects
        Oral Health 40

Section 4.1

Keeping Your Child's Teeth Healthy

When should I schedule my child's first trip to the dentist? Should my 3-year-old be flossing? How do I know if my child needs braces? Many parents have a difficult time judging how much dental care their children need. They know they want to prevent cavities, but they don't always know the best way to do so.

When should I start caring for my child's teeth?

Proper dental care begins even before a baby's first tooth appears. Remember that just because you can't see the teeth doesn't mean they aren't there. Teeth actually begin to form in the second trimester of pregnancy. At birth your baby has 20 primary teeth, some of which are fully developed in the jaw.

Running a damp washcloth over your baby's gums following feedings can prevent buildup of damaging bacteria. Once your child has a few teeth showing, you can brush them with a soft child's toothbrush or rub them with gauze at the end of the day.

Even babies can have problems with dental decay when parents do not practice good feeding habits at home. Putting your baby to sleep with a bottle in his or her mouth may be convenient in the short term—but it can harm the baby's teeth. When the sugars from juice or milk remain on a baby's teeth for hours, they may eat away at the enamel, creating a condition known as bottle mouth. Pocked, pitted, or discolored front teeth are signs of bottle mouth. Severe cases result in cavities and the need to pull all the front teeth until the permanent ones grow in. Parents and child care providers should also help young children develop set times for drinking during the day as well because sucking on a bottle throughout the day can be equally damaging to young teeth.

What kind of dentist should my child see?

You may want to take your child to a dentist who specializes in treating kids. Pediatric dentists are trained to handle the wide range of issues associated with kids' dental health. They also know when to refer you to a different type of specialist such as an orthodontist to correct an overbite or an oral surgeon for jaw realignment.

A pediatric dentist's primary goals are prevention, heading off potential oral health problems before they occur, and maintenance, ensuring through routine checkups and proper daily care that teeth and gums stay healthy.

How can I prevent cavities?

The American Dental Association recommends that your child's first visit to the dentist take place by the first birthday. At this visit, the dentist will explain proper brushing and flossing techniques (you need to floss once your baby has two teeth that touch) and conduct a modified exam while your baby sits on your lap.

Such visits can help in the early detection of potential problems, and help kids become accustomed to visiting the dentist so they'll have less fear about going as they grow older.

When all of your child's primary teeth have come in (usually around age 2 1/2) your dentist may start applying topical fluoride. Fluoride hardens the tooth enamel, helping to ward off the most common childhood oral disease, dental caries, or cavities. Cavities are caused by bacteria and food that are left on the teeth after eating. When these are not brushed away, acid collects on a tooth, softening its enamel until a hole—or cavity—forms. Regular use of fluoride toughens the enamel, making it more difficult for acid to penetrate.

Although many municipalities require tap water to be fluoridated, other communities have no such regulations. If the water supply is not fluoridated, or if your family uses purified water, ask your dentist for fluoride supplements. Even though most toothpastes contain fluoride, toothpaste alone will not fully protect a child's mouth. Be careful, however, since too much fluoride can cause tooth discoloration. Check with your dentist before supplementing.

Discoloration can also occur as a result of prolonged use of antibiotics, as some children's medications contain a large amount of sugar.

Parents should encourage children to brush after they take their medicine, particularly if the prescription will be long-term.

Brushing at least twice a day and routine flossing will help maintain a healthy mouth. Kids as young as age 2 or 3 can begin to use toothpaste when brushing, as long as they are supervised. Kids should not ingest large amounts of toothpaste—a pea-sized amount for toddlers is just right. Parents should always make sure the child spits the toothpaste out instead of swallowing.

As your child's permanent teeth grow in, the dentist can help seal out decay by applying a thin wash of resin to the back teeth, where most chewing occurs. Known as a sealant, this protective coating keeps bacteria from settling in the hard-to-reach crevices of the molars.

Although dental research has resulted in increasingly sophisticated preventative techniques, including fillings and sealants that seep fluoride, a dentist's care is only part of the equation. Follow-up at home plays an equally important role. For example, sealants on the teeth do not mean that a child can eat sweets uncontrollably or slack off on the daily brushing and flossing—parents must work with kids to teach good oral health habits.

What should I do if my child has a problem?

If you are prone to tooth decay or gum disease, your child may be at higher risk as well. Therefore, sometimes even the most diligent brushing and flossing will not prevent a cavity. Be sure to call your dentist if your child complains of tooth pain. The pain could be a sign of a cavity that needs to be treated.

New materials have given the pediatric dentist more filling and repair options than ever before. Silver remains the substance of choice for the majority of fillings in permanent teeth. Other materials, such as composite resins, also are gaining popularity. Composite resins bond to the teeth so the filling won't pop out, and they can be used to rebuild teeth damaged through injury or conditions such as cleft palate.

Tooth-colored resins are also more attractive. But in cases of fracture, extensive decay, or malformation of baby teeth, dentists often opt for stainless steel crowns. Crowns maintain the tooth while preventing the decay from spreading.

As kids grow older, their bite and the straightness of their teeth can become an issue. Orthodontic treatment begins earlier now than it once did, but what once was a symbol of preteen anguish—a mouth filled with metal wires and braces—is a relic of the past. Kids as young as age 7 now sport corrective appliances. Efficient, plastic-based materials have replaced old-fashioned metal contraptions. Dentists now understand that manipulation of teeth at a younger age can be easier and more effective in the long run. Younger children's teeth can be positioned with relatively minor orthodontia, thus preventing major orthodontia later on.

In some rare instances, usually when a more complicated dental procedure is to be performed, a dentist will recommend general anesthesia be used.

Parents should make sure that the professional who administers the medicine is a trained anesthesiologist or oral surgeon before agreeing to the procedure. Don't be afraid to question the dentist. Giving your child an early start on checkups and good dental hygiene is an effective way to help prevent this kind of extensive dental work. Encouraging your child to use a mouth guard during sports can also prevent serious dental injuries.

As your child grows, plan on routine dental checkups anywhere from once every 3 months to once a year, depending on the dentist's recommendations. Limiting intake of sugary foods and regular brushing and flossing all contribute to your child's dental health. Your partnership with the dentist will help ensure healthy teeth and a beautiful smile.

Section 4.2

Your Child's Nutrition and How It Affects Oral Health

"Diet and Snacking," © 2008 American Academy of Pediatric Dentistry (www.aapd.org). Reprinted with permission.

What is a healthy diet for my child?

A healthy diet is a balanced diet that naturally supplies all the nutrients your child needs to grow. And what's a balanced diet? One that includes the following major food groups every day: fruits and vegetables; breads and cereals; milk and dairy products; meat, fish, and eggs.

How does my child's diet affect her dental health?

She must have a balanced diet for her teeth to develop properly. She also needs a balanced diet for healthy gum tissue around the teeth. Equally important, a diet high in certain kinds of carbohydrates, such as sugar and starches, may place your child at extra risk of tooth decay.

How do I make my child's diet safe for his teeth?

First, be sure he has a balanced diet. Then, check how frequently he eats foods with sugar or starch in them. Foods with starch include breads, crackers, pasta, and such snacks as pretzels and potato chips. When checking for sugar, look beyond the sugar bowl and candy dish. A variety of foods contain one or more types of sugar, and all types of sugars can promote dental decay. Fruits, a few vegetables, and most milk products have at least one type of sugar.

Sugar can be found in many processed foods, even some that do not taste sweet. For example, a peanut butter and jelly sandwich not only has sugar in the jelly, but may have sugar added to the peanut butter. Sugar is also added to such condiments as catsup and salad dressings.

Should my child give up all foods with sugar or starch?

Certainly not. Many provide nutrients your child needs. You simply need to select and serve them wisely. A food with sugar or starch is safer for teeth if it's eaten with a meal, not as a snack. Sticky foods, such as dried fruit or toffee, are not easily washed away from the teeth by saliva, water or milk. So, they have more cavity-causing potential than foods more rapidly cleared from the teeth. Talk to your pediatric dentist about selecting and serving foods that protect your child's dental health.

Does a balanced diet assure that my child is getting enough fluoride?

No. A balanced diet does not guarantee the proper amount of fluoride for the development and maintenance of your child's teeth. If you do not live in a fluoridated community or have an ideal amount of naturally occurring fluoride in your well water, your child needs a fluoride supplement during the years of tooth development. Your pediatric dentist can help assess how much supplemental fluoride your child needs, based upon the amount of fluoride in your drinking water and your child's age and weight.

My youngest isn't on solid foods yet. Do you have suggestions for her?

Don't nurse your daughter to sleep or put her to bed with a bottle of milk, formula, juice, or sweetened liquid. While she sleeps, any unswallowed liquid in the mouth supports bacteria that produce acids and attack the teeth. Protect your child from severe tooth decay by putting her to bed with nothing more than a pacifier or bottle of water.

Any final advice?

Yes. Here are tips for your child's diet and dental health.

- Ask your pediatric dentist to help you assess your child's diet.
- Shop smart. Do not routinely stock your pantry with sugary or starchy snacks. Buy "fun foods" just for special times.
- Limit the number of snack times; choose nutritious snacks.
- Provide a balanced diet, and save foods with sugar or starch for mealtimes.

- Don't put your young child to bed with a bottle of milk, formula, or juice.

- If your child chews gum or sips soda, choose those without sugar.

Chapter 5

Oral Health in Adolescents

Chapter Contents

Section 5.1—Oral Health Advice for Teens 44
Section 5.2—Oral Piercings: What Problems Can They
            Cause? 49

Section 5.1

Oral Health Advice for Teens

"Taking Care of Your Teeth," July 2005, reprinted with permission from www.kidshealth.org. Copyright © 2005 The Nemours Foundation. This information was provided by KidsHealth, one of the largest resources online for medically reviewed health information written for parents, kids, and teens. For more articles like this one, visit www.KidsHealth.org, or www.TeensHealth.org. Reviewed by Garrett B. Lyons, Sr., D.D.S., and Lisa A. Goss, R.D.H., B.S.

Dentists say that the most important part of tooth care happens at home. Brushing and flossing properly, along with regular dental checkups, can help prevent tooth decay and gum disease.

If you're like most people, you don't exactly look forward to facing a dentist's drill. So wouldn't it be better to prevent cavities before they begin?

Giving Plaque the Brush-Off

To prevent cavities, you need to remove plaque, the transparent layer of bacteria that coats the teeth. The best way to do this is by brushing your teeth twice a day and flossing at least once a day. Brushing also stimulates the gums, which helps to keep them healthy and prevent gum disease. Brushing and flossing are the most important things that you can do to keep your teeth and gums healthy.

Toothpastes contain abrasives, detergents, and foaming agents. Fluoride, the most common active ingredient in toothpaste, is what prevents cavities. So you should always be sure your toothpaste contains fluoride.

About one person in 10 has a tendency to accumulate tartar quickly. Tartar is plaque in a hardened form that is more damaging and difficult to remove. Using antitartar toothpastes and mouthwashes, as well as spending extra time brushing the teeth near the salivary glands (the inside of the lower front teeth and the outside of the upper back teeth), may slow the development of new tartar.

If you have teeth that are sensitive to heat, cold, and pressure, you may want to try a special toothpaste for sensitive teeth. But you'll still need to talk to your dentist about your sensitivity because it may indicate a more serious problem, such as a cavity or nerve inflammation (irritation).

Tips on Proper Brushing

Dentists say that the minimum time you should spend brushing your teeth is 2 minutes twice a day. Here are some tips on how to brush properly:

- Hold your brush at a 45-degree angle against your gumline. Gently brush from where the tooth and gum meet to the chewing surface in short (about half-a-tooth-wide) strokes. Brushing too hard can cause receding gums, tooth sensitivity, and, over time, loose teeth.

- Use the same method to brush all outside and inside surfaces of your teeth.

- To clean the chewing surfaces of your teeth, use short sweeping strokes, tipping the bristles into the pits and crevices.

- To clean the inside surfaces of your top and bottom front teeth and gums, hold the brush almost vertical. With back and forth motions, bring the front part of the brush over the teeth and gums.

- Using a forward-sweeping motion, gently brush your tongue and the roof of your mouth to remove the decay-causing bacteria that exist in these places.

- Use an egg timer or play a favorite song while brushing your teeth to get used to brushing for a full 2 to 3 minutes. Some electronic toothbrushes have timers that let you know when 2 minutes are up.

Facts on Flossing

Brushing is important but it won't remove the plaque and particles of food between your teeth, under the gumline, or under braces.

You'll need to floss these spaces at least once a day. The type of floss you choose depends on how much space you have between your teeth. Dentists usually recommend unwaxed floss because it's thinner and easier to slide through small spaces. However, studies have shown that there is no major difference in the effectiveness based on the type of floss used.

With any floss, you should be careful to avoid injuring your gums. Follow these instructions:

- Carefully insert the floss between two teeth, using a back and forth motion. Gently bring the floss to the gumline, but don't force it under the gums. Curve the floss around the edge of your tooth in the shape of the letter "C" and slide it up and down the side of each tooth.

- Repeat this process between all your teeth, and remember to floss the back sides of your back teeth.

Tooth-Whitening Products

Some toothpastes claim to whiten teeth. There's nothing wrong with using whitening toothpastes as long as they also contain fluoride and ingredients that fight plaque and tartar. But these toothpastes alone don't contain much in the way of whitening ingredients and probably won't noticeably change the color of your teeth.

It's easy to be lured by ads telling people they need gleaming white teeth. But these ads are really targeted to older people. The truth is that most teens don't need tooth whitening because teeth usually yellow as a person gets older. If you think your teeth aren't white enough, though, talk to your dentist before you try any over-the-counter whitening products. Your dentist may be able to offer you professional treatment, which will be suited to your unique needs and will work better than over-the-counter products.

Be careful when buying over-the-counter whitening products. Some bleaching agents may damage your gums and mouth. So always follow the instructions on any whitening product you use.

The Nutrition Connection

Eating sugar, as you probably already know, is a major cause of tooth decay. But it's not just how much sugar you eat—when and how you eat it can be just as important to keeping teeth healthy.

When you eat sugary foods or drink sodas frequently throughout the day, the enamel that protects your teeth is constantly exposed to acids. Hard candies, cough drops, and breath mints that contain sugar are especially harmful because they dissolve slowly in your mouth. Many experts suggest that you take a 3-hour break between eating foods containing sugar.

Sugary or starchy foods eaten with a meal are less harmful to your teeth than when they're eaten alone, possibly because the production of saliva, which washes away the sugar and bacteria, is increased. Eating sugary foods before you go to bed can be the most damaging (especially if you don't brush your teeth afterward) because you don't produce as much saliva when you sleep.

For most people, it's hard to cut out sweets completely, so try to follow these more realistic guidelines:

- Eat carbohydrates (sugars and starches) with a meal.

- If you can't brush your teeth after eating, rinse your mouth with water or mouthwash, or chew sugarless gum.

- Don't eat sugary foods between meals.

- If you snack, eat nonsugary foods, such as cheese, popcorn, raw veggies, or yogurt.

Going to the Dentist

The main reason for going to the dentist regularly—every 6 months—is prevention. The goal is to prevent tooth decay, gum disease, and other disorders that put the health of your teeth and mouth at risk.

Your first consultation with a dentist will probably consist of three main parts: a dental and medical history (where the dentist or dental hygienist asks you questions about your tooth care and reviews any dental records), a dental examination, and a professional cleaning.

The dentist will examine your teeth, gums, and other mouth tissues. He or she may also examine the joints of your jaws. The dentist will use a mirror and probe (a metal pick-like instrument) to check the crown (visible part) of each tooth for plaque and evidence of looseness or decay. The dentist also will check your bite and the way your teeth fit together (also called occlusion).

Your dentist will examine the general condition of your gums, which should be firm and pink, not soft, swollen, or inflamed. He or she (or an assistant) will use the probe to check the depth of the sulcus, the slight depression where each tooth meets the gum. Deep depressions, called pockets, are evidence of gum disease.

After examining the visible parts of your teeth and mouth, your dentist will take x-rays that might reveal tooth decay, abscesses (collections of pus surrounded by swollen tissue), or impacted wisdom teeth.

Professional cleaning is usually performed by a dental hygienist, a specially trained and licensed dental professional. Cleaning consists mainly of removing hard deposits using a scaler (a scraping instrument) or an ultrasonic machine, which uses high-frequency sound waves to loosen plaque deposits. The particles are then rinsed off with water.

After cleaning, the dental hygienist will polish your teeth. The process cleans and smoothes the surfaces of the teeth, removing stains and making it harder for plaque to stick to the teeth. Finally, the hygienist may treat your teeth with a fluoride compound or a sealant to help prevent decay.

At the end of your visit, the dentist will let you know if you need to return to fill a cavity. Your dentist also may refer you to an orthodontist if he or she thinks you may need braces or have other issues.

More Dental Problems

Dental caries (tooth decay) can attack the teeth at any age. In fact, 84% of 17-year-olds have the disease. Left untreated, caries can cause severe pain and result in tooth loss. Losing teeth affects how you look and feel about yourself as well as your ability to chew and speak. Treating caries is also expensive. So prevention and early treatment are important.

It may surprise you to know that 60% of 15-year-olds experience gingivitis, the first stage of gum disease. Gingivitis, which involves the gums but not the underlying bone and ligament, is almost always caused by an accumulation of plaque. As with caries, treatment can be expensive. If you remove plaque regularly and follow good oral hygiene habits, your gums usually will return to their healthy state. However, more serious gum disease can cause gums to swell, turn red, and bleed, and sometimes causes discomfort. How dentists treat gum disease depends on the extent of the disease.

Section 5.2

Oral Piercings:
What Problems Can They Cause?

Excerpted from "Oral Piercing and Soldiers," by the
U.S. Army Center for Health Promotion and Preventive Medicine
(usachppm.apgea.army.mil/dhpw), 2006.

Body piercing has become viewed as a form of self-expression in today's society. Piercing areas of the face or mouth is especially popular.

Dangers of Oral Piercing

Piercers who do not follow infection control procedures place clients at risk of diseases such as hepatitis, HIV [human immunodeficiency virus], herpes, Epstein-Barr, or tetanus.

Oral piercing has a high risk of complications because it is usually performed by someone who is unlicensed or self-trained. Common problems following oral piercing include the following:

- pain;
- swelling;
- prolonged bleeding;
- infection;
- increased salivation;
- interference with speaking, chewing, and swallowing;
- scar tissue formation;
- hypersensitivity or allergy to metals;
- collection of debris in the pierced site; and
- inhalation of pieces of jewelry.

Damage from Oral Piercing

The most common problems caused by oral piercing are damage to the teeth and gums. Metal objects fastened to the tongue or lips

49

are often accidentally bitten. As a result, teeth become chipped, cracked, and even broken. These injuries can be quite painful and expensive to repair. The metal objects can also rub on the gums. The gums can become injured or even stripped away from the teeth.

Chapter 6

Adult Oral Health

Chapter Contents

Section 6.1—What Adults Can Do to Maintain Good Oral
Health 52

Section 6.2—Dental Concerns in Women 54

Section 6.3—Menstrual Cycle Affects Periodontal Health 57

Section 6.4—What Your Gums Can Expect When You're
Expecting 58

Section 6.5—Why Is Dental Care Important for Men? 60

Section 6.1

What Adults Can Do to Maintain Good Oral Health

"Oral Health for Adults," from the Centers for Disease Control and Prevention (CDC, www.cdc.gov), Division of Oral Health, December 2006.

The baby boomer generation will be the first where the majority will maintain their natural teeth over their entire lifetime, having benefited from water fluoridation and fluoride toothpastes.

Over the past 10 years, the number of adults missing all their natural teeth has declined from 31 percent to 25 percent for those aged 60 years and older, and from 9 percent to 5 percent for those adults between 40 and 59 years. However, 5 percent means a surprising 1 out of 20 middle-aged adults are missing all their teeth.

Over 40 percent of poor adults (20 years and older) have at least one untreated decayed tooth compared to 16 percent of non-poor adults.

Toothaches are the most common pain of the mouth or face reported by adults. This pain can interfere with vital functions such as eating, swallowing, and talking. Almost 1 of every 4 adults reported some form of facial pain in the past 6 months.

Most adults show signs of gum disease. Severe gum disease affects about 14 percent of adults aged 45 to 54 years.

Signs and symptoms of soft tissue diseases such as cold sores are common in adults and affect about 19 percent of those aged 25 to 44 years.

Chronic disabling diseases such as jaw joint diseases (temporomandibular disorders, or TMD), diabetes, and osteoporosis affect millions of Americans and compromise oral health and functioning.

Women report certain painful mouth and facial conditions (TMD, migraine headaches, and burning mouth syndrome) more often than men.

Every year more than 400,000 cancer patients undergoing chemotherapy suffer from oral problems such as painful mouth ulcers, impaired taste, and dry mouth.

Patients with weakened immune systems, such as those infected with HIV [human immunodeficiency virus] and other medical conditions (organ transplants) and who use some medications (e.g., steroids), are at higher risk for some oral problems.

Employed adults lose more than 164 million hours of work each year due to oral health problems or dental visits. Customer service industry employees lose 2 to 4 times more work hours than executives or professional workers.

For every adult 19 years or older without medical insurance, there are three without dental insurance.

Seventy percent of adults reported visiting a dentist in the past 12 months. Those with incomes at or above the poverty level are much more likely to report a visit to a dentist in the past 12 months as those with lower incomes.

What You Can Do to Maintain Good Oral Health

- Drink fluoridated water and use a fluoride toothpaste. Fluoride's protection against tooth decay works at all ages.

- Take care of your teeth and gums. Thorough tooth brushing and flossing to reduce dental plaque can prevent gingivitis—the mildest form of gum disease.

- Avoid tobacco. In addition to the general health risks posed by tobacco, smokers have four times the risk of developing gum disease compared to non-smokers. Tobacco use in any form—cigarette, pipes, and smokeless (spit) tobacco—increases the risk for gum disease, oral and throat cancers, and oral fungal infection (candidiasis). Spit tobacco containing sugar increases the risk of tooth decay.

- Limit alcohol. Heavy use of alcohol is also a risk factor for oral and throat cancers. When used alone, alcohol and tobacco are risk factors for oral cancers, but when used in combination the effects of alcohol and tobacco are even greater.

- Eat wisely. Adults should avoid snacks full of sugars and starches. Limit the number of snacks eaten throughout the day. The recommended five-a-day helping of fiber-rich fruits and vegetables stimulates salivary flow to aid remineralization of tooth surfaces with early stages of tooth decay.

- Visit the dentist regularly. Checkups can detect early signs of oral health problems and can lead to treatments that will prevent further damage, and in some cases, reverse the problem. Professional tooth cleaning (prophylaxis) also is important for preventing oral problems, especially when self-care is difficult.

- Diabetic patients should work to maintain control of their disease. This will help prevent the complications of diabetes, including an increased risk of gum disease.

- If medications produce a dry mouth, ask your doctor if there are other drugs that can be substituted. If dry mouth cannot be avoided, drink plenty of water, chew sugarless gum, and avoid tobacco and alcohol.

- Have an oral health checkup before beginning cancer treatment. Radiation to the head or neck and/or chemotherapy may cause problems for your teeth and gums. Treating existing oral health problems before cancer therapy may help prevent or limit oral complications or tissue damage.

Section 6.2

Dental Concerns in Women

"Protecting Oral Health Throughout Your Life," © 2004 American
Academy of Periodontology (www.perio.org). Reprinted with permission.

As a woman, you know that your health needs are unique. You also know that at specific times in your life, you need to take extra care of yourself. Times when you mature and change, for example, puberty or menopause, and times when you have special health needs, such as menstruation or pregnancy. Did you know that your oral health needs also change at these times?

While women tend to take better care of their oral health than men do, women's oral health is not markedly better than men's. This is because hormonal fluctuations throughout a woman's life can affect many tissues, including gum tissue.

A study published in the January 1999 issue of the *Journal of Periodontology* reports that at least 23 percent of women ages 30 to 54 have periodontitis (an advanced state of periodontal disease in which there is active destruction of the periodontal supporting tissues). And, 44 percent of women ages 55 to 90 who still have their teeth have periodontitis.

Because periodontal disease is often a "silent" disease, many women do not realize they have it until it reaches an advanced state. However, at each stage of your life, you can take steps to protect your oral health.

Puberty

During puberty, an increased level of sex hormones, such as progesterone and possibly estrogen, causes increased blood circulation to the gums. This may cause an increase in the gum's sensitivity and lead to a greater reaction to any irritation, including food particles and plaque. During this time, the gums may become swollen, turn red, and feel tender.

As a young woman progresses through puberty, the tendency for her gums to swell in response to irritants will lessen. However, during puberty, it is important to follow a good at-home oral hygiene regimen, including regular brushing and flossing, and regular dental care. In some cases, a dental professional may recommend periodontal therapy to help prevent damage to the tissues and bone surrounding the teeth.

Menstruation

Occasionally, some women experience menstruation gingivitis. Women with this condition may experience bleeding gums, bright red and swollen gums, and sores on the inside of the cheek. Menstruation gingivitis typically occurs right before a woman's period and clears up once her period has started.

Pregnancy

Women may experience increased gingivitis or pregnancy gingivitis beginning in the second or third month of pregnancy that increases in severity throughout the eighth month. During this time, some women may notice swelling, bleeding, redness, or tenderness in the gum tissue.

In some cases, gums swollen by pregnancy gingivitis can react strongly to irritants and form large lumps. These growths, called pregnancy tumors, are not cancerous and are generally painless. If the tumor persists, it may require removal by a periodontist.

Studies have shown a relationship between periodontal disease and preterm, low-birthweight babies. Any infection, including periodontal infection, is cause for concern during pregnancy. In fact, pregnant women who have periodontal disease may be seven times more likely to have a baby that is born too early and too small. If you are planning to become pregnant, be sure to include a periodontal evaluation as part of your prenatal care.

Women who use oral contraceptives may be susceptible to the same oral health conditions that affect pregnant women. They may experience red, bleeding, and swollen gums. Women who use oral contraceptives should know that taking drugs sometimes used to help treat periodontal disease, such as antibiotics, may lessen the effect of an oral contraceptive.

Menopause and Postmenopause

Women who are menopausal or postmenopausal may experience changes in their mouths. They may notice discomfort in the mouth, including dry mouth, pain, and burning sensations in the gum tissue and altered taste, especially salty, peppery, or sour.

In addition, menopausal gingivostomatitis affects a small percentage of women. Gums that look dry or shiny, bleed easily, and range from abnormally pale to deep red mark this condition. Most women find that estrogen supplements help to relieve these symptoms.

Bone loss is associated with both periodontal disease and osteoporosis. Research is being done to determine whether the two are related. Women considering Hormone Replacement Therapy (HRT) to help fight osteoporosis should note that this may help protect their teeth as well as other parts of the body.

Steps to Protect Oral Health

Careful periodontal monitoring and excellent oral hygiene is especially important for women who may be noticing changes in their mouths during times of hormonal fluctuation. To help ensure good oral (and overall) health, be sure to:

- See a dental professional for cleaning at least twice a year.

- See a periodontist in your area if you or your dentist notice problems with your gum tissue. Problems may include:

    - Red, swollen, or tender gums

    - Gums that have pulled away from the teeth

    - Persistent bad breath

- Pus between the teeth and gums
- Loose or separating teeth
- A change in the way your teeth fit together when you bite
- A change in the fit of your dentures

- Keep your dental professionals informed about any medications you are taking and any changes in your health history.

- Brush and floss properly every day. Review your techniques with a dental professional or view a free American Academy of Periodontology brochure sample [http://www.perio.org/consumer/request.htm] on how to brush and floss.

Section 6.3

Menstrual Cycle Affects Periodontal Health

Many women report an increase in gingival inflammation and discomfort associated with their menstrual cycle, according to findings published in the March [2004] *Journal of Periodontology*. This is the first time this well-known phenomenon has ever been studied.

"What we found is that several women reported considerable oral symptoms prior to menses," said Eli E. Machtei, D.M.D., Unit of Periodontology Department of Maxillofacial Surgery, Rambam Medical Center and Technion Faculty of Medicine.

The symptoms included a slight burning sensation, bleeding with minor irritation, redness to the gums, oral ulcers, and general pain and discomfort in the gums.

In this study, researchers compared the gingival and periodontal status of 18 premenopausal women between the ages of 20 to 50 years at different time points of their menstrual cycles. The time points were ovulation, premenstruation, and menstruation. During the examination, researchers measured plaque index, gingival index, probing depth, gingival recession and clinical attachment level.

"Gingival inflammation was lower during menstruation than during ovulation and premenstruation," said Machtei. "This may be attributed to the hormone known as serum estradiol, which is a natural form of estrogen that peaks and drops during ovulation and premenstruation."

"Further studies will be required to explore the mechanism by which this phenomenon occurs, and to examine whether these transitional changes have any lasting negative effects on the periodontium," said Michael P. Rethman, D.D.S., MS, and president of the American Academy of Periodontology. "In the meantime, patients should remember the importance of telling their dental professionals about what is going on in their bodies including any prescription or over-the-counter medications they are taking. This way dental professionals can explain any effects it has on periodontal health."

Section 6.4

What Your Gums Can Expect When You're Expecting

Good oral health is always important. However, it may be especially important for expectant mothers, as recent research suggests that pregnant women with periodontal diseases may be up to seven times more likely to have a baby that's born too early and too small. Preterm births are dangerous for both baby and mother. They are the leading cause of neonatal death and can lead to life-long health problems such as cerebral palsy, mental retardation, and difficulties with blindness and lung disease.

What Causes the Connection?

The likely culprit of this possible connection is a labor-inducing chemical called prostaglandin found in oral bacteria. Very high levels of prostaglandin are present in women with severe cases of periodontal disease. In addition, other research has identified bacteria commonly found in the mouth and associated with periodontal diseases in the amniotic fluid of some pregnant women. Amniotic fluid is the liquid that surrounds an unborn baby during pregnancy. Any disruptions in the amniotic fluid, such as a bacterial infection, could potentially be dangerous to both the mother and baby.

What Should You Do?

Don't panic. Take your concerns to your dental professional. If you're diagnosed with periodontal disease, your periodontist might recommend a common nonsurgical procedure called scaling and root planing. During this procedure, your tooth-root surfaces are cleaned to remove plaque and tartar from deep periodontal pockets and to smooth the root to remove bacterial toxins. Research suggests that scaling and root planing may reduce the risk of preterm birth in pregnant women with periodontal disease by up to 84 percent.

Attention, Women of All Ages

It isn't just pregnant women who should pay special attention to their periodontal health; women of all ages should take action.
Consider the following results of two recent studies:

- Women taking oral contraceptive pills were found to have more gingival bleeding during probing and deeper periodontal pockets than those who were not using oral contraception. It is important for women to alert their dental practitioners if they are taking medications such as oral contraceptive pills that may affect oral health.

- Postmenopausal women with periodontal bacteria in their mouths were also more likely to have bone loss in the oral cavity, a condition which can lead to tooth loss if not treated.

Section 6.5

Why Is Dental Care Important for Men?

"Why is Oral Health Important for Men?"
© 2007 Academy of General Dentistry (www.agd.org).
Reprinted with permission.

Men are less likely than women to take care of their physical health and, according to surveys and studies, their oral health is equally ignored. Good oral health recently has been linked with longevity. Yet, one of the most common factors associated with infrequent dental checkups is just being male. Men are less likely than women to seek preventive dental care and often neglect their oral health for years, visiting a dentist only when a problem arises. When it comes to oral health, statistics show that the average man brushes his teeth 1.9 times a day and will lose 5.4 teeth by age 72. If he smokes, he can plan on losing 12 teeth by age 72. Men are also more likely to develop oral and throat cancer and periodontal (gum) disease.

Why Is Periodontal Disease a Problem?

Periodontal disease is a result of plaque, which hardens into a rough, porous substance called tartar. The acids produced and released by bacteria found in tartar irritate gums. These acids cause the breakdown of fibers that anchor the gums tightly to the teeth, creating periodontal pockets that fill with even more bacteria. Researchers have found a connection between gum disease and cardiovascular disease, which can place people at risk for heart attacks and strokes. See your dentist if you have any of these symptoms:

- Bleeding gums during brushing
- Red, swollen, or tender gums
- Persistent bad breath
- Loose or separating teeth
- Do you take medications?

Since men are more likely to suffer from heart attacks, they also are more likely to be on medications that can cause dry mouth. If you take medication for the heart or blood pressure, or if you take anti-depressants, your salivary flow could be inhibited, increasing the risk for cavities. Saliva helps to reduce the cavity-causing bacteria found in your mouth.

Do You Use Tobacco?

If you smoke or chew, you have a greater risk for gum disease and oral cancer. Men are affected twice as often as women, and 95% of oral cancers occur in those over 40 years of age.

The most frequent oral cancer sites are the tongue, the floor of the mouth, and soft palate tissues in back of the tongue, lips, and gums. If not diagnosed and treated in its early stages, oral cancer can spread, leading to chronic pain, loss of function, and irreparable facial and oral disfigurement following surgery and even death. More than 8,000 people die each year from oral and pharyngeal diseases. If you use tobacco, it is important to see a dentist frequently for cleanings and to ensure your mouth remains healthy. Your general dentist can perform a thorough screening for oral cancer.

Do You Play Sports?

If you participate in sports, you have a greater potential for trauma to your mouth and teeth. If you play contact sports, such as football, soccer, basketball, and even baseball, it is important to use a mouth-guard, which is a flexible appliance made of plastic that protects teeth from trauma. If you ride bicycles or motorcycles, wear a helmet.

Taking Care of Your Teeth

To take better care of your oral health, it is important to floss daily, brush your teeth with fluoride toothpaste twice daily, and visit your dentist at least twice a year for cleanings. Here are some tips to better dental health:

- Use a soft-bristled toothbrush to reach every surface of each tooth. If the bristles on your toothbrush are bent or frayed, buy a new one.

- Replace your toothbrush every three months or after you've been sick.

- Choose a toothpaste with fluoride. This can reduce tooth decay by as much as 40%.

- Brush properly. To clean the outside surfaces of your teeth, position the brush at a 45-degree angle where your gums and teeth meet. Gently move the brush in a circular motion using short, gentle strokes. To clean the inside surfaces of the upper and lower front teeth, hold the brush vertically. Make several gentle strokes over each tooth and its surrounding gum tissue. Spend at least three minutes brushing.

- Floss properly. Gently insert floss between teeth using a back-and-forth motion. Do not force the floss or snap it into place. Curve the floss into a C-shape against one tooth and then the other.

Chapter 7

Oral Health Concerns in the Elderly

Chapter Contents

Section 7.1—Overview of Oral Health Concerns in Older
          Americans 64
Section 7.2—Taking Care of Your Teeth and Mouth as
          You Age 67

Section 7.1

Overview of Oral Health Concerns in Older Americans

"Oral Health for Older Americans,"
from the Centers for Disease Control and Prevention
(CDC, www.cdc.gov), Division of Oral Health, December 2006.

Older Americans make up a growing percentage of the U.S. population; according to the 2000 U.S. Census, nearly 35 million are 65 years or older. By 2050, that number is expected to increase to 48 million. Oral diseases and conditions are common among these Americans who grew up without the benefit of community water fluoridation and other fluoride products.

Older Americans with the poorest oral health are those who are economically disadvantaged, lack insurance, and are members of racial and ethnic minorities. Being disabled, homebound, or institutionalized also increases the risk of poor oral health.

Many older Americans do not have dental insurance. Often these benefits are lost when they retire. The situation may be worse for older women, who generally have lower incomes and may never have had dental insurance.

Medicaid, the jointly-funded federal-state health insurance program for certain low-income and needy people, funds dental care for low income and disabled elderly in some states, but reimbursements for this care are low. Medicare, which provides health insurance for people over age 65 and people with certain illnesses and disabilities, was not designed to provide routine dental care.

About 25 percent of adults 60 years old and older no longer have any natural teeth. Interestingly, toothlessness varies greatly by state. Roughly 42 percent of Americans over age 65 living in West Virginia are toothless, compared to only 13 percent of those living in California. Having missing teeth can affect nutrition, since people without teeth often prefer soft, easily chewed foods. Because dentures are not as efficient for chewing food as natural teeth, denture wearers also may choose soft foods and avoid fresh fruits and vegetables.

Periodontal (gum) disease or tooth decay (cavities) are the most frequent causes of tooth loss. Older Americans continue to experience dental decay on the crowns of teeth (coronal caries) and on tooth roots (because of gum recession). In fact, older adults may have new tooth decay at higher rates than children.

Severity of periodontal (gum) disease increases with age. About 23 percent of 65- to 74-year-olds have severe disease, which is measured by 6 mm loss of attachment of the tooth to the adjacent gum tissue. At all ages men are more likely than women to have more severe disease. At all ages, people at the lowest socioeconomic level have the most severe periodontal disease.

Oral and pharyngeal cancers, which are diagnosed in some 31,000 Americans each year, result in about 7,400 deaths each year. These cancers are primarily diagnosed in the elderly. Prognosis is poor. The five-year survival rate for white patients is 56 percent and for African American patients is only 34 percent.

Most older Americans take both prescription and over-the-counter drugs. Over 400 commonly used medications can be the cause of a dry mouth. Reduction of the flow of saliva increases the risk for oral disease, since saliva contains antimicrobial components as well as minerals that help rebuild tooth enamel attacked by decay-causing bacteria. Individuals in long-term care facilities—about 5 percent of the elderly—take an average of eight drugs each day.

Painful conditions that affect the facial nerves are more common among the elderly and can be severely debilitating. These conditions can affect mood, sleep, and oral-motor functions such as chewing and swallowing. Neurological diseases associated with age, such as Parkinson disease, Alzheimer disease, Huntington disease, and stroke also affect oral sensory and motor functions, in addition to limiting the ability to care for oneself.

What Can I Do to Maintain My Oral Health?

- Drink fluoridated water and use fluoride toothpaste; fluoride provides protection against dental decay at all ages.

- Practice good oral hygiene. Careful tooth brushing and flossing to reduce dental plaque can help prevent periodontal disease.

- It is important to see your dentist on a regular basis, even if you have no natural teeth and have dentures. Professional care helps to maintain the overall health of the teeth and mouth, and provides for early detection of precancerous or cancerous lesions.

- Avoid tobacco. In addition to the general health risks posed by tobacco use, smokers have seven times the risk of developing periodontal disease compared to non-smokers. Tobacco used in any form—cigarettes, cigars, pipes, and smokeless (spit) tobacco—increases the risk for periodontal disease, oral and throat cancers, and oral fungal infection (candidiasis). Spit tobacco containing sugar also increases the risk of cavities.

- Limit alcohol. Drinking a high amount of alcoholic beverages is a risk factor for oral and throat cancers. Alcohol and tobacco used together are the primary risk factors for these cancers.

- Make sure that you or your loved one gets dental care prior to having cancer chemotherapy or radiation to the head or neck. These therapies can damage or destroy oral tissues and can result in severe irritation of the oral tissues and mouth ulcers, loss of salivary function, rampant tooth decay, and destruction of bone.

- Caregivers should reinforce the daily oral hygiene routines of elders who are unable to perform these activities independently.

- Sudden changes in taste and smell should not be considered signs of aging, but should be a sign to seek professional care.

- If medications produce a dry mouth, ask your doctor if there are other drugs that can be substituted. If dry mouth cannot be avoided, drink plenty of water, chew sugarless gum, and avoid tobacco and alcohol.

Section 7.2

Taking Care of Your Teeth and Mouth as You Age

Excerpted from "Taking Care of Your Teeth and Mouth," from the National Institute on Aging (NIA, www.nia.nih.gov), part of the National Institutes of Health, March 7, 2007.

No matter how old you are, you need to take care of your teeth and mouth. When your mouth is healthy, you can eat the foods you need for good nutrition. You will also feel better about smiling, talking, and laughing. Teeth are meant to last a lifetime. By taking good care of your teeth and gums, you can protect them for many years.

Tooth Decay

Teeth are covered in a hard, outer coating called enamel. Every day, a thin film of bacteria builds up on your teeth. Over time, the bacteria can cause holes in the enamel. These holes are called cavities. Brushing and flossing your teeth can protect you from decay, but once a cavity happens, a dentist has to fix it.

You can protect your teeth from decay by using fluoride toothpaste. If you have a lot of tooth decay, your dentist or dental hygienist may give you a fluoride treatment during an office visit. Or, the dentist may tell you to use a fluoride gel or mouth rinse at home.

Gum Diseases

Gum disease begins when plaque builds up along and under the gum line. This plaque causes infections that hurt the gum and bone that hold teeth in place. Sometimes gum disease makes your gums tender and more likely to bleed. This problem, called gingivitis, can often be fixed by daily brushing and flossing.

Other gum diseases need to be treated by a dentist. If not treated, these infections can ruin the bones, gums, and other tissues that support your teeth. Over time, your teeth may have to be removed.

To prevent gum disease:

- Brush your teeth twice a day with fluoride toothpaste.
- Floss once a day.
- Visit your dentist regularly for a checkup and cleaning.
- Eat a well-balanced diet.
- Quit smoking. Smoking increases your risk for gum disease.

Cleaning Your Teeth and Gums

There is a right way to brush and floss your teeth. Every day:

- Gently brush your teeth on all sides with a soft-bristle brush and fluoride toothpaste.
- Use small circular motions and short back-and-forth strokes.
- Take the time to brush carefully and gently along the gum line.
- Lightly brush your tongue to help keep your mouth clean.

You also need to clean around your teeth with dental floss every day. Careful flossing will take off plaque and leftover food that a toothbrush can't reach. Be sure to rinse after you floss.

See your dentist if brushing or flossing causes your gums to bleed or hurts your mouth. If you have trouble flossing, a floss holder may help. Ask your dentist to show you the right way to floss.

People with arthritis or other conditions that limit hand motion may find it hard to hold a toothbrush. Some helpful ideas are:

- Slide a bicycle grip or foam tube over the handle of the toothbrush.
- Buy a toothbrush with a larger handle.
- Attach the toothbrush handle to your hand with a wide elastic band.

Dentures

Sometimes, dentures (false teeth) are needed to replace badly damaged teeth. Dentures may feel strange at first. In the beginning, your dentist may want to see you often to make sure the dentures fit. Over time, your mouth will change and your dentures may need to be adjusted or replaced. Be sure to let your dentist handle these adjustments.

When you are learning to eat with dentures, it may be easier if you:

- Start with soft, non-sticky food.
- Cut your food into small pieces.
- Chew slowly using both sides of your mouth.

Be careful when wearing dentures because they may make it harder for you to feel hot foods and liquids. Also, you may not notice things like bones in your mouth.

Keep your dentures clean and free from food that can cause stains, bad breath, or swollen gums. Brush them every day with a denture care product. Take your dentures out of your mouth at night and put them in water or a denture cleansing liquid. Partial dentures are used to fill in one or more missing teeth. Take care of them in the same way as dentures.

Dry Mouth

Dry mouth happens when you don't have enough saliva, or spit, to keep your mouth wet. That can make it hard to eat, swallow, taste, and even speak. Dry mouth can cause tooth decay and other infections of the mouth.

Many common medicines can cause dry mouth. Try sipping water or sugarless drinks. Stay away from drinks with caffeine. Don't smoke and avoid alcohol. Some people are helped by sucking sugarless hard candy or chewing sugarless gum. Talk to your dentist or doctor for other ideas on how to cope with dry mouth.

Oral Cancer

Oral cancer most often happens in people over age 40. Treatment works best before the disease spreads. Pain is not usually an early symptom of the disease. A dental checkup is a good time for your dentist to look for signs of oral cancer. Even if you have lost all your natural teeth, you should still see your dentist for regular oral cancer exams.

You can lower your risk of getting oral cancer in a few ways:

- Do not use tobacco products—cigarettes, chewing tobacco, snuff, pipes, or cigars.
- If you drink alcohol, do so only in moderation.
- Use lip balm with sunscreen.

Finding Low Cost Dental Care

The following resources may be helpful in finding low cost dental care:

- See if local dental schools have student clinics. Visit www.nidcr .nih.gov/FindingDentalCare/ReducedCost/FLCDC.htm.

- Contact your county or state health department to find dental clinics near you that charge based on income.

- Visit www.ask.hrsa.gov/pc to locate a community health center near you that offers dental services.

- Check your State or local dental association at www.ada.org/ ada/organizations/searchcons1.asp to find dentists in your area who have lower fees for older adults.

Chapter 8

Oral Care for People with Disabilities or Special Needs

Chapter Contents

Section 8.1—Who Needs Special Dental Care? 72
Section 8.2—Helping Someone Care for Their Teeth and
            Mouth: A Caregiver's Guide 73

Section 8.1

Who Needs Special Dental Care?

From "Special Care in Oral Health," National Institute of Dental and Craniofacial Research (NIDCR, www.nidcr.nih.gov), part of the National Institutes of Health, November 14, 2007.

What is special care?

It is an approach to oral health management tailored to the individual needs of people with a variety of medical conditions or limitations that require more than routine delivery of oral care. Special care encompasses preventive, diagnostic, and treatment services.

A person with diabetes who is at increased risk of gum disease, a young child who needs dentures because of a genetic disorder, or a person with arthritis who cannot hold a toothbrush require special care. Standard treatment procedures can be adapted to fit most patients' needs and abilities. While some patients require more specialized care, most can be treated successfully in general dental practices.

Why do patients need special care?

Some patients need routine oral health care, but have medical conditions or limitations that require delivery of care beyond the routine. The dental team, for example, may need to learn to transfer a patient with cerebral palsy from the wheelchair to the dental chair, to use some sign language to communicate with deaf patients, or to adapt oral hygiene devices so a patient can use them.

Other patients have medical and oral conditions that call for extraordinary care and require oral health professionals to have specialized knowledge. Surgical treatment of oral cancer or genetic craniofacial defects, such as cleft lip and palate, often require extensive reconstruction that involves many health specialists. Further, disorders such as ectodermal dysplasia and osteogenesis imperfecta directly affect tooth and facial development and demand specialized treatment.

In addition, many systemic diseases and certain medical treatments have oral health implications. Dental professionals may need to develop a treatment strategy for a patient who has received an organ transplant, determine the best anesthetic alternative for a patient who has heart disease, or develop an oral health plan for a patient who must undergo treatment for cancer.

Disability status also plays a role in special care and contributes to disparities in the oral health of affected Americans. The oral health of special care patients may be neglected because of a demanding disease, conditions such as developmental disabilities, or limited access to oral health care. The coordination of care and an understanding of special care issues in oral health are essential for all members of a patient's health care team, including medical and dental professionals and caregivers.

Section 8.2

Helping Someone Care for Their Teeth and Mouth: A Caregiver's Guide

From "Dental Care Every Day: A Caregiver's Guide," by the National Institute of Dental and Craniofacial Research (NIDCR, www.nidcr.nih.gov), part of the National Institutes of Health, November 9, 2007.

As a caregiver, you play an important role in maintaining the oral health of your client or family member. Helping someone with brushing and flossing, however, isn't always easy. But there are steps you can take to make daily dental care a good experience. The key ingredients are patience and preparation: pick a place in the house where the person is comfortable; allow time for him or her to adjust to the dental care; have a set routine; and reward cooperation. Remember, a healthy mouth can make a big difference in the quality of life for the person in your care.

Taking care of someone with a developmental disability requires patience and skill. As a caregiver, you know this as well as anyone does. You also know how challenging it is to help that person with dental care. It takes planning, time, and the ability to manage physical, mental, and behavioral problems. Dental care isn't always easy, but you can make it work for you and the person you help. This information will show you how to help someone brush, floss, and have a healthy mouth.

Everyone needs dental care every day. Brushing and flossing are crucial activities that affect our health. In fact, dental care is just as important to your client's health and daily routine as taking medications and getting physical exercise. A healthy mouth helps people eat well, avoid pain and tooth loss, and feel good about themselves.

Getting Started

Location: The bathroom isn't the only place to brush someone's teeth. For example, the kitchen or dining room may be more comfortable. Instead of standing next to a bathroom sink, allow the person to sit at a table. Place the toothbrush, toothpaste, floss, and a bowl and glass of water on the table within easy reach.

No matter what location you choose, make sure you have good light. You can't help someone brush unless you can see inside that person's mouth. Positioning your body lists ideas on how to sit or stand when you help someone brush and floss.

Behavior: Problem behavior can make dental care difficult. Try these ideas and see what works for you.

- At first, dental care can be frightening to some people. Try the "tell-show-do" approach to deal with this natural reaction. Tell your client about each step before you do it. For example, explain how you'll help him or her brush and what it feels like. Show how you're going to do each step before you do it. Also, it might help to let your client hold and feel the toothbrush and floss. Do the steps in the same way that you've explained them.

- Give your client time to adjust to dental care. Be patient as that person learns to trust you working in and around his or her mouth.

- Use your voice and body to communicate that you care. Give positive feedback often to reinforce good behavior.

- Have a routine for dental care. Use the same technique at the same time and place every day. Many people with developmental disabilities accept dental care when it's familiar. A routine might soothe fears or help eliminate problem behavior.

- Be creative. Some caregivers allow their client to hold a favorite toy or special item for comfort. Others make dental care a game or play a person's favorite music. If none of these ideas helps, ask your client's dentist or dental hygienist for advice.

Three Steps to a Healthy Mouth

Like everyone else, people with developmental disabilities can have a healthy mouth if these three steps are followed:

- Brush every day.
- Floss every day.
- Visit a dentist regularly.

Brush Every Day

If the person you care for is unable to brush, these suggestions might be helpful.

- First, wash your hands and put on disposable gloves. Sit or stand where you can see all of the surfaces of the teeth.
- Be sure to use a regular or power toothbrush with soft bristles.
- Use a pea-size amount of toothpaste with fluoride, or none at all. Toothpaste bothers people who have swallowing problems. If this is the case for the person you care for, brush with water instead.
- Brush the front, back, and top of each tooth. Gently brush back and forth in short strokes.
- Gently brush the tongue after you brush the teeth.
- Help the person rinse with plain water. Give people who can't rinse a drink of water or consider sweeping the mouth with a finger wrapped in gauze.

If the person you care for can brush but needs some help, the following ideas might work for you. You may think of other creative ways to solve brushing problems based on your client's special needs.

A power toothbrush might make brushing easier. Take the time to help your client get used to one.

Guide the toothbrush. Help brush by placing your hand very gently over your client's hand and guiding the toothbrush. If that doesn't work, you may need to brush the teeth yourself.

Floss Every Day

Flossing cleans between the teeth where a toothbrush can't reach. Many people with disabilities need a caregiver to help them floss. Flossing is a tough job that takes a lot of practice. Waxed, unwaxed, flavored, or plain floss all do the same thing. The person you care for might like one more than another, or a certain type might be easier to use.

- Use a string of floss 18 inches long. Wrap that piece around the middle finger of each hand.

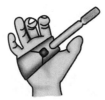

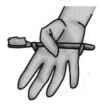

Figure 8.1. *The same kind of Velcro® strap used to hold food utensils is helpful for some people.*

Figure 8.2. *Others attach the brush to the hand with a wide elastic or rubber band. Make sure the band isn't too tight.*

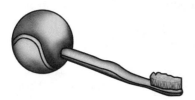

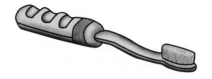

Figure 8.3. *You can also cut a small slit in the side of a tennis ball and slide it onto the handle of the toothbrush.*

Figure 8.4. *You can buy a toothbrush with a large handle, or you can slide a bicycle grip onto the handle. Attaching foam tubing, available from home health care catalogs, is also helpful.*

- Grip the floss between the thumb and index finger of each hand.

- Start with the lower front teeth, then floss the upper front teeth. Next, work your way around to all the other teeth.

- Work the floss gently between the teeth until it reaches the gumline. Curve the floss around each tooth and slip it under the gum. Slide the floss up and down. Do this for both sides of every tooth, one side at a time.

- Adjust the floss a little as you move from tooth to tooth so the floss is clean for each one.

- If you have trouble flossing, try using a floss holder instead of holding the floss with your fingers.

The dentist may prescribe a special rinse for your client. Fluoride rinses can help prevent cavities. Chlorhexidine rinses fight germs that cause gum disease. Follow the dentist's instructions and tell your client not to swallow any of the rinse. Ask the dentist for creative ways to use rinses for a client with swallowing problems.

Positioning Your Body: Where to Sit or Stand

Keeping people safe when you clean their mouth is important. Experts in providing dental care for people with developmental disabilities recommend the following positions for caregivers. If you work in a group home or related facility, get permission from your supervisor before trying any of these positions.

- If the person you're helping is in a wheelchair, sit behind it. Lock the wheels, then tilt the chair into your lap.

- Stand behind the person or lean against a wall for additional support. Use your arm to hold the person's head gently against your body.

Visit a Dentist Regularly

Your client should have regular dental appointments. Professional cleanings are just as important as brushing and flossing every day. Regular examinations can identify problems before they cause unnecessary pain.

As is the case with dental care at home, it may take time for the person you care for to become comfortable at the dental office. A "get acquainted" visit with no treatment provided might help: The person can meet the dental team, sit in the dental chair if he or she wishes, and receive instructions on how to brush and floss. Such a visit can go a long way toward making dental appointments easier.

Prepare for Every Dental Visit: Your Role

Be prepared for every appointment. You're an important source of information for the dentist. If you have questions about what the dentist will need to know, call the office before the appointment.

- Know the person's dental history. Keep a record of what happens at each visit. Talk to the dentist about what occurred at the last appointment. Remind the dental team of what worked and what didn't.

- Bring a complete medical history. The dentist needs each patient's medical history before treatment can begin. Bring a list of all the medications the person you care for is taking and all known allergies.

- Bring all insurance, billing, and legal information. Know who is responsible for payment. The dentist may need permission, or legal consent, before treatment can begin. Know who can legally give consent.

- Be on time.

Remember

Brushing and flossing every day and seeing the dentist regularly can make a big difference in the quality of life of the person you care for. If you have questions or need more information, talk to a dentist.

Chapter 9

Recent Research in Dental Care and Oral Health

Chapter Contents

Section 9.1—Researchers Report Initial Success in
          Promising Approach to Prevent Tooth Decay 80

Section 9.2—Salivary Diagnostic Device Shows Promise 83

Section 9.3—New Vaccine May Decrease Risk of Oral
          Cancers 86

Section 9.4—The Phenomenon of Dental Tourism 88

Section 9.1

Researchers Report Initial Success in Promising Approach to Prevent Tooth Decay

From the National Institute of Dental and Craniofacial Research
(NIDCR, www.nidcr.nih.gov), part of the National Institutes of Health,
October 23, 2006.

Preventing cavities could one day involve the dental equivalent of a military surgical strike. A team of researchers supported by the National Institute of Dental and Craniofacial Research report they have created a new smart antimicrobial treatment that can be chemically programmed in the laboratory to seek out and kill a specific cavity-causing species of bacteria, leaving the good bacteria untouched.

The experimental treatment, reported online in the journal *Antimicrobial Agents and Chemotherapy,* is called a STAMP. The acronym stands for "specifically targeted antimicrobial peptides" and, like its postal namesake, STAMPs have a two-sided structure. The first is the short homing sequence of a pheromone, a signaling chemical that can be as unique as a fingerprint to a bacterium and assures the STAMP will find its target. The second is a small antimicrobial bomb that is chemically linked to the homing sequence and kills the bacterium upon delivery.

While scientists have succeeded in the past in targeting specific bacteria in the laboratory, this report is unique because of the STAMPs themselves. They generally consist of less than 25 amino acids, a relative pipsqueak compared to the bulky, bacteria-seeking antibodies that have fascinated scientists for years. Because of their streamlined design, STAMPs also can be efficiently and rapidly produced on automated solid-phase chemistry machines designed to synthesize small molecules under 100 amino acids, called peptides.

The first-generation STAMPs also proved extremely effective in the initial laboratory work. As reported in the paper, the scientists found they could eliminate the cavity-associated oral bacterium *Streptococcus mutans* within 30 seconds from an oral biofilm without any collateral damage to related but non pathogenic species attached nearby.

Biofilms are complex, multi-layered microbial communities that routinely form on our teeth and organs throughout the body. According to one estimate, biofilms may be involved to varying degrees in up to 80 percent of human infections. "We've already moved the *S. mutans* STAMP into human studies, where it can be applied as part of a paste or mouth rinse," said Dr. Wenyuan Shi, senior author on the paper and a scientist at the University of California at Los Angeles School of Dentistry. "We're also developing other dental STAMPs that target the specific oral microbes involved in periodontal disease and possibly even halitosis. Thereafter, we hope to pursue possible medical applications of this technology."

Shi said his group's work on a targeted dental therapy began about eight years ago with the recognition that everyday dental care had reached a crossroads. "The standard way to combat bacterial infections is through vaccination, antibiotics, and/or hygienic care," said Shi. "They represent three of the greatest public-health discoveries of the 20th century, but each has its limitations in the mouth. Take vaccination. We can generate antibodies in the blood against *S. mutans*. But in the mouth, where *S. mutans* lives and our innate immunity is much weaker, generating a strong immune response has been challenging."

According to Shi, a major limitation of antibiotics and standard dental hygiene is their lack of selectivity. "At least 700 bacterial species are now known to inhabit the mouth," said Shi. "The good bacteria are mixed in with the bad ones, and our current treatments simply clear everything away. That can be a problem because we have data to show that the pathogens grow back first. They're extremely competitive, and that's what makes them pathogenic."

To illustrate this point, Shi offered an analogy. "Think of a lawn infested with dandelions," he said. "If you use a general herbicide and kill everything there, the dandelions will come back first. But if you use a dandelion-specific killer and let the grass fill in the lawn, the dandelions won't come back."

Hoping to solve the selectivity issue, Shi and his colleagues began attaching toxins to the homing region of antibodies. They borrowed the concept from immunotherapy, an area of cancer research in which toxin-toting antibodies are programmed to kill tumor cells and leave the nearby normal cells alone.

Despite some success in killing specific bacteria in the oral biofilm, Shi said his group soon encountered the same technical difficulty that cancer researchers initially ran into with immunotherapy. Their targeting antibodies were large and bulky, making them unstable, therapeutically inefficient, and expensive to produce. "That's when we decided to get higher tech," said Dr. Randal Eckert, a UCLA scientist and lead author on the study.

Or, as Eckert noted, that's when they turned to the power of genomics, or the comparative study of DNA among species. Eckert and colleagues clicked onto an online database that contains the complete DNA sequence of *S. mutans*. They identified a 21-peptide pheromone called "competence stimulating peptide," or CSP, that was specific to the bacterium. From there, they typed instructions into an automated solid-phase chemistry machine to synthesize at once the full-length CSP and a 16-peptide antimicrobial sequence, and out came their first batch of STAMPs.

After some trial and error, Eckert said he and his colleagues decided "to get even shorter." They ultimately generated a STAMP with the same antimicrobial agent but with a signature eight-peptide CSP sequence to target *S. mutans*. "We pooled saliva from five people and created an oral biofilm in the laboratory that included a couple hundred species of bacteria," said Eckert. "We applied the STAMP, and it took only about 30 seconds to eliminate the *S. mutans* in the mixture, while leaving the other bacteria in tact."

As dentists sometimes wonder, what would happen if *S. mutans* is eliminated from the oral biofilm? Does another equally or more destructive species fill its void, creating a new set of oral problems? Shi said nature already provides a good answer. "About 10 to 15 percent of people don't have *S. mutans* in their biofilms, and they do just fine without it," he said. "Besides, *S. mutans* is not a dominant species in the biofilm. It only becomes a problem when we eat a lot of carbohydrates."

Looking to the future, Shi said new STAMPs that seek out other potentially harmful bacterial species could be generated in a matter of days. He said all that is needed is the full DNA sequence of a microbe, a unique homing sequence from a pheromone, and an appropriate antimicrobial peptide. "We have a collection of antimicrobial peptides that we usually screen the bacterium through first in the laboratory," said Shi. "We can employ the antimicrobial equivalent of either a 2,000-ton bomb or a 200-pound bomb. Our choice is usually somewhere in the middle. If the antimicrobial peptide is too strong, it will also kill the surrounding bacteria, so we have to be very careful."

This research also was supported by a University of California Discovery Grant, Delta Dental of Washington, Delta Dental of Wisconsin, and C3 Jian Corporation. The National Institute of Dental and Craniofacial Research is the nation's leading funder of research on oral, dental, and craniofacial health.

Section 9.2

Salivary Diagnostic Device Shows Promise

From the National Institute of Dental and Craniofacial Research
(NIDCR, www.nidcr.nih.gov), part of the National Institutes of Health,
April 11, 2007.

Researchers supported by the National Institute of Dental and Craniofacial Research (NIDCR), part of the National Institutes of Health, have engineered a portable, phone-sized test that in minutes measures proteins in saliva that may indicate a developing disease in the mouth or possibly elsewhere in the body.

The point-of-care test, one of several saliva-based diagnostic devices now under development with NIDCR support, one day in the future could become a common sight in the dentist's office. As envisioned by the researchers, a dentist would collect a small saliva sample with a patient's consent, load it into the diagnostic cartridge, start the assay, and have a read out waiting after a cleaning or a dental procedure has been completed.

Called IMPOD, the device is described in the March 27 [2007] issue of the *Proceedings of the National Academy of Sciences.* In the report, the scientists offer the results of proof of principle experiments in which IMPOD reliably measured the concentrations of MMP-8, an enzyme associated with chronic inflammation of the gums called periodontitis.

"The IMPOD is designed to measure up to 20 analytes, or biochemicals, at once," said Dr. Anup Singh, a chemical engineer at the Sandia National Laboratories in Livermore, California, and senior author on the paper. "We haven't scaled up to that point, but we are doing multi-analyte analyses in the laboratory. Our greatest need right now is validated biomarkers to enable further clinical studies. The basic engineering of the device has been completed."

According to Singh, he and his colleagues were intrigued a few years ago by the many potential advantages of saliva as a diagnostic fluid. These include easy collection, no painful needle sticks, portability of the tests, and potentially a lower cost to patients than blood assays.

But they were initially daunted by the research task at hand. "Saliva is a mirror of blood, but with a caveat," said Singh. "It's not an exact mirror, meaning everything that is present in blood is present in saliva but at concentrations 1,000 to 10,000 times lower. It's diluted by saliva and the other secretions in the mouth. So we needed sensitivity 1,000 to 10,000 times better than we'd need if we were screening serum samples." Sensitivity refers to the lowest amount of an analyte that a test can detect.

Singh said he and his colleagues chose to use a lab-on-a-chip device. The term refers in this case to a microchip, roughly the size of a laboratory slide, containing networks of tiny channels and chambers in which the salivary assay, or biochemical test, is performed. For the researchers, the challenge was to design the entire assay to fit into the microchip. The scientists also had to miniaturize the components required to run the microchip, such as the power supply and optical detection unit, and integrate them into a rapid, fully automated diagnostic system.

The result is the IMPOD, short for Integrated Microfluidic Platform for Oral Diagnostics. The process begins with a series of microwells, each as distinct as fingers on a hand. One well holds the saliva sample, while the other wells contain cleansing buffering solution and antibodies that are preprogrammed to bind the specific protein of interest in saliva. The antibodies are tagged with a fluorescent dye that can be illuminated and measured at the end of the assay.

With the punch of a button, the contents of the wells are released and merge into a single channel about 40 microns wide, or roughly the width of a human hair. As the mixture flows in these tight quarters, the antibodies readily find the proteins of interest, tag them, and continue forward to be trapped on a porous gel membrane that serves as a filter.

"The bound proteins stack against the membrane because they are too big to squeeze through the pores," said Dr. Amy Herr, also at Sandia National Laboratories and lead author on the paper. "Conversely, the many smaller molecules in saliva flow right through the pores and are filtered out and routed to a waste chamber."

Thereafter, a voltage reversal releases the trapped proteins from the gel. They continue down a channel, where a standard diode laser shines onto the fluorescent tags and quantifies the concentration of the protein in the sample. The dentist reads the result and determines whether the protein levels correlate with a given disease.

To put their lab on a chip to the test, they collected saliva from 23 people—14 with periodontitis and nine in good oral health. Loading roughly one-tenth of a drop of saliva for analysis, the IMPOD processed the samples and produced a result in less than five minutes. The results showed that on average those in good oral health had lower concentrations of MMP, while people with periodontitis on average had elevated levels of the tissue-damaging enzyme. The results were confirmed with a standard ELISA blood test, currently the gold standard.

"The data correlate nicely with those from other types of studies that show that MMP-8 is indicative of periodontitis," said Dr. William Giannobile, a researcher at the University of Michigan School of Dentistry in Ann Arbor. "There is every reason to believe additional biomarkers for periodontitis can be identified, as the work to catalogue salivary genes and proteins nears completion and our understanding of periodontal disease continues to advance."

The researchers noted that IMPOD, although developed for saliva, could be used to test other diagnostic fluids such as blood and urine.

The National Institute of Dental and Craniofacial Research is the nation's leading funder of research on oral, dental, and craniofacial health.

Section 9.3

New Vaccine May Decrease Risk of Oral Cancers

"The Oral Cancer Foundation Urges HPV Vaccination for Males,"
© 2007 Oral Cancer Foundation. Reprinted with permission.

On the heels of a study published in the October 2007 issue of the journal *Cancer,* and recent supporting science related to HPV and oral cancer in the *New England Journal of Medicine,* the Oral Cancer Foundation is urging researchers to expedite investigations on the safety of human papillomavirus (HPV) vaccinations for males, and the FDA [U.S. Food and Drug Administration] to fast track the approval once scientific due diligence has been accomplished.

"The study affirms what we have long believed, namely that the vaccine can reduce oral cancer rates if given to both males and females," says Brian Hill, Founder and Executive Director of the foundation.

Currently, the vaccine, which shields against HPV strains 6, 11, 16 and 18, is administered to girls and adolescent females to protect against cervical cancer.

Deaths from cervical cancer, which number about 3,700 annually, have steadily declined due to improved methods of early detection, and a population that knows the importance of annual screenings. Oral cancer also lends itself to early detection through a simple visual and tactile examination which could easily be implemented, but does not have a nationally adopted program of public awareness and compliant professionals engaged in such a screening process. In the United States, 93 people per day will develop oral cancer, and one person will die from it every hour. This is more than double the death rate of cervical cancers, and is higher than that of many other cancers we commonly hear about. Because it is frequently painless and goes unnoticed in its early stages, the cancer is usually not found until late stages, when prognosis is poor. Opportunistic screenings like those done for cervical cancer could change this were they being done routinely.

In fact, oral cancer, which occurs in those very visible parts of the mouth that we all are familiar with, but also includes the tonsils, base of the tongue, soft palate, and side and back of the throat (oropharynx), is one of the few cancers on the rise in the United States, despite years of declining tobacco use. Tobacco use has been historically considered the most significant risk factor for the disease.

"Fewer people are using tobacco, but more people are getting oral cancer," Hill says. "What seems like a paradox actually illuminates the expanding role HPV-16 plays in acquiring this disease."

HPV is the most common sexually transmitted disease in the United States. About 20 million men and women currently have the disease, and close to 80 percent of sexually active adults will acquire the virus at some point in their lives. The virus can be transmitted either through genital or oral-genital contact.

HPV-16, one of the most destructive strains out of over 100 versions of the virus, was first linked to oral cancer more than a decade ago, but research since 2001 has removed any ambiguity about its role as a causative factor in oral cancer in both men and women. "Widespread use of the vaccine for both males and females, even if just in relationship to cervical cancer, will reduce the reservoir of the virus in the United States, and in slightly more than a decade we could begin to see the positive collateral benefits in the oral and head and neck cancer world," Hill says. Vaccinating males will also eliminate them as a vector for the virus.

On the other hand, the foundation cautions that while Pharma giants Merck and GlaxoSmithKline are doing studies on the current vaccines and males, delaying research and subsequent FDA approvals will likely come at a cost: As our society's sexual behaviors change, adolescents have engaged in oral-genital sex at younger ages, and transmission of HPV will increase and the attendant risks for cancer of the mouth, cervix, vulva, vagina, anus and penis will increase exponentially. "Significant pre approval research was done on these vaccines and proper due diligence review conducted by the FDA prior to approvals. There is no scientific evidence that indicates that this virus behaves differently at the cellular level in males than in females," says Hill.

He further stated, "What we know about HPV-16 as a cancer-causer is just the tip of the iceberg," Hill says, "These vaccines are the first major breakthrough against a cause of cancer in decades. We must act now."

The Oral Cancer Foundation, founded in 2000, is a national IRS 501c3 non-profit based in California. The foundation advocates for better public understanding of the disease and engages the medical and scientific communities to develop more effective methods of early detection. The foundation conducts screenings across the country and maintains a website with information for patients, the public and health care providers at www.oralcancer.org.

Section 9.4

The Phenomenon of Dental Tourism

"The phenomenon of dental tourism," ADA News Today, August 23, 2006, http://www.ada.org/prof/resources/pubs/adanews/adanewsarticle.asp ?articleid=2064. © 2006 American Dental Association. All rights reserved. Reprinted with permission.

Google the term "dental tourism" and the vaunted internet search engine serves up nearly 9.4 million listings, most of them links to other websites that offer a dizzying array of options for dental patients willing to cross borders or even oceans in pursuit of cut-rate dental care.

Globalization and Its Implications for Dentistry

Promising low cost and high quality, dental service outlets in Mexico, Hungary, Bulgaria, Austria, India, Australia, the Philippines and uncounted points in between are pitching their services to relatively affluent, yet cost-conscious health care consumers in Western Europe and the United States.

The Sahaj Dental Clinic in New Delhi, India, for example, tells website visitors that U.S. and European dentists "can charge $300 to $400" for a single caries restoration that "costs only $20 to $40 in India."

Never mind that even a discounted round-trip ticket to New Delhi from, say, Chicago would set the traveler back more than $1,400, a booking agent at "Goindiatravel" reported July 3.

Americans obviously are not trekking to India or Eastern Europe for single routine restorations. Most who go the extra miles need extensive care that, as they see it, justifies the added expense, particularly when a dental visit is combined with an exotic vacation.

Health care tourism has emerged in recent years as "a fast-growing phenomenon in which travelers, typically from wealthier countries, visit less-developed nations for medical care mixed with vacation, all at cut-rate prices," *USA Today* reported in July 2005.

The newspaper described towns in Hungary and other Eastern European countries where "brass plaques and molar-shaped signs bearing easy-to-grasp names like 'Eurodent' and 'Happy Dent' line the streets along a central shopping district."

The website "dentaltourism.org" lures visitors to the Hungarian capital of Budapest, which it claims has emerged as a center of health care service for tourists "now that the communist system has expired." The site boasts that the "Hungarian medical level of training compares to the [United Kingdom] or Irish practitioners."

Random spot checks with state dental leaders for this report suggest that for most, particularly in the northern regions, dental tourism is not high on their list of pressing concerns, and for good reason. It's not a major issue with a lot of their members, at least for now.

"Nobody's called me to grouse about it or to express amazement at it," said Peter Taylor, executive director of the Vermont State Dental Society.

Further south, however, that some patients leave the country for dental treatment is a larger issue, though it hardly qualifies as news.

"The term 'dental tourism' may be new, but certainly what we see happening is not new," said Dr. John S. Findley, who represents the 15th District (Texas) on the ADA Board of Trustees. "I don't think it's new anywhere, but it's especially not new in Texas."

Dr. Findley said he's heard estimates that, in the state's lower Rio Grande Valley, as much as 30 percent of the population will cross the border for dental care in a given year, a percentage that he said includes people who winter in the area.

"But it's not really a Texas or border-state problem," he added. "Disappearing borders and the ease of air travel today make a flat world a shrinking world. It's easy to travel anywhere."

Dr. Ivan E. Rodriguez, immediate past president of the Rio Grande Valley District Dental Society in Brownsville, Texas, noted that literally hundreds of dental offices and clinics are crowded into the cities and towns south of the border. "I'm told the area has the highest number of dentists per capita in the world," he said.

(The town of Nuevo Progreso, for example, advertises itself as the border "crossing point of choice" and boasts that the community is home to 90 to 100 dental offices.)

Some dentists interviewed for this report blamed employers and insurers for allegedly encouraging patients to travel in pursuit of reduced-fee treatments. But Dr. Frank Ceja of National City, California, about

15 miles from the border with Mexico, said that insurance may not be the driving force.

"Most of the people who go down there don't have insurance," he said. "That's why they go down there."

Dr. Ceja recounted the harrowing story of a woman who entered his office one day complaining of pain. She claimed she had been to Mexico where she spent nearly three hours in a dental chair as one practitioner, then another, attempted unsuccessfully to extract a tooth.

Finally, she said, a third practitioner—whether any of them were dentists is unknown—used a handpiece to grind down the tooth. "They ground the tooth down to below the gum line but left the root," recalled Dr. Ceja, who removed the root and relieved the woman's pain.

Kent Cravens, executive director of the New Mexico Dental Association and a native of the state, recalled hearing reports 30 years ago of patients crossing the border into Mexico for dental care.

"Some ended up with dentistry that was adequate," he said. "Some were not so fortunate."

Dr. Lee Cain, a general dentist in Albuquerque and a past president of the state dental association, tells the story of one patient who was not so fortunate.

"I had a young woman in her early 20s, a patient with me for about a year or less," he recalled. "I examined her and recommended numerous dental restorations."

Instead of accepting Dr. Cain's treatment plan, the woman crossed the border into Mexico where composite resins were applied to her teeth.

"It was as if someone took a handpiece, ran it down the grooves and over the marginal ridges and then put composite down the middle of it," he said. "There was no separation between the teeth. She couldn't floss. There had been no actual caries removal, no preparation of the teeth."

Dr. Cain advised the woman that the "restorations" would have to be redone. He noted, too, that she had developed a severe case of gingivitis. Adding to her woes, the woman had used up her dental benefits for the year.

"She's in a situation where she can't afford to have anything done" at least until next year, said Dr. Cain. "The saddest part of this is that she is so very young."

The anecdotal experiences of random patients are not indictments of dental care in Mexico or, for that matter, anywhere else on the planet. Capable dentists and quality care can be found the world over. The question is what becomes of patients who fall prey to incompetence.

Dr. Thomas J. Schripsema, also from Albuquerque and a member of the ADA Council on Dental Benefit Programs [CDBP], said there has been talk in his trustee district about asking the Association to open a dialogue with insurers on what can be done to help patients like the one Dr. Cain described.

The objective, he said, would be to "make sure that patients were receiving quality care and that they weren't having to pay for things twice."

He said his district caucus (Trustee District 14) may ask the ADA House of Delegates to urge the appropriate Association agency, most likely CDBP, to communicate with insurers on what might be done for such patients.

"It was my feeling that this was something that would be in the insurers' interests as well," said Dr. Schripsema. "It's a good place for us to cooperate, I think, in terms of helping patients get quality care and not have to go through rehabilitation."

Dr. Joel F. Glover, ADA trustee for the 14th District, said he was "aware and fully supportive of" the push to bring the matter to the ADA House.

In a June report to the ADA Board, Dr. Albert Guay, the Association's chief policy advisor, said health care tourism is limited to "a small number of people now, but has the potential to expand."

Driving expansion, he said, is the travel industry itself, adding a "new dimension to health care advertising" by bringing "a non-health care third party" into the health care system.

"The potential for mischief is great and may be difficult to control," Dr. Guay told the Board.

Dr. Kathleen Roth, ADA president-elect, visited the Texas border region in August "to be educated on the issues" as seen through the eyes of local dentists.

"The key," she said, "is educating patients to understand that optimal dental health is not a tour-bus stop, not a one-time visit, but a lifetime of joint effort involving the patient and the dental team."

She added, "We want what's best for our patients. Freedom of choice has certainly been one of our hallmarks. We believe that a patient should be able to choose his or her provider, but we want them to make informed choices."

The ADA is keeping an eye on the phenomenon of dental tourism as just one element of globalization—a wide range of economic, social and geopolitical factors affecting the way of life for millions around the world, including U.S. dentists and the patients they serve.

The next installment of this series will explore the insurance industry's views on dental tourism.

Part Two

Dental Hygiene at Home

Chapter 10

Toothbrushes, Toothpaste, and Other Home Dental Care Products

Chapter Contents

Section 10.1—Choosing Dental Care Materials 96

Section 10.2—The Use and Handling of Toothbrushes 99

Section 10.3—Why Is Brushing with Toothpaste
Important? 102

Section 10.4—Concerns over Imported Toothpastes 104

Section 10.5—Oral Irrigation Devices 107

Section 10.6—Mouth Rinses 113

Section 10.7—Denture Cleansers 115

Section 10.1

Choosing Dental Care Materials

"Choosing Dental Care Products," © 2008 The Cleveland Clinic Foundation, 9500 Euclid Avenue, Cleveland, OH 44195, www.clevelandclinic.org. Additional information is available from the Cleveland Clinic Health Information Center, 216-444-3771, toll-free 800-223-2273 extension 43771, or at http://www.clevelandclinic.org/health.

With so many dental care products (competing toothpastes, toothbrushes, mouthwashes, etc.) on the market today, how should you decide which product to use? This chapter provides information to help guide your decision-making among the various types of available products.

Toothpastes

When purchasing a toothpaste for you or your child, select one that contains fluoride. Toothpastes containing fluoride have been shown to prevent cavities. One word of caution: check the manufacturer's label. Some toothpastes are not recommended for children under age 6. This is because young children swallow toothpaste, and swallowing too much fluoride can lead to tooth discoloration in permanent teeth.

It is also wise to select a product approved by the American Dental Association (ADA). The ADA's Seal of Acceptance means that the product has met ADA criteria for safety and effectiveness, and that packaging and advertising claims are scientifically supported. Some manufacturers choose not to seek the ADA's Seal of Acceptance. Although these products might be safe and effective, these products' performance have not been evaluated or endorsed by the ADA.

Types of toothpaste (beyond containing fluoride)—whitening toothpastes, tartar-control, gum care, desensitizing, etc.: With the number and types of available toothpastes on the market, the best strategy to selecting among these products might be to simply ask your dental hygienist or dentist what the greatest concerns are for your mouth. Also, be aware that your needs will likely change as you get older. After consulting with your dentist or hygienist about your oral health's greatest needs, look for products within that category (for example, within the tartar control brands or within the desensitizing toothpaste brands) that have received the ADA Seal of Acceptance. Finally, some degree of personal preference comes into play. Choose the toothpaste that tastes and feels best. Gel or paste, wintergreen or spearmint all work alike. If you find that certain ingredients are irritating to your teeth, cheeks, or lips, or if your teeth have become more sensitive, or if your mouth is irritated after brushing, try changing toothpastes. If the problem continues, see your dentist.

Manual Toothbrushes

The main criterion to look for in manual toothbrushes is soft bristles. Both adults and children should use a toothbrush that has soft bristles. Harder bristles might cause gum tissue to pull back from teeth, which can expose the tooth root and lead to increased sensitivity to hot, cold, and sweet foods and beverages. Even worse, receding gum tissue can ultimately lead to tooth loss if not prevented or treated.

Be sure to select a toothbrush head size that can easily fit into the mouth and is capable of brushing one to two teeth at a time. With this guideline in mind, be sure to select a toothbrush with a very small head for a very young child or infant.

If you are unsure of what features to look for or the best bristle head design for cleaning your teeth's unique contours and alignment, be sure to ask your dentist or hygienist for assistance.

Toothbrushes should be replaced about every 4 months or earlier if the bristles begin to look worn or frayed. (Bristles that fan out or spread is one sign of wear.)

Manual Versus Powered Toothbrushes

Is there any advantage to using a powered (electric or sonic) toothbrush compared with a manual toothbrush? Not necessarily. The key to good oral hygiene is correct and effective use of a toothbrush rather than simply an issue of powered versus manual operation.

One of the main advantages of powered toothbrushes is that they provide a means to consistently brush using an adequate technique. Beyond this point, however, there are certain other situations where use of a powered toothbrush might make sense:

- Powered toothbrushes can ease the chore of tooth brushing in individuals with medical conditions that limit manual dexterity (such as arthritis), or who are elderly or physically handicapped, or who have oral conditions (such as misaligned teeth or teeth with uneven surfaces) that make thorough cleaning of all tooth surfaces difficult.

- They can ease the chore of tooth brushing in individuals with orthodontic appliances (such as bands, brackets, and wires).

- They motivate those who don't brush their teeth regularly. Use of a powered toothbrush might be considered "fun" or "different" such that it encourages tooth brushing. Others might be motivated to brush longer or correctly because of the money spent on purchasing the toothbrush.

- They better fight gum disease. At least one study has shown that the long-term (four to six months) use of powered toothbrushes produces significant reductions in the amount of dental plaque on the teeth—and therefore improves the oral health—of patients with periodontal disease.

- They minimize or eliminate tooth staining. The scrubbing effect of powered toothbrushes might be superior to manual toothbrushes in possibly reducing or even totally removing surface stains on teeth.

A complete list of toothbrushes that have received the ADA's Seal of Acceptance can be found at this website: http://www.ada.org/ada/seal/sealsrch.asp?searchtype=Category&keyword=toothbrushes.

Water Pik Devices

Water piks, otherwise known as water irrigating devices, are usually unnecessary for most people. Individuals who can benefit the most from these devices are those with braces or other orthodontics who need help removing food between teeth and within the orthodontic appliance. It is important to keep in mind that these devices do not remove plaque. Only tooth brushing with toothpaste and flossing can do that.

Mouthwashes

Mouthwashes simply freshen breath; they do not clean teeth. Most of these products contain alcohol and are not appropriate for children under 6 years of age because they can swallow it.

Fluoride Mouth Rinses

Fluoride mouth rinses coat the teeth with cavity-preventing fluoride. These rinses are typically recommended for cavity-prone individuals and can be used in children as young as 7 if they know how to spit out a liquid without swallowing it. Ask your dentist or hygienist to recommend the type of rinse that would be best for you.

Section 10.2

The Use and Handling of Toothbrushes

From "The Use and Handling of Toothbrushes," a fact sheet from the Centers for Disease Control and Prevention (CDC, www.cdc.gov), Division of Oral Health, April 26, 2007.

Tooth brushing with a fluoride toothpaste is a simple, widely recommended and widely practiced method of caring for one's teeth. When done routinely and properly, tooth brushing can reduce the amount of plaque which contains the bacteria associated with gum disease and tooth decay, as well as provide the cavity-preventing benefits of fluoride.

To date, the Centers for Disease Control and Prevention is unaware of any adverse health effects directly related to toothbrush use, although people with bleeding disorders and those severely immunodepressed may suffer trauma from tooth brushing and may need to seek alternate means of oral hygiene. The mouth is home to millions of microorganisms (germs). In removing plaque and other soft debris from the teeth, toothbrushes become contaminated with bacteria, blood, saliva, oral debris, and toothpaste. Because of this contamination, a common recommendation is to rinse one's toothbrush thoroughly with tap water following brushing. Limited research has suggested that even after being rinsed visibly clean, toothbrushes can remain contaminated with potentially pathogenic organisms. In response to this, various means of cleaning, disinfecting, or sterilizing toothbrushes between uses have been developed. To date, however, no published research data documents that brushing with a contaminated toothbrush has led to recontamination of a user's mouth, oral infections, or other adverse health effects.

Recommended Toothbrush Care

- Do not share toothbrushes. The exchange of body fluids that such sharing would foster places toothbrush sharers at an increased risk for infections, a particularly important consideration for persons with compromised immune systems or infectious diseases.

- After brushing, rinse your toothbrush thoroughly with tap water to ensure the removal of toothpaste and debris, allow it to air-dry, and store it in an upright position. If multiple brushes are stored in the same holder, do not allow them to contact each other.

- It is not necessary to soak toothbrushes in disinfecting solutions or mouthwash. This practice actually may lead to cross-contamination of toothbrushes if the same disinfectant solution is used over a period of time or by multiple users.

- It is also unnecessary to use dishwashers, microwaves, or ultra-violet devices to disinfect toothbrushes. These measures may damage the toothbrush.

- Do not routinely cover toothbrushes or store them in closed containers. Such conditions (a humid environment) are more conducive to bacterial growth than the open air.

- Replace your toothbrush every 3–4 months, or sooner if the bristles appear worn or splayed. This recommendation of the American Dental Association is based on the expected wear of the toothbrush and its subsequent loss of mechanical effectiveness, not on its bacterial contamination.

A decision to purchase or use products for toothbrush disinfection requires careful consideration, as the scientific literature does not support this practice at the present time.

Tooth Brushing Programs in Schools and Group Settings

Tooth brushing in group settings should always be supervised to ensure that toothbrushes are not shared and that they are handled properly. The likelihood of toothbrush cross-contamination in these environments is very high, either through children playing with them or toothbrushes being stored improperly. In addition a small chance exists that toothbrushes could become contaminated with blood during brushing. Although the risk for disease transmission through toothbrushes is still minimal, it is a potential cause for concern. Therefore, officials in charge of tooth brushing programs in these settings should evaluate their programs carefully.

Recommended measures for hygienic tooth brushing in schools:

- Ensure that each child has his or her own toothbrush, clearly marked with identification. Do not allow children to share or borrow toothbrushes.

- To prevent cross-contamination of the toothpaste tube, ensure that a pea-sized amount of toothpaste is always dispensed onto a piece of wax paper before dispensing any onto the toothbrush.

- After the children finish brushing, ensure that they rinse their toothbrushes thoroughly with tap water, allow them to air dry, and store them in an upright position so they cannot contact those of other children.

- Provide children with paper cups to use for rinsing after they finish brushing. Do not allow them to share cups, and ensure that they dispose of the cups properly after a single use.

Section 10.3

Why Is Brushing with Toothpaste Important?

Brushing with toothpaste is important for several reasons. First and foremost, a toothpaste and a correct brushing action work to remove plaque, a sticky, harmful film of bacteria that grows on your teeth that causes cavities, gum disease, and eventual tooth loss if not controlled.

Second, toothpaste contains fluoride, which makes the entire tooth structure more resistant to decay and promotes remineralization, which aids in repairing early decay before the damage can even be seen. Third, special ingredients in toothpaste help to clean and polish the teeth and remove stains over time. Fourth, toothpastes help freshen breath and leave your mouth with a clean feeling.

What type of toothpaste should I use?

As long as your toothpaste contains fluoride, the brand you buy really does not matter, neither does whether or not it is in paste, gel, or even powder form, or containing a certain flavor. All fluoride toothpastes work effectively to fight plaque and cavities and clean and polish tooth enamel. Your toothpaste brand should bear the ADA (American Dental Association) seal of approval on the container, which means that adequate evidence of safety and efficacy have been demonstrated in controlled, clinical trials.

If your teeth are hypersensitive to hot or cold, consider trying a toothpaste designed for sensitive teeth. These "desensitizing" toothpastes, which contain strontium chloride or potassium nitrate, protect exposed dentin by blocking the tubes in the teeth that are connected to nerves. Desensitizing pastes must be used for at least one month before any therapeutic effects are felt.

Toothpastes containing baking soda and/or hydrogen peroxide (which are both good cleansing agents) give the teeth and mouth a clean, fresh, pleasant feeling that can offer an incentive to brush more, but fluoride is the true active ingredient at work protecting your teeth. Some prefer a tartar-control toothpaste containing pyrophosphates to prevent the buildup of soft calculus (tartar) deposits on their teeth. New pastes offer advanced whitening formulas aimed at safely removing stains to make teeth brighter and shinier, although they can't nearly match the effectiveness of a professional bleaching formula administered or prescribed by a dentist.

How much should I use?

Contrary to what toothpaste commercials show, the amount of paste or gel needed on your brush for effective cleaning does not have to be a heaping amount. Simply squeeze a pea-sized dab of paste on the top half of your brush. If you brush correctly, holding the toothbrush at a 45-degree angle and brush inside, outside and between your teeth, the paste should foam enough to cover all of your teeth. Children under age 6, however, should be given a very small, baby pea-sized dab of toothpaste on their brush.

Is brushing with toothpaste enough to fight cavities and gum disease?

No. Although brushing thoroughly after each meal helps, flossing your teeth every day to remove plaque and food particles between teeth and at the gumline is just as important. Studies show that plaque will regrow on teeth that are completely clean within three to four hours of brushing.

Section 10.4

Concerns over Imported Toothpastes

From "How to Recognize Potentially Unsafe Imported Toothpastes,"
from the U.S. Food and Drug Administration (FDA, www.fda.gov), 2007.

On June 1, 2007, FDA warned consumers to avoid using tubes of toothpaste labeled as made in China because of concerns that the toothpaste may contain the poisonous chemical diethylene glycol (DEG), an ingredient used in antifreeze.

FDA has also identified toothpaste products from South Africa that contain DEG. FDA is working to stop the import of toothpaste containing DEG. The agency issued an import alert to prevent toothpaste containing DEG from entering the United States from any country. FDA's scrutiny of toothpastes has uncovered other problems. Some imported toothpastes do not contain DEG, but they do not meet the requirements of FDA regulations for other reasons. These toothpastes, typically sold at low-cost, "bargain" retail outlets, may not be safe.

FDA advises consumers to examine imported toothpaste packages carefully before purchasing them, using the information below to help identify unacceptable imported toothpastes. To find out if a toothpaste is imported, look at the label for the manufacturer's or distributor's name, followed by the city and state. If this information is not there, or the label states another country name, it's most likely imported.

Diethylene Glycol (DEG) in Toothpaste

DEG is not allowed in any toothpaste marketed in the United States. Some of the toothpastes FDA has found to contain DEG have labels that identify the ingredient either as diethylene glycol or diglycol. FDA has also found DEG in imported toothpastes that did not declare the ingredient on the label. FDA is taking steps to identify toothpastes that may contain undeclared DEG in order to prevent their distribution and sale in the United States.

Although FDA is not aware of any U.S. reports of poisonings from toothpaste containing DEG, the agency is concerned about potential risks from chronic exposure to DEG and exposure to DEG in certain populations, such as children and people with kidney or liver disease.

On July 11, 2007, China's government banned the export of DEG-containing toothpaste products. FDA commends this action, but continues to advise consumers to avoid using toothpaste from China at this time. Toothpaste currently on store shelves may have arrived in the United States prior to the ban and may contain DEG. In addition, some manufacturers in China may not yet have reformulated their toothpastes to comply with the ban. FDA will continue to monitor toothpaste from China and update its advice if appropriate.

Advice to consumers:

- Look at the list of ingredients on the toothpaste label. If diethylene glycol or diglycol are listed, do not use it. Throw it away or return it to the store where you bought it.

- Avoid using toothpaste labeled as made in China.

Counterfeit and "Gray Market" Products

Even with the precautions taken by FDA, illegal toothpaste products may still reach consumers, particularly through discount stores and flea markets. Some of these toothpaste products are considered "counterfeit" or "gray market" goods.

Counterfeit toothpaste is marketed under a product name without the permission of the company that has the legal right to use that name. These products are not legally marketed in the United States and they may not have the same ingredients, or the same quality of ingredients, as the original products.

Imported "gray market" toothpastes are products that are authorized for production and marketing in other countries. These products are not intended for the U.S. market, but are sold in the United States through unauthorized channels.

FDA specifically prohibits the marketing of counterfeit drugs. Gray market drugs do not usually meet FDA requirements, particularly with respect to labeling and fluoride content. FDA cannot assure the safety or effectiveness of counterfeit toothpastes, gray market toothpastes, and toothpastes that do not otherwise meet FDA regulatory requirements.

Advice to consumers:

- Do not use counterfeit toothpastes, which may sometimes be identified by spelling mistakes and uneven spacing between letters and words on the product label.

- Do not use gray market toothpastes, which may sometimes be identified by foreign language labeling and, for toothpastes that are drugs, by labeling that is not consistent with the "Drug Facts" format described below.

Regulated as Drugs or Cosmetics

FDA regulates toothpastes as drugs or cosmetics, depending on their ingredients and purpose. Toothpastes are drugs if they contain fluoride, are intended to prevent or lessen diseases like tooth decay, or affect the structure of the body or how it functions. Toothpastes that do not contain fluoride and that claim only to cleanse teeth are considered cosmetics and are not regulated as drugs.

Understanding the requirements for drug and cosmetic toothpaste labeling may help consumers identify potentially unsafe toothpastes.

Drug Toothpaste Labeling

Over-the-counter toothpaste that is not sold as a cosmetic must be labeled in "Drug Facts" format, which means a standard "box" format on the side or back panels of the outer carton or on the tube of toothpaste if there is no outer carton. This format is easy to recognize:

- The panels are labeled with the heading "Drug Facts."

- Information in the panel is printed in a single color against a white or contrasting background.

- Information in the box is separated by horizontal lines.

- Information is under the headings "Active ingredient(s)," "Use," "Warnings," "Directions," "Other information," "Inactive ingredients," and "Questions" in that order.

Advice to consumers:

If a drug toothpaste does not show the "Drug Facts" information above, do not use it. It is not legally marketed in the United States.

- If any toothpaste does not list ingredients on the label, do not use it.

- Cosmetic toothpastes are not required to have all the drug labeling information, but must still list all ingredients on the label.

- If any toothpaste does not have information on the label in English, do not use it. Both cosmetic and drug toothpastes must have information on the label in English to meet U.S. standards. The toothpaste can also include required information in a foreign language if it also provides this information in English.

Section 10.5

Oral Irrigation Devices

"Oral Irrigation" by Denise Parker, R.D.H.
© 2003 PennWell Corporation. Reprinted with permission.

Recently, there has been a renewed interest in oral irrigation. Numerous studies have supported the hypothesis that daily irrigation with a pulsed water-jet device improves oral health. Maximum benefit appears to be achieved with initial to moderate periodontal patients whose traditional mechanical methods of oral hygiene may be less than ideal. There have also been studies evaluating the efficacy of different antimicrobial agents added to the irrigation unit's reservoir. These studies have met with varying results, and the literature will be examined to determine current recommendations and expected clinical outcomes. Another area of research is the professional delivery of antimicrobial agents. The most promising agents and techniques for delivering antimicrobial agents in the dental office will be reviewed to enable the clinician to make informed decisions regarding patient therapy.

In 1962, the Waterpik® oral irrigator was introduced as a homecare aid to help with removal of plaque and debris. Early studies showed a reduction in gingivitis but not in the plaque (biofilm) index. This led to confusion as clinicians felt that if plaque was not mechanically removed, then the Waterpik oral irrigator was not an effective homecare device. For many years, the oral irrigation device was reserved for orthodontic patients and for patients with food impaction or tooth positioning problems. Currently, research has focused on plaque alteration and host modulation. One of the areas that researchers focused on in the past was the possibility of oral irrigation forcing bacteria into the blood stream, where it could cause infection or damage to bodily organs. Research has found little evidence to suggest that daily irrigation causes significant bacteremia, at least not more than other oral hygiene practices such as toothbrushing or flossing. In 1988, Cobb found that irrigated areas reduced pathogenic bacteria up to 6 mm and was non-injurious to the tissue. In fact, the risk of bacteremia is significantly higher in those individuals who have poor oral hygiene, thus controlling oral infection is of utmost importance in reducing the incidence of bacteremia. Studies have shown that using an oral irrigation device can substantially improve tissue health and thus can be an effective tool for daily use.

The primary purpose of oral irrigation is to reduce harmful bacteria and therefore the risk and severity of periodontal disease. Studies have shown that daily oral irrigation has the potential to suppress periodontal pathogens located within the pocket. Oral irrigation has demonstrated a reduction in proinflammatory mediators. Periodontal disease causing bacteria cause an increase in cytokine levels, which leads to bone resorption. Daily oral irrigation leads to a reduction in pro-inflammatory cytokines that leads to a slight, but significant, improvement in mild to moderate periodontal disease. In addition, oral irrigation has demonstrated a significant reduction in bleeding, gingivitis, periodontal pathogens, and probing depths. The reduction in probing depth was minimal and may not be clinically relevant.. Thus it appears that oral irrigation is a useful adjunct in suppressing and controlling periodontal disease.

Patients who may benefit from oral irrigation include those with orthodontic appliances, implants, crown and bridge, diabetes, periodontal maintenance, gingivitis, and those whose traditional oral hygiene may be less than ideal.

Daily Irrigation

There are several types of oral irrigators, but like all self-care devices they require daily use for maximum efficacy. The most common type for home use is a pulsed flow irrigator. There are also direct flow or steady stream irrigators. Most of the studies completed on oral irrigation were done using pulsed irrigators by Waterpik Technologies. Results cannot be extrapolated to other pulsating devices or direct flow irrigators. Another type of oral irrigator is the pulsed flow, magnetized irrigator. The hypothesis is that the charged water decreases calculus formation as well as achieves the benefits found with non-magnetic irrigators. Two studies have shown a decrease in calculus on lower anterior teeth only with magnetization but no greater reductions in bleeding or gingivitis.

There is also a type of irrigator that incorporates micro-bubbles of air into the water stream. These bubbles produced by the Braun Oral B OxyJet, are designed to enhance plaque disruption and thereby reduce gingival inflammation. However, in a study by Frascella et. al. the OxyJet was found to be safe but there was not difference in the reduction of clinical parameters compared to the non-irrigation group.

There are several tips for use on the market today. The most prevalent is the jet tip or standard tip, which is designed for supragingival placement. This standard tip can deliver an irrigant to an average of 50 percent of the pocket depth. Another tip that can be very helpful for periodontal patients is the Pik Pocket™ subgingival irrigation tip by Waterpik Technologies. This is a soft latex free rubber tip designed to fit Waterpik oral irrigators. The Pik Pocket tip has been found to penetrate 90 percent of the depth of the pocket. This can be a very effective tool to flush out periodontal pockets or to deliver antimicrobials to the depth of the pocket. Ora-tec also manufactures a uniquely designed tip that can be used for both standard and sulcus irrigation with their Via-Jet home irrigator. In addition, a few manufacturers supply cannula tips to be used with their irrigators. Cannula tips have not been tested for safety or efficacy for home use by the patient.

There are several reasons why daily irrigation is beneficial for oral health. One reason is to remove unattached plaque and dilute toxins. A second reason is to control gingivitis, especially in those patients who do not or cannot perform adequate interproximal hygiene. The oral irrigator appears to "pick up the slack" in patients whose home care is less than ideal. A third reason that oral irrigation is beneficial is that it can improve bad breath by reducing the pathogenic bacteria or by using a specially designed tongue cleaner attachment. This can be an effective tool in motivating patients to irrigate. For patients who do not receive the desired result with traditional home care methods, irrigation can be most effective in helping them to gain good oral health.

Patients should be instructed to direct the tip at a 90-degree angle to the long axis of the tooth, and about 3 mm away from the gingival margin. Then, follow the gingival margin and stop at each interproximal area for five or six seconds, irrigating both the lingual and buccal aspect of the teeth. For moderate to advanced periodontal disease, daily subgingival irrigation can be very beneficial in helping to achieve adequate home care.

It is well established that traditional brushing and flossing or rinsing with antimicrobials does not penetrate more than a millimeter or two subgingivally. Since most of the active periodontal disease process occurs subgingivally, the necessity of cleaning to the base of the pocket becomes apparent. Fortunately, the Pik Pocket tip attachment for the Waterpik oral irrigator is easy to use and is safe and effective. In a study by Braun and Ciancio, it was discovered that the subgingival tip was able to reach 90 percent of moderate (4–6 mm) pockets, and 64 percent of deeper pockets (7 mm or above). One final method of irrigation that can be an effective method for delivering an antimicrobial to deeper areas is the cannula. This method requires commitment, easy access, an isolated area, and high dexterity on the part of the patient.

Some researchers have investigated the efficacy of irrigating with an antimicrobial. Several studies assessed the efficacy of supragingival irrigation with 0.06 percent chlorhexidine (1 part water to 1 part CHX [chlorhexidine]) and demonstrated a significant reduction in gingivitis and bleeding. It is important to mention that water also significantly reduced gingivitis and bleeding and the differences between the groups if statistically significant may be clinically insignificant. A 1990 study used a 3:1 ratio (0.04 percent CHX concentration) with the Pik Pocket tip. Again both the CHX irrigation group and the water irrigation groups show significant reductions in GI [gingival index] along with reduction in the pocket probing depths. Higher concentrations of CHX (0.2 percent) have been studied with positive results but is not available in the United States.

Other irrigants that have been used for home irrigation include stannous fluoride, Listerine® antiseptic, acetylsalicylic acid, hydrogen peroxide, and sodium hypochlorite. Listerine antiseptic is a phenolic compound that has shown antibacterial properties. Listerine antiseptic has only been studied full strength and demonstrated significant reductions in plaque, gingivitis, bleeding, and pathogenic bacteria. Jorgensen and Slots recommend irrigating two to three times a week with a teaspoon of 5.25 percent plain household bleach added to the 300 ml of water. This regimen has never been studied for clinical efficacy or safety.

In-Office Irrigation

Recently there has been much attention paid to using antimicrobials to combat periodontal disease. Since periodontal disease is a bacterial infection, the practice of using antimicrobials and antibiotics to control the disease makes sense. Many offices have incorporated irrigation to deliver antimicrobials subgingivally, especially after periodontal treatments.

Collectively, studies show that most single applications of antimicrobials have not increased the efficacy of scaling and root planing.

To be of benefit, it is believed that the agent must be applied with enough frequency and duration to keep the bacterial count down. Typically, bacterial counts return to baseline one to eight weeks following a single episode of irrigation. Clearly, the need for additional studies to clarify guidelines and procedures for subgingival irrigation as an adjunct to periodontal therapy are needed but with the introduction of controlled and sustained released delivery systems this area of study may be moot.

Many different agents have been utilized for irrigation for in office application. The most widely studied agent is chlorhexidine. Another irrigant used for in office irrigation is 10 percent povidone iodine solution (Betadine). The use of povidone-iodine as an antimicrobial has been found to be effective at reducing the number of bacteria in periodontal pockets.

In fact, in an article by Slots, he stated that irrigating with undiluted povidone-iodine might reduce the number of cultivable bacteria by as much as 98 percent. Iodine exhibits rapid antimicrobial action, so is an effective topical agent. Slots also recommends incorporating a 10 percent iodine solution as the irrigant when performing ultrasonic debridement.

Other agents that have been tested for irrigation include stannous fluoride, saline solution, tetracycline, metronidazole, and hydrogen peroxide. There are many new promising products on the market that deliver a chemotherapeutic agent to the pocket, and maintain effective drug concentrations for at least two weeks. These include Arestin™, which incorporates minocycline into microspheres that can then be injected into the pocket. Another product that may be effective for treating many pockets at a time is the doxycycline gel, Atridox™. Thus, there are a wide variety of options available to help treat periodontal disease and this is beneficial to the clinician and the patient in their battle against the disease.

Oral irrigation in the dental office can be achieved by several methods. Of course, power scalers provide the easiest and most effective method for irrigating in the office. Using water as the irrigant is helpful to flush out pockets. Most of the newer units are available with optional reservoirs that can hold antimicrobials to be used as the irrigant. These provide an easy and efficient way to irrigate with antimicrobials in the dental office. Another type of in-office oral irrigator is a freestanding model by Ora-tec, the Via-jet Professional model. This unit comes with a heated reservoir and the handpiece facilitates delivery of antimicrobial agents subgingivally with a cannula.

Perhaps the biggest advantage of daily irrigation is that it helps patients to maintain a reduced bacterial count in the oral cavity. This in turn leads to fewer bleeding points, more shallow probing depths, and improved gingival health.

The key to success with oral irrigation seems to be consistency, as the bacteria must be continually "knocked down" to achieve maximum benefit. Still, irrigation is only one component of a comprehensive dental care program. Patients must also perform daily thorough toothbrushing, flossing, and any other adjuncts the dental professional deems appropriate. During dental office visits, thorough debridement is still paramount to achieving oral health.

In conclusion, home irrigation can be a key part of treatment planning to care for patients by reducing the numbers of harmful bacteria in the oral cavity, and thus reducing the severity of periodontal disease. Professional irrigation may be limited but new sustained or controlled release devices have shown efficacy when used with scaling and root planing.

Denise Parker, RDH, is a practicing dental hygienist in California. She is a May 2003 graduate from the University of New Mexico. References available upon request.

Section 10.6

Mouth Rinses

From "Choose Your Weapon: Mouth Rinses," from the
U.S. Army Center for Health Promotion and Preventive Medicine
(chppm-www.apgea.army.mil/dhpw), 2006.

Can I Just Rinse?

A mouth rinse is not a substitute for good oral hygiene. The American Dental Association recommends regular brushing and flossing as the best defense against cavities and gum disease.

Do I Need to Use a Mouth Rinse?

Mouth rinses can freshen breath for up to three hours and help remove food particles from the mouth. Most people do not need to use a rinse regularly unless they have an oral problem. Bad breath or unpleasant taste can be a sign of gum disease, cavities, or some other problem. Ask your dentist if you think you might benefit from using a mouth rinse. If you have a more severe problem such as multiple cavities, gum disease, xerostomia (dry mouth), or halitosis (bad breath), your dentist may prescribe a special rinse for you. Otherwise, they may recommend that you use an over-the-counter (OTC) rinse.

Using Mouth Rinses Correctly

Children under the age of six should not use mouthwashes. They have trouble controlling their swallowing reflex. Older children who use a rinse should be supervised by an adult.

Take the proper amount of liquid as directed by the dentist or on the bottle. With your mouth closed, swish the front and sides of your mouth forcefully using your tongue and cheeks for 30 seconds. For fluoride rinses swish for one minute. Do not swallow the mouth rinse. Spit it out.

Side Effects of Rinses

Routine or excessive use of antiseptic mouth rinses may cause:

Table 10.1. Over-the-Counter Mouth Rinses

Over-the-counter (OTC) Rinses	Examples	Functions	Ingredients
Antibacterial Rinses: Antiseptic Rinses	Listerine or equivalent brands	Prevents and reduces plaque and bacteria (germs), even between teeth; prevents and reduces gingivitis (bleeding gums) and gum disease	Thymol, eucalyptol, menthol, and methylsalicylate; 22% alcohol (or more); Benzoic or boric acid
Antibacterial Rinses: Enzymatic Rinses	Biotene or equivalent brands	Natural enzymes fight bacteria; moisturizes dry mouth; protects sore mouth tissues	Lysozyme, lactoferrin; glucose oxidase; lactoperoxidase
Anticavity Rinses	Examples: ACT, Fluorigard, Oral B Anticavity Rinse, or equivalent brands	Prevent cavities; blocks bacterial acid production; strengthens weakened areas of the teeth	.05% sodium fluoride
Other Rinses	Examples: Scope, Cepacol, Signal, Lavoris, or equivalent brands	Temporarily mask bad breath; help remove oral debris before or after brushing	14–15% alcohol; astringents (zinc chloride)

- a burning sensation in the cheeks, teeth, and gums; or
- painful ulcers, soreness, or numbness.

Table 10.2. Homemade Mouth Rinses

Type	Functions	Ingredients
Salt water	Aid healing; soothe sore mouth tissues	1/2 tsp. of salt; 8 oz. of water
Sodium bicarbonate	Neutralize acid reflux (stomach acid); freshen breath	1/2 tsp. of baking soda; 8 oz. water

Section 10.7

Denture Cleansers

"Advice for Patients: Denture Cleansers" is from the
U.S. Food and Drug Administration (FDA, www.fda.gov), Center
for Devices and Radiological Health, February 14, 2008.

FDA is asking the manufacturers of denture cleansers to revise labeling and to consider appropriate alternatives to an ingredient in their products. This action is in response to reports of 73 severe reactions linked to these cleansers, including at least one death.

The ingredient, persulfate, which is known to cause allergic reactions, is the most likely cause of the problem according to literature and research. Persulfates are used in these products as part of the cleaning and bleaching process.

Other reactions may be due to product misuse. The labeling revisions are needed to ensure that denture wearers clearly understand that these products are to clean dentures in a container—not while still in the mouth. For example, some cleansers that contain mouthwash are described as minty fresh, or they may have graphics such as fizzing bubbles. This may mislead consumers by implying that the product may be chewed, gargled, or swallowed.

Who is at risk?

- **People who are allergic to persulfates:** (All users should be aware that this kind of allergic reaction may not occur after the first use or even until many years of use. Also some symptoms may not appear for several minutes or even hours after actual use.)

- **People who are unable to read or understand the product label:** Examples include those with poor eyesight or with a condition such as Alzheimer disease, which compromises cognitive ability.

What are the symptoms of reaction?

Allergic reactions can occur with both proper and improper use of these cleansers. Reactions may become more frequent and severe with repeated use of the product.

Symptoms of an allergic reaction may include:

- irritation;
- tissue damage;
- rash;
- hives;
- gum tenderness;
- breathing problems; and
- low blood pressure.

Symptoms from product misuse may include:

- damage to the esophagus;
- abdominal pain;
- burns;
- breathing problems;
- low blood pressure;
- seizures;
- bleaching of tissue;
- blood in the urine;
- internal bleeding; and
- vomiting.

What should denture wearers do?

- Read all instructions carefully.
- Never chew, swallow, or gargle with denture cleansers.
- Always thoroughly rinse dentures and other dental appliances before placing in the mouth.
- Remember that reactions might not occur right away.
- If symptoms do occur, remove dentures and contact the prescribing dentist.
- Ask the prescribing dentist about using an alternative method for cleaning dentures.

Chapter 11

Cleaning Your Teeth and Gums

To have good dental health, you need a mix of personal dental care and the care of your dentist.

Flossing

Flossing removes plaque and bacteria that you cannot reach with your toothbrush. If you don't floss, you are missing more than one-third of your tooth surface. Plaque is the main cause of gum disease. It is an invisible bacterial film that develops on your teeth every day.

Within 24 to 36 hours, plaque hardens into tartar (also called calculus), which can only be removed by professional cleaning. Floss at least once a day, and plaque never gets the chance to harden into tartar. Getting into the habit of daily flossing is easier when you floss while doing something else like watching TV or listening to music, for example.

How to Floss Your Teeth

- **Step 1:** Take a length of floss equal to the distance from your hand to your shoulder. Wrap it around your index and middle fingers, leaving about 2 inches between your hands.

- **Step 2:** Slide the floss between your teeth and wrap it into a "C" shape around the base of the tooth and gently under the gumline. Wipe the tooth from base to tip two or three times.

"Flossing and Brushing" © 2007 Canadian Dental Association. Reprinted with permission.

- **Step 3:** Be sure to floss both sides of every tooth. Don't forget the backs of your last molars. Go to a new section of the floss as it wears and picks up particles.

- **Step 4:** Brush your teeth after you floss—it is a more effective method of preventing tooth decay and gum disease.

Flossing Problems and Solutions

Gums sometimes bleed when you first begin to floss. Bleeding usually stops after a few days. If bleeding does not stop, see your dentist. Floss can shred if you snag it on an old filling or on the ragged edge of a tooth.

Try another type of floss or dental tape. Ask your dentist or dental hygienist for advice. If your floss still shreds, see your dentist.

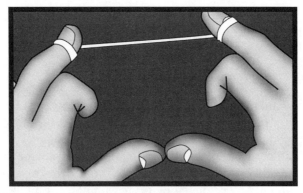

Figure 11.1. *The first step when flossing your teeth.*

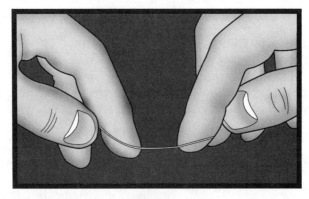

Figure 11.2. *Leave about 2 inches of floss between your hands.*

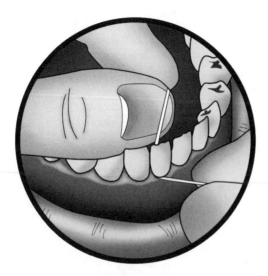

Figure 11.3. The second step when flossing your teeth.

Brushing

Regular, thorough brushing is a very important step in preventing tooth decay and gum disease. Brushing removes the bacteria that promote tooth decay and the plaque that can cause gum disease.

Ideally, you should brush after every meal, because the bacterial attack on teeth begins minutes after eating. At the very least, brush once a day and always before you go to bed. Brushing your teeth isn't complicated, but there is a right and a wrong way.

How to Brush Your Teeth

- **Step 1:** Brush at a 45-degree angle to your teeth. Direct the bristles to where your gums and teeth meet. Use a gentle, circular, massaging motion, up and down. Don't scrub. Gums that recede visibly are often a result of years of brushing too hard.

- **Step 2:** Clean every surface of every tooth. The chewing surface, the cheek side, and the tongue side.

- **Step 3:** Don't rush your brush. A thorough brushing should take at least 2 to 3 minutes. Try timing yourself.

- **Step 4:** Change your usual brushing pattern. Most people brush their teeth the same way all the time. That means they miss the same spots all the time. Try reversing your usual pattern.

• **Step 5:** Use a soft brush with rounded bristles. The right toothbrush cleans better. Choose a size and shape that allow you to reach all the way to your back teeth. There are many different types of brushes, so ask your dentist to suggest the best one for you. The Canadian Dental Association recommends you replace your toothbrush every 3 months.

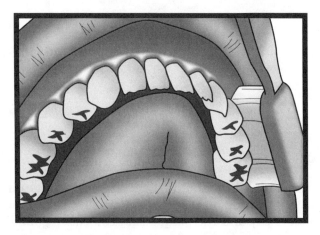

Figure 11.4. The first step when brushing your teeth.

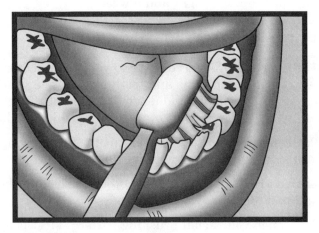

Figure 11.5. The second step when brushing your teeth.

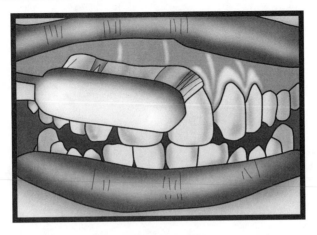

Figure 11.6. *The fourth step when brushing your teeth.*

Chapter 12

Good Nutrition Linked to Healthy Mouths

Chapter Contents

Section 12.1—Vitamins and Minerals Needed for Oral
            Health 126
Section 12.2—Oral Health and Calcium 128
Section 12.3—Gum Chewers Have Reason to Smile 129
Section 12.4—Snack Smart for Healthy Teeth 132
Section 12.5—Soft Drinks and Oral Health 135

Section 12.1

Vitamins and Minerals Needed for Oral Health

From "Nutrition and Oral Health," from the
U.S. Army Center for Health Promotion and Preventive
Medicine (http://chppm-www.apgea.army.mil/dhpw), 2006.

People who have oral health problems often have pain or difficulty chewing. People with chewing difficulties are less likely to eat balanced diets. This can result in poor nutrition.

Poor nutrition can cause a breakdown in your oral health:

- Decreased intake of vitamins and minerals can lead to mouth sores, breakdown of your gums, and oral cancer.

- A diet that is high in starch or sugar promotes tooth decay.

- Poor diet affects how well your immune system functions. It affects your ability to resist bacteria that cause gum disease.

- Eat foods that provide the vitamins and minerals needed for good oral health.

Table 12.1. Vitamins and Minerals Needed for Oral Health (continued on next page)

Vitamin	How it affects your mouth	Found in these foods
Vitamin A (carotene)	Prevents dry mouth and oral cancer	Broccoli, Brussels sprouts, green leafy vegetables (spinach, collard greens, kale, etc.)
Vitamin C (ascorbic acid)	Prevents soft, bleeding gums, and loose teeth; prevents oral cancer	Citrus fruits, cantaloupe, strawberries, green leafy vegetables, bell peppers
Vitamin D	Promotes strong teeth and jaw bones	Oily fish, milk, eggs, cereals, sunshine
Vitamin E	Prevents growth of thick white patches in the mouth (leukoplakia); prevents oral cancer	Vegetable oil, nuts, peanut butter, wheat germ

Table 12.1. (continued) Vitamins and Minerals Needed for Oral Health

Vitamin	How it affects your mouth	Found in these foods
B2, Niacin, B6, B12	Prevents soreness, redness and bleeding of the gums, cracking and sores in the corners of the mouth and on the tongue	Salmon, beef, liver, chicken, fish, yogurt, nuts, and beans
Folic acid	Prevents soreness, redness and bleeding of the gums, cracking and sores in the corners of the mouth and on the tongue	Breakfast cereals, spinach, navy beans, orange juice, pasta, rice
Calcium, Phosphorous, Magnesium	Needed for tooth development, prevents loss of jaw bone and teeth, rebuilds hard surface of the teeth (enamel)	Milk, cheese, yogurt, seafood, dark green leafy vegetables
Fluoride	Prevents tooth decay, helps repair enamel	Fluoridated water, black tea, sardines
Zinc	Needed for digestion, healing cold and canker sores	Liver, various meats, eggs, seafood, whole-grain cereals
Iodine	Needed for tooth development	Iodized salt, seafood, kelp, saltwater fish
Copper	Absorbs iron. Helps produce blood and nerve fibers	Liver, kidney, seafood, nuts, seeds, tap water
Iron	Protects against oral cancer and helps the immune system	Liver, eggs, fish, seafood, various other meats, enriched breads and cereals, green leafy vegetables
Potassium	Needed for nerve function and muscle contractions	Vegetables, legumes, fruits, milk, cheese, various meats, whole grains

Keep your mouth healthy so you can eat nutritious foods. Choose the right foods to protect or improve your oral health.

Section 12.2

Oral Health and Calcium

From the National Institute of Child Health and Human Development
(NICHD, www.nichd.nih.gov), part of the National Institutes of Health,
February 19, 2007.

What is calcium?

Calcium is a mineral your body needs to help build strong bones
and healthy teeth. Low-fat and fat-free milk and dairy products are
especially good sources of calcium.

How does calcium help keep mouths healthy?

- Even before baby teeth and adult teeth come in, they need calcium.

- And after teeth come in, they continue to take in calcium so
  they can develop fully.

- Calcium makes gums healthy. Getting enough calcium as a
  young adult may help prevent gum disease later in life.

- Calcium makes jawbones strong and healthy too. Jawbones
  need to be strong—they hold the teeth in place!

How else can I help my child have a healthy mouth?

Besides teaching your children to drink milk and eat other calcium-
rich foods, there are a number of ways you can help keep your child's
mouth healthy.

Section 12.3

Gum Chewers Have Reason to Smile

"Chew for Health," reprinted with
permission from Science News for Kids, © 2007.

Most schools ban chewing gum, but in a few years they might consider changing that rule. Why? Scientists are finding evidence that gum chewing may be good for your health. It may even help boost your test scores.

This exciting research is just beginning. And in the meantime, companies are also experimenting with adding vitamins, minerals, medicines, and other substances that could give gum the power to cure headaches and fight everything from serious diseases to bad breath.

These enhanced gums are part of the growing number of foods and drinks that contain health-boosting ingredients. If you're already a gum fan, that's probably welcome news.

Making Gum

People have been chewing gum for thousands of years. Ancient Greeks, Mayas, and Native Americans, for example, chewed on the sap, or resin, of certain types of trees.

Today, gum is a little more complicated, says Ron Ream, a food scientist in Plano, Ill. Gum manufacturers start by mixing resin, wax, and a molecule called polyvinyl acetate to make a gum base. By varying the types and amounts of these ingredients, scientists can make thousands of formulations.

Giant mixers then combine vats of melted gum base with powders, syrups, and sweeteners. Other machines roll the goo into sticks or press them into pellets. Packaging is the final step.

Americans chew about 1.8 pounds of gum per person each year, according to the U.S. Census Bureau. By showing that gum chewing can be healthy, companies that make and sell gum hope that we'll chew even more.

Just what can gum do for your health? Many studies show that chewing gum after meals fights cavities by stimulating the production of saliva. Saliva helps wash away bacteria that damage our teeth. (It also offers other benefits.)

An ingredient called xylitol, which is added to some gums, provides an extra dose of cavity-fighting power. This is good for more than just the teeth. Research suggests that good oral health decreases the risk of heart disease, diabetes, and other serious diseases.

Nutritionist Gil Leveille, executive director of the Wrigley Science Institute, says that chewing gum might also be good for your brain. One Japanese study of nine participants, he says, found that chewing gum boosted the flow of blood to participants' brains by up to 40 percent. Blood carries oxygen, which fuels brain cells.

Other small studies have found that people perform better on memory tests while chewing gum. And a study in the United Kingdom found that people who chewed gum while memorizing a list of words did about 25 percent better at recalling those words than people who didn't chew gum.

"It certainly makes sense," Leveille says, "that increased blood flow would be related to increased alertness."

Additional studies, with longer follow-up, are needed to confirm that chewing gum has benefits, he adds. So far, results of studies about memory have been mixed. Not all tests have had similarly encouraging results. What's more, many of the studies that show gum's benefits are funded by gum companies.

Medicine Gumballs

Other researchers are finding that gum might work better than a pill to deliver medicines and other substances into the bloodstream. That's because the lining of our cheeks can absorb certain substances more quickly than our stomachs and intestines can.

In 2006, Danish scientists found that people absorbed nearly three times as much of an allergy medicine when they chewed it in gum as when they swallowed it in tablet form. The researchers found that 40 percent of the medicine entered the bloodstream directly through the cheeks of the gum-chewing patients.

That discovery could help other researchers develop medicine-containing gums that fight colds, relieve headaches, battle nervousness, and more. Scientists might even create antimicrobial gums that cure bad breath.

Those projects may take years, but gum scientists have already had at least one recent success: They've created a gum that could help us stay awake.

Researchers at the Walter Reed Army Institute of Research (WRAIR) in Silver Spring, Md., manufactured a caffeine-laced gum called Stay Alert. Each stick has as much caffeine as a cup of coffee.

It can take an hour for the caffeine in coffee to have its full effect, but the caffeine in Stay Alert hits in just a few minutes, says WRAIR research physiologist Gary Kamimori.

Chewing Stay Alert is "like pouring coffee directly into your bloodstream," he says.

The military helped invent the product because it wants to be sure that soldiers stay awake during long, tiring night shifts. Kamimori's studies show that soldiers who chew Stay Alert can function well for up to 72 hours without sleep.

The gum is easy to transport and it's stable in cold and hot climates, Kamimori says. Unlike a pill, it doesn't require water to swallow. Those qualities make it easy for soldiers to use.

For now, Stay Alert is available only to the military, Kamimori says. The manufacturer may one day offer it for sale to the public. People who work at night, such as truck drivers and medical personnel who ride in ambulances, might benefit from a product such as Stay Alert.

Some caffeine gums are already available in stores, but they haven't been as rigorously tested or regulated as Stay Alert has, says Kamimori. Testing is essential because untested products might be harmful to health, or they simply might not do what they claim to do.

Let the Chewer Beware

For now, chew with caution. Too much chewing can damage the jaw joint. And chewing too much of a gum that contains vitamins, caffeine, or a medicine could lead to an overdose, warns Gayl Canfield, a registered dietitian at the Pritikin Longevity Center & Spa in Aventura, Fla. What's more, no matter how healthy gum chewing proves to be, she adds, it will never be a match for a healthy lifestyle.

"Nothing like a gum or a vitamin is going to cure a bad dietary habit or a bad exercise habit," Canfield says. "It's not a magic bullet."

Section 12.4

Snack Smart for Healthy Teeth

From the National Institute of Dental and Craniofacial Research (NIDCR, www.nidcr.nih.gov), part of the National Institutes of Health, November 13, 2007.

What's wrong with sugary snacks, anyway?

Sugary snacks taste so good—but they aren't so good for your teeth or your body. The candies, cakes, cookies, and other sugary foods that kids love to eat between meals can cause tooth decay. Some sugary foods have a lot of fat in them, too.

Kids who consume sugary snacks eat many different kinds of sugar every day, including table sugar (sucrose) and corn sweeteners (fructose). Starchy snacks can also break down into sugars once they're in your mouth.

Did you know that the average American eats about 147 pounds of sugars a year? That's a big pile of sugar! No wonder the average 17-year-old in this country has more than three decayed teeth!

How do sugars attack your teeth?

Invisible germs called bacteria live in your mouth all the time. Some of these bacteria form a sticky material called plaque on the surface of the teeth. When you put sugar in your mouth, the bacteria in the plaque gobble up the sweet stuff and turn it into acids. These acids are powerful enough to dissolve the hard enamel that covers your teeth. That's how cavities get started. If you don't eat much sugar, the bacteria can't produce as much of the acid that eats away enamel.

How can I snack smart to protect myself from tooth decay?

Before you start munching on a snack, ask yourself what's in the food you've chosen. Is it loaded with sugar? If it is, think again. Another choice would be better for your teeth. And keep in mind that certain kinds of sweets can do more damage than others. Gooey or chewy sweets spend more time sticking to the surface of your teeth.

Because sticky snacks stay in your mouth longer than foods that you quickly chew and swallow, they give your teeth a longer sugar bath.

You should also think about when and how often you eat snacks. Do you nibble on sugary snacks many times throughout the day, or do you usually just have dessert after dinner? Damaging acids form in your mouth every time you eat a sugary snack. The acids continue to affect your teeth for at least 20 minutes before they are neutralized and can't do any more harm. So, the more times you eat sugary snacks during the day, the more often you feed bacteria the fuel they need to cause tooth decay.

If you eat sweets, it's best to eat them as dessert after a main meal instead of several times a day between meals. Whenever you eat sweets—in any meal or snack—brush your teeth well with a fluoride toothpaste afterward.

When you're deciding about snacks, think about:

- the number of times a day you eat sugary snacks;
- how long the sugary food stays in your mouth; and
- the texture of the sugary food (chewy? sticky?).

If you snack after school, before bedtime, or other times during the day, choose something without a lot of sugar or fat. There are lots of tasty, filling snacks that are less harmful to your teeth—and the rest of your body—than foods loaded with sugars and low in nutritional value. Snack smart!

Low-fat choices like raw vegetables, fresh fruits, or whole-grain crackers or bread are smart choices. Eating the right foods can help protect you from tooth decay and other diseases. Next time you reach for a snack, pick a food from the list inside or make up your own menu of non-sugary, low-fat snack foods from the basic food groups.

Snack Smart Food List

Pick a variety of foods from these groups.
Fresh fruits and raw vegetables:

- berries
- oranges
- grapefruit
- melons
- pineapple
- pears

- tangerines
- broccoli
- celery
- carrots
- cucumbers
- tomatoes

- unsweetened fruit and vegetable juices
- canned fruits in natural juices

Grains:

- bread
- plain bagels
- unsweetened cereals
- unbuttered popcorn
- tortilla chips (baked, not fried)
- pretzels (low-salt)
- pasta
- plain crackers

Milk and dairy products:

- low- or nonfat milk
- low- or nonfat yogurt
- low- or nonfat cheeses
- low- or nonfat cottage cheese

Meat, nuts, and seeds:

- chicken
- turkey
- sliced meats
- pumpkin seeds
- sunflower seeds
- nuts

Others (these snacks combine foods from the different groups):

- pizza
- tacos

Remember to:

- choose sugary foods less often;
- avoid sweets between meals;
- eat a variety of low- or nonfat foods from the basic groups; and
- brush your teeth with fluoride toothpaste after snacks and meals.

Note to Parents

The foods listed in this text have not all been tested for their decay-causing potential. However, knowledge to date indicates that they are less likely to promote tooth decay than are some of the heavily sugared foods children often eat between meals.

Candy bars aren't the only culprits. Foods such as pizza, breads, and hamburger buns may also contain sugars. Check the label. The new food labels identify sugars and fats on the Nutrition Facts panel on the package. Keep in mind that brown sugar, honey, molasses, and syrups also react with bacteria to produce acids, just as refined table sugar does. These foods also are potentially damaging to teeth.

Your child's meals and snacks should include a variety of foods from the basic food groups, including fruits and vegetables; grains, including breads and cereals; milk and dairy products; and meat, nuts, and seeds. Some snack foods have greater nutritional value than others and will better promote your child's growth and development. However, be aware that even some fresh fruits, if eaten in excess, may promote tooth decay. Children should brush their teeth with fluoride toothpaste after snacks and meals. (So should you!)

Please note: These general recommendations may need to be adapted for children on special diets because of diseases or conditions that interfere with normal nutrition.

Section 12.5

Soft Drinks and Oral Health

"Soft Drinks and Oral Health,"
© 2008 Mississippi State Department of Health
(www.msdh.state.ms.us). Reprinted with permission.

Soft drink consumption is one of several leading causes of tooth decay. Carbonation, sugar, and acids in soft drinks weaken tooth enamel and encourage the growth of bacteria that contribute to tooth decay. This information will help you reduce the impact of soft drinks on your and your kids' teeth and health.

Get the facts on how tooth decay starts and what you can do to prevent it.

How Tooth Decay Starts

- Sugar in soda combines with bacteria in your mouth to form acid.

- This acid, plus the extra acid from soft drinks, attacks the teeth. Each acid attack lasts about 20 minutes, and acid attacks start over again with every sip.

- Ongoing acid attacks weaken tooth enamel.

- Cavities begin when tooth enamel is damaged.
- Remember, diet or "sugar-free" soda still has acid that can harm your teeth. Although fruit drinks aren't carbonated like soda, they too have acid and sugar that can cause decay.

Reduce the Risk

- Drink carbonated beverages (soft drinks, soda pop) in moderation.
- Give infants and toddlers these beverages in a regular cup. Sucking on a bottle or sippy cup filled with these beverages promotes tooth decay.
- Use a straw to help keep sugar away from your teeth while drinking.
- Choose fluoridated water instead of fizzy drinks.
- Avoid drinking soft drinks and fruit juice before bedtime.
- Rinse your mouth with water or brush your teeth soon after using either of these.
- Get regular dental checkups and cleanings.

Table 12.2. Acid and Sugar in Soft Drinks

	Acidity	**Sugar Amount**
Battery Acid	6	0
Pepsi	4.5	9.8 tsp
Coca-Cola	4.5	9.3 tsp
Minute Maid Orange Soda	4.2	11.2 tsp
Dr. Pepper	4	9.5 tsp
Gatorade	4	3.3 tsp
Nestea	4	5.0 tsp
Diet Pepsi	4	0
Mountain Dew	3.7	11.0 tsp
Minute Maid Grape Soda	3.7	11.9 tsp
Diet Coke	3.6	0
Diet Dr. Pepper	3.6	0
Sprite	3.6	9.0 tsp
Barq's	2.4	10.7 tsp
Pure Water	0	0

Chapter 13

Fluoride: Its Role in Cavity Prevention

Chapter Contents

Section 13.1—Fluoridated Water: Questions and Answers 138

Section 13.2—Your Child's Fluoride Needs 140

Section 13.3—Bottled Water Users: Are You Getting
Enough Fluoride? 145

Section 13.4—Excess Fluoride Consumption: Enamel
Fluorosis 152

Section 13.1

Fluoridated Water: Questions and Answers

From the National Cancer Institute
(NCI, www.cancer.gov), part of the National Institutes of Health,
June 29, 2005.

What is fluoride?

Fluoride is the name given to a group of compounds that are composed of the naturally occurring element fluorine and one or more other elements. Fluorides are present naturally in water and soil.

What is fluoridated water?

Virtually all water contains some amount of fluoride. Water fluoridation is the process of adding fluoride to the water supply so that the level reaches approximately 1 part fluoride per million parts water (ppm) or 1 milligram fluoride per liter of water (mg/L); this is the optimal level for preventing tooth decay.

Why fluoridate water?

In the early 1940s, scientists discovered that people who lived where drinking water supplies had naturally occurring fluoride levels of approximately 1.0 ppm had fewer dental caries (cavities). Many more recent studies have supported this finding.

Fluoride can prevent and even reverse tooth decay by enhancing remineralization, the process by which fluoride "rebuilds" tooth enamel that is beginning to decay.

When did water fluoridation begin in the United States?

In 1945, Grand Rapids, Michigan, adjusted the fluoride content of its water supply to 1.0 ppm and thus became the first city to implement community water fluoridation. By 1992, more than 60 percent of the U.S. population served by public water systems had access to water fluoridated at approximately 1.0 ppm, the optimal level to prevent tooth decay.

The Centers for Disease Control and Prevention (CDC) considers fluoridation of water one of the greatest achievements in public health in the 20th century.

Can fluoridated water cause cancer?

The possible relationship between fluoridated water and cancer has been debated at length. The debate resurfaced in 1990 when a study by the National Toxicology Program, part of the National Institute of Environmental Health Sciences, showed an increased number of osteosarcomas (bone tumors) in male rats given water high in fluoride for 2 years. However, other studies in humans and in animals have not shown an association between fluoridated water and cancer.

In a February 1991 Public Health Service (PHS) report, the agency said it found no evidence of an association between fluoride and cancer in humans. The report, based on a review of more than 50 human epidemiological (population) studies produced over the past 40 years, concluded that optimal fluoridation of drinking water "does not pose a detectable cancer risk to humans" as evidenced by extensive human epidemiological data reported to date.

In one of the studies reviewed for the PHS report, scientists at the National Cancer Institute evaluated the relationship between the fluoridation of drinking water and the number of deaths due to cancer in the United States during a 36-year period, and the relationship between water fluoridation and number of new cases of cancer during a 15-year period. After examining more than 2.2 million cancer death records and 125,000 cancer case records in counties using fluoridated water, the researchers found no indication of increased cancer risk associated with fluoridated drinking water.

In 1993, the Subcommittee on Health Effects of Ingested Fluoride of the National Research Council, part of the National Academy of Sciences, conducted an extensive literature review concerning the association between fluoridated drinking water and increased cancer risk. The review included data from more than 50 human epidemiological studies and six animal studies. The Subcommittee concluded that none of the data demonstrated an association between fluoridated drinking water and cancer. A 1999 report by the CDC supported these findings. The report concluded that studies to date have produced "no credible evidence" of an association between fluoridated drinking water and an increased risk for cancer.

Where can people find additional information on fluoridated water?

The CDC website has information on standards for and surveillance of current fluoridated water supplies in the United States. Visit http://www.cdc.gov and search for "fluoridation."

The Environmental Protection Agency (EPA) website has more information about drinking water and health. It includes information about drinking water quality and standards. This website is located at http://www.epa.gov/safewater/ on the internet.

Section 13.2

Your Child's Fluoride Needs

"Fluoride and Water," September 2005, reprinted with permission from www.kidshealth.org. Copyright © 2005 The Nemours Foundation. This information was provided by KidsHealth, one of the largest resources online for medically reviewed health information written for parents, kids, and teens. For more articles like this one, visit www.KidsHealth.org, or www.TeensHealth.org. Reviewed by: Lisa Goss, R.D.H., B.S., and Garrett B. Lyons Sr., D.D.S.

Keeping your child's teeth healthy requires more than just daily brushing. During a routine well-child exam, you may be surprised to find the doctor examining your child's teeth and asking you about your water supply. That's because fluoride, a substance that's found naturally in water, plays an important role in healthy tooth development and cavity prevention.

What Is Fluoride?

Fluoride exists naturally in water sources and is derived from fluorine, the thirteenth most common element in the Earth's crust. It is well known that fluoride helps prevent and even reverse the early stages of tooth decay.

Tooth decay occurs when bacteria—found in the plaque that dentists try so hard to get rid of—break down sugars in food. This process produces damaging acids that dissolve the hard enamel surfaces of teeth. If the damage is not stopped or treated, the bacteria can penetrate through the enamel to the underlying tissues of the teeth, causing cavities (also called caries). Cavities weaken teeth and cause pain, tooth loss, or even widespread infection in the most severe cases.

Fluoride combats tooth decay in two ways. It strengthens tooth enamel, a hard and shiny substance that protects the teeth, so that it can better resist the acid formed by plaque. Fluoride also allows teeth damaged by acid to repair, or remineralize, themselves. Fluoride cannot repair cavities, but it can reverse low levels of tooth decay and thus prevent new cavities from forming.

Though fluoride benefits adults, it is especially critical to the health of developing teeth in children. And despite all the good news about dental health, tooth decay remains one of the most common diseases of childhood. According to 2000 statistics from the U.S. Surgeon General, more than half of children ages 5 to 9 years have had at least one cavity or filling, and tooth decay has affected 78% of 17-year-olds.

Fluoride and the Water Supply

As of 2002, the Centers for Disease Control and Prevention (CDC) statistics show that almost 66% of the U.S. population receives fluoridated water through the taps in their homes. Some communities have naturally occurring fluoride in their water; others add it at water-processing plants.

Some parents purchase bottled water for their children to drink instead of tap water. The growing bottled water industry claims that bottled water is safer, purer, mineral-free, and better tasting, and that may be true in some cases. But most bottled waters also lack fluoride. Fluoridated bottled water is one exception—it can sometimes be found in the baby-food aisle at the grocery store, usually labeled as baby water or nursery water.

Your child's doctor or dentist may know whether local water supplies contain adequate levels of fluoride (between 0.7 and 1.2 parts fluoride per million parts of water). If your water comes from a public system, you could also call your local water authority or public health department, or check online at the Environmental Protection Agency's (EPA) database of local water safety reports. If you use well water or water from a private source, fluoride levels should be checked by a laboratory or public health department.

The Controversy over Fluoride

You may have heard that the addition of fluoride to the water supply is dangerous and damaging. Some advocacy groups publish reports on the hazards of fluoridation, and they point to toxicity warnings on toothpaste, concluding that any substance needing such careful dosage must be dangerous.

In response to claims that water fluoridation is dangerous, the National Institutes of Health (NIH) reviewed research on dental cavities prevention and public policy, including fluoridation. It agreed with antifluoride activists that many studies in this area are of poor quality. However, the NIH panel concluded that the unevenness of research does not invalidate the clear benefits of fluoride. The NIH believes that the dramatic reductions in tooth decay in the past 30 years are due to fluoridation of the water supply, and parents and health professionals should continue to ensure that kids receive enough fluoride to prevent cavities.

Your Child's Fluoride Needs

So how much fluoride does your child need? In general, children under the age of 6 months do not need fluoride. Your child's 6-month checkup offers a great chance to discuss fluoride needs with a health professional.

If you live in a nonfluoridated area, your child's doctor or dentist may prescribe fluoride drops, tablets, or vitamins after your baby is 6 months old. The American Academy of Pediatrics recommends that these fluoride supplements be given daily to children between the ages of 6 months and 16 years. The dosage will change as your child grows. Only children living in nonfluoridated areas or children who drink only nonfluoridated bottled water should receive supplements.

What about toothpastes, mouth rinses, and other products that contain fluoride? Here are a few tips for parents:

- Because children younger than 3 can't spit effectively, they may swallow too much toothpaste while brushing, and should be helped with their twice-daily brushings.

- Ask your child's dentist about the type of toothpaste your child under 3 should use. Many dental professionals recommend using toothpastes specially formulated for infants and toddlers.

- Children over age 3 should use a fluoride-containing toothpaste that carries the American Dental Association's (ADA) seal of acceptance.

- Kids should use only a pea-sized amount of toothpaste and spit out as much as possible after brushing. Even a small amount of toothpaste supplies enough fluoride for tooth protection but minimizes the chances of side effects from too much fluoride.

- Only mouth rinses clearly labeled "anticavity with fluoride" contain fluoride. They are regulated by the U.S. Food and Drug Administration (FDA) and are approved by the ADA. Children under age 6 should never use these rinses, as their spitting abilities haven't fully developed by that age. However, older children at high risk for tooth decay may benefit from fluoride-containing rinses. Your child's dentist can talk with you about risk factors such as a family history of dental disease, recent periodontal surgery or disease, or a physical impediment to brushing regularly and thoroughly.

Children over age 3 are at lowest risk for cavities if they regularly get fluoride from drinking naturally fluoridated or supplemented water, in addition to routinely brushing with fluoridated toothpaste. Consult your child's dentist before using any fluoridated mouth rinses or other products besides toothpaste.

Your family dentist or pediatric dentist (one who specializes in the care of children's teeth) is a great resource for information about your child's dental care and fluoride needs. A dentist can help you understand more about how fluoride affects the teeth, and once all of your child's primary teeth have come in, may further strengthen them by applying regular topical fluoride during visits.

Overexposure to Fluoride

If some fluoride is good, why not give children as much fluoride as possible? As with most minerals and vitamins, overexposure can be harmful. Most children get the right amount of fluoride through a combination of fluoridated toothpaste and fluoridated water or supplements.

Too much fluoride before 8 years of age can cause enamel fluorosis, a discoloration or mottling of the permanent teeth. This condition is unsightly but harmless and often can be treated with cosmetic procedures.

Most cases of fluorosis occur in children who take unnecessary daily fluoride supplements even though they brush regularly with fluoridated toothpaste and their home's tap water contains good levels of fluoride. Misuse of fluoride products, including rinses and toothpaste, also can contribute to fluorosis, but this is less common.

Very rarely, fluoride toxicity can occur when large amounts of fluoride are ingested during a short period of time. Children under age 6 account for more than 80% of reports of suspected overingestion. Although outcomes are generally not serious, fluoride toxicity sends several hundred children to emergency rooms each year.

Symptoms of fluoride toxicity may include nausea, diarrhea, vomiting, abdominal pain, increased salivation, or increased thirst. Symptoms begin 30 minutes after ingestion and can last up to 24 hours. If you suspect your child may have eaten a substantial amount of a fluoridated product or supplement, call the poison control center or 911.

Be sure to keep toothpaste, supplements, mouth rinses, and other fluoride-containing products out of children's reach or in a locked cabinet. You should also supervise your young child's toothbrushing sessions to prevent swallowing of toothpaste or other fluoridated products.

If you have any questions about your water's fluoride content, the fluoridated products your child uses, or whether your child is receiving too much or too little fluoride, talk to your child's doctor or dentist.

Section 13.3

Bottled Water Users: Are You Getting Enough Fluoride?

"Bottled Water: Better Than the Tap?" by Anne Christiansen Bullers, from the *FDA Consumer* magazine, U.S. Food and Drug Administration (FDA, www.fda.gov), July-August 2002. This document was reviewed by David A. Cooke, M.D., May 11, 2008.

It's a rare day that Kelly Harrison, a mother of five from Tulsa, Oklahoma, doesn't find herself chauffeuring kids to some kind of sports practice or school activity. As she checks to see that each child is seat-belted into the family's minivan, Harrison also makes sure they've got the essentials: the right sports equipment, the right clothes, and what she considers to be the right drink—bottled water.

When she was growing up, Harrison, 34, might have grabbed a soft drink or juice on her way out the door. But for her kids, Harrison insists on what she thinks is a healthier choice—water. She says her children's young bodies need water as they play in the Oklahoma sun. Bottled water also contains no caffeine, no calories, and no sugar. Plus, bottled water comes in convenient bottles, easy to tote from home to wherever the busy family goes.

"I really think this is best for a lot of different reasons," says Harrison, who often tucks a bottle for herself into the basket in her minivan that contains other on-the-go mom necessities, such as a paperback book and her cell phone.

Once, most Americans got their water only from the tap. Now, like Harrison, they're often buying their water in a bottle. At work, after a workout, or just about any time, Americans are drinking bottled water in record numbers—a whopping 5 billion gallons in 2001, according to the International Bottled Water Association (IBWA), an industry trade group. That's about the same amount of water that falls from the American Falls at Niagara Falls in two hours.

Explosive growth in the industry for more than a decade has placed bottled water in nearly every supermarket, convenience store, and vending machine from coast to coast, where dozens of brands compete for consumers' dollars. In four years, industry experts anticipate that bottled water will be second only to soda pop as America's beverage of choice.

Water, of course, is essential to human health. Drinking enough water to replace whatever is lost through bodily functions is important. But surveys indicate that most of us might not be drinking enough. Is bottled water part of the answer? To decide, consumers need to arm themselves with knowledge about what they're buying before they grab the next bottle of Dasani, Evian, or Perrier off the shelf. "It really pays to do your homework," says Stew Thornley, a water quality health educator with the Minnesota Department of Health.

Different Varieties

Bottled water may seem like a relatively new idea—one born during the heightened awareness of fitness and potential water pollution during the last two or three decades. However, water has been bottled and sold far from its source for thousands of years. In Europe, water from mineral springs was often thought to have curative and sometimes religious powers. Pioneers trekking west across the United States during the 19th century also typically considered drinkable (potable) water a staple to be purchased in anticipation of the long trip across the arid West.

Today, of course, there are dozens of brands of bottled water and many different kinds, including flavored or fizzy, to choose from.

Federal Regulations

The Food and Drug Administration regulates bottled water products that are in interstate commerce under the Federal Food, Drug, and Cosmetic Act (FD&C Act).

Under the FD&C Act, manufacturers are responsible for producing safe, wholesome, and truthfully labeled food products, including bottled water products. It is a violation of the law to introduce into interstate commerce adulterated or misbranded products that violate the various provisions of the FD&C Act.

The FDA also has established regulations specifically for bottled water, including standard of identity regulations, which define different types of bottled water, and standard of quality regulations, which set maximum levels of contaminants (chemical, physical, microbial, and radiological) allowed in bottled water.

From a regulatory standpoint, the FDA describes bottled water as water that is intended for human consumption and that is sealed in bottles or other containers with no added ingredients, except that it may contain a safe and suitable antimicrobial agent. Fluoride may also be added within the limits set by the FDA.

High Standards

Is the extra expense of bottled water worth it? One thing consumers can depend on is that the FDA sets regulations specifically for bottled water to ensure that the bottled water they buy is safe, according to Henry Kim, Ph.D., a supervisory chemist at the FDA's Center for Food Safety and Applied Nutrition, Office of Plant and Dairy Foods and Beverages. Kim, whose office oversees the agency's regulatory program for bottled water, says that major changes have been made since 1974, when the Safe Drinking Water Act (SDWA) first gave regulatory oversight of public drinking water (tap water) to the U.S. Environmental Protection Agency (EPA). Each time the EPA establishes a standard for a chemical or microbial contaminant, the FDA either adopts it for bottled water or makes a finding that the standard is not necessary for bottled water in order to protect the public health.

"Generally, over the years, the FDA has adopted EPA standards for tap water as standards for bottled water," Kim says. As a result, standards for contaminants in tap water and bottled water are very similar.

However, in some instances, standards for bottled water are different than for tap water. Kim cites lead as an example. Because lead can leach from pipes as water travels from water utilities to home faucets, the EPA set an action level of 15 parts per billion (ppb) in tap water. This means that when lead levels are above 15 ppb in tap water that reaches home faucets, water utilities must treat the water to reduce the lead levels to below 15 ppb. In bottled water, where lead pipes are not used, the lead limit is set at 5 ppb. Based on FDA survey information, bottlers can readily produce bottled water products with lead levels below 5 ppb. This action was consistent with the FDA's goal of reducing consumers' exposure to lead in drinking water to the extent practicable.

Production of bottled water also must follow the current good manufacturing practices (CGMP) regulations set up and enforced by the FDA. Water must be sampled, analyzed, and found to be safe and sanitary. These regulations also require proper plant and equipment design, bottling procedures, and recordkeeping.

The FDA also oversees inspections of the bottling plants. Kim says, "Because the FDA's experience over the years has shown that bottled water poses no significant public health risk, we consider bottled water not to be a high risk food." Nevertheless, the FDA inspects bottled water plants under its general food safety program and also contracts with the states to perform some bottled water plant inspections. In addition, some states require bottled water firms to be licensed annually.

Members of the IBWA also agree to adhere to the association's Model Code, a set of standards that is more stringent than federal regulations in some areas. Bottling plants that adopt the IBWA Model Code agree to one unannounced annual inspection by an independent firm.

The FDA also classifies some bottled water according to its origin.

- **Artesian well water:** Water from a well that taps an aquifer— layers of porous rock, sand, and earth that contain water—which is under pressure from surrounding upper layers of rock or clay. When tapped, the pressure in the aquifer, commonly called artesian pressure, pushes the water above the level of the aquifer, sometimes to the surface. Other means may be used to help bring the water to the surface. According to the EPA, water from artesian aquifers often is more pure because the confining layers of rock and clay impede the movement of contamination. However, despite the claims of some bottlers, there is no guarantee that artesian waters are any cleaner than ground water from an unconfined aquifer, the EPA says.

- **Mineral water:** Water from an underground source that contains at least 250 parts per million total dissolved solids. Minerals and trace elements must come from the source of the underground water. They cannot be added later.

- **Spring water:** Derived from an underground formation from which water flows naturally to the earth's surface. Spring water must be collected only at the spring or through a borehole tapping the underground formation feeding the spring. If some external force is used to collect the water through a borehole, the water must have the same composition and quality as the water that naturally flows to the surface.

- **Well water:** Water from a hole bored or drilled into the ground, which taps into an aquifer.

Bottled water may be used as an ingredient in beverages, such as diluted juices or flavored bottled waters. However, beverages labeled as containing "sparkling water," "seltzer water," "soda water," "tonic water," or "club soda" are not included as bottled water under the FDA's regulations, because these beverages have historically been considered soft drinks.

Some bottled water also comes from municipal sources—in other words—the tap. Municipal water is usually treated before it is bottled. Examples of water treatments include:

- **Distillation:** In this process, water is turned into a vapor. Since minerals are too heavy to vaporize, they are left behind, and the vapors are condensed into water again.

- **Reverse osmosis:** Water is forced through membranes to remove minerals in the water.

- **Absolute 1 micron filtration:** Water flows through filters that remove particles larger than one micron in size, such as *Cryptosporidium,* a parasitic protozoan.

- **Ozonation:** Bottlers of all types of waters typically use ozone gas, an antimicrobial agent, to disinfect the water instead of chlorine, since chlorine can leave residual taste and odor to the water.

Bottled water that has been treated by distillation, reverse osmosis, or other suitable process and that meets the definition of "purified water" in the U.S. Pharmacopeia can be labeled as "purified water."

Bottled Versus Tap

Whether bottled water is better than tap water, and justifies its expense, remains under debate. Stephen Kay, vice president of the IBWA, says member bottlers are selling the quality, consistency, and safety that bottled water promises, and providing a service for those whose municipal systems do not provide good quality drinking water.

"Bottled water is produced and regulated exclusively for human consumption," Kay says. "Some people in their municipal markets have the luxury of good water. Others do not."

Thornley, of the Minnesota Department of Health, agrees that consumers can depend on bottled water's safety and quality. But he says consumers should feel the same way about the quality of their tap water. Tap water may sometimes look or taste differently, he says, but that doesn't mean it's unsafe. In fact, the most dangerous contaminants are those that consumers cannot see, smell, or taste, he says. But consumers don't need to worry about their presence, he adds. Municipal water systems serving 25 people or more are subject to the federal Safe Drinking Water Act. As such, the water is constantly and thoroughly tested for harmful substances, he says. If there is a problem, consumers will be warned through the media or other outlets.

"In lieu of being told otherwise, consumers should feel confident of the safety of their water," Thornley says.

Dr. Robert Ophaug, a professor of oral health at the University of Minnesota School of Dentistry, notes that tap water has another advantage many people don't think about: It typically contains fluoride. Many communities have elected to add fluoride to drinking water to promote strong teeth and prevent tooth decay in residents, though some groups continue to oppose this practice and believe it's detrimental to health.

Ophaug says bottled water often does not have fluoride added to it. Or, if it has been purified through reverse osmosis or distillation, the fluoride may have been removed. People who drink mostly bottled water, especially those who have children, need to be aware of this, he says. They may need to use supplemental fluoride that is available by prescription from dentists or doctors. The supplements are usually recommended for children ages 7 to 16. Fluoride supplements cost around $15 for a three-month supply.

"At the least, inform the children's dentist or doctor that you are relying on bottled water," Ophaug says.

The IBWA says there are more than 20 brands of bottled water with added fluoride available to consumers today. When fluoride is added to bottled water, the FDA requires that the term "fluoridated," "fluoride added," or "with added fluoride" be used on the label. Consumers interested in how much fluoride bottled water contains can usually find out by contacting individual companies directly.

Surging Sales

Consumers don't appear ready to give up their bottled water any time soon. Younger, health-oriented people are driving the market's growth, according to industry officials. "They've grown up with bottled water, and it doesn't seem like such a stretch to them to buy water," says Kay.

Jeremy Buccellato, 31, of Ramsey, Minnesota, says he's heard the arguments that tap water is just as good if not better than bottled water. A glass from his own tap, however, provides water that's discolored, chlorinated, and tastes like "pool water." Buccellato says the extra money he spends on bottles of Dasani water is worth it.

"It tastes better and looks better, plus it's easy to take with me," says Buccellato. "What's not to like?"

Harrison agrees that there's nothing like a refreshing cool bottle of water to beat the heat during an Oklahoma summer.

"It's a product that fits our needs and our lifestyle," she says.

To Filter or Not to Filter?

Consumers can buy purified water. They also have the option of doing it at home.

Numerous companies sell filtration systems. Some attach to the faucet and filter the water as it comes through the tap. Others are containers that filter the water in them. Among the best-known manufacturers are PUR and Brita.

Water purified with these products typically costs less than buying bottled water. According to Brita, its high-end faucet filter system provides water for 18 cents a gallon, a considerable saving from $1 or more typically charged for an 8- to 12-ounce bottle of water.

John B. Ferguson, communications manager/executive editor with the Water Quality Association, says that consumers can feel confident about the water quality provided by brand name home-filtration systems.

Stew Thornley of the Minnesota Department of Health agrees that home filtration systems can improve the taste or appearance of tap water at a minimal cost. However, Thornley points out that consumers need to be careful about maintaining these filters. Typically, specific instructions are included with the purchase of the product. Without proper maintenance, he says, it's possible bacteria or other contaminants can build up in the products.

Section 13.4

Excess Fluoride Consumption: Enamel Fluorosis

"Enamel Fluorosis," from the Centers for Disease
Control and Prevention (CDC, www.cdc.gov), November 21, 2007.

The proper amount of fluoride helps prevent and control tooth decay. Fluoride works both before the tooth erupts into the mouth (i.e., while the teeth are developing) and every day once the teeth have erupted. Fluoride consumed during tooth development can also result in a range of changes in the enamel surface of the tooth. These changes have been broadly termed enamel fluorosis.

What is enamel fluorosis?

Enamel fluorosis is a hypomineralization of the enamel surface of the tooth that develops during tooth formation. Clinically this appears as a range of cosmetic changes varying from barely noticeable white spots to pitting and staining. Severe forms can occur when young children consume excess fluoride, from any source, during critical periods of tooth development.

Who is at risk for enamel fluorosis?

- Only children 8 years old and younger are at risk, because this is the time when permanent teeth are developing under the gums.

- Once the teeth erupt (emerge through the gums), they are no longer at risk for fluorosis.

- Adults, adolescents, and children older than 8 years cannot develop enamel fluorosis.

What does enamel fluorosis look like?

- Very mild and mild forms may have scattered white flecks, white tips of teeth, or fine, lacy chalklike lines. Most people with fluorosis have these barely noticeable forms.

- Moderate and severe forms may have stains and rough, irregular enamel surfaces. These rarely occurring forms may be considered cosmetically objectionable.

What causes enamel fluorosis?

The occurrence of enamel fluorosis is reported to be most strongly associated with fluoride intake during enamel development, with the severity of the condition depending on the dose, duration, and timing of fluoride intake.

The transition and early maturation stages of enamel development appear to be most susceptible to the effects of fluoride; these stages occur at varying times for different tooth types. The risk for enamel fluorosis, even for posterior (back of mouth) teeth that do not show, ends when children reach age 8, because the pre-eruptive maturation of the tooth is complete and the enamel is no longer susceptible.

What are the sources of fluoride?

- Toothpaste
- Drinking water
- Processed beverages and food
- Dietary supplements that include fluoride (tablets or drops)
- Other dental products (mouth rinses, gels, and foams)

What accounts for most of the fluoride intake?

In the United States, water and processed beverages (e.g., soft drinks and fruit juices) can provide approximately 75% of a person's fluoride intake. Inadvertent swallowing of toothpaste and inappropriate use of other dental products containing fluoride can result in greater intake than desired.

In which communities can enamel fluorosis be found?

Enamel fluorosis occurs among some persons in all communities, even in communities with a low natural concentration of fluoride.

Part Three

At the Dentist's Office

Chapter 14

Finding and Choosing a Dentist

Chapter Contents

Section 14.1—What Are the Dental Specialties? 158

Section 14.2—The Pediatric Dentist: Teaching Kids and
Teens to Care for Their Teeth 161

Section 14.3—Choosing a Dentist 164

Section 14.4—Dental Insurance: What You Need to Know 169

Section 14.1

What Are the Dental Specialties?

The American Dental Association defines dentistry as the evaluation, diagnosis, prevention, and/or treatment (nonsurgical, surgical, or related procedures) of diseases, disorders, and/or conditions of the oral cavity, maxillofacial area, and/or the adjacent and associated structures of their impact on the human body; provided by a dentist, within the scope of his/her education, training, and experience, in accordance with the ethics of the profession and applicable law.

Overview of Responsibilities

Dentists have earned at minimum a doctorate degree in dental surgery (D.D.S.) and receive extensive training and education on the diagnosis and treatment of dental disease. Dental school education and training qualifies them to perform a variety of surgical procedures on the teeth, gums, lips, and jaws. It helps them detect diseases such as oral cancer and educate patients about good dental health.

To maintain the highest quality of oral health care, the dentist must be the primary oral health care provider. All patients should receive the same standard of care, beginning with a qualified diagnosis by a licensed dentist.

The goal of dentistry is to prevent and control dental diseases, the vast majority of which are infectious, irreversible, and destructive. These diseases can only be diagnosed and successfully treated with the intervention of a licensed dentist and a qualified dental team.

Dental Specialties

Most practicing dentists are general practitioners, yet some go for an additional two years of school (in addition to four years of dental school) to become a dental specialist.

There are nine specialties in dentistry recognized by the American Dental Association (ADA). They are:

- **Dental public health:** Prevent and control disease. Promote dental health through organized community efforts.

- **Endodontics:** Diagnose and treat oral conditions caused by problems with the dental pulp (i.e., root canals).

- **Oral and maxillofacial pathology:** Study the nature of diseases affecting the mouth.

- **Oral and maxillofacial radiology:** A new dental specialty. These specialists use imaging and associated technology for the diagnosis and management of a range of diseases affecting the mouth, jaws, and related areas of the head and neck.

- **Oral and maxillofacial surgery:** Diagnose, surgically and otherwise treat diseases, injuries, and defects of the mouth's tissues.

- **Orthodontics and dentofacial orthopedics:** Supervise, guide, and correct the growth of teeth and facial bones.

- **Pediatric dentistry:** Provide both primary and comprehensive preventive and therapeutic oral health care for infants and children through adolescence, including those with special health care needs.

- **Periodontics:** Diagnose and treat diseases of the gums.

- **Prosthodontics:** Restore and maintain the oral functions, comfort, appearance, and health of patients by restoring natural teeth and/or replacing missing teeth with artificial substitutes (i.e., dentures).

Education

In order to become a dentist, although the steps may vary, you generally will need to do the following:

- Earn a college degree and take predental courses in biology, chemistry, and physics.

- Take and earn a good score on the Dental Admissions Test (DAT).

- Complete four years of dental school. An additional two years or more may be necessary if you choose to specialize.

- Take and pass national board exams and state licensure exams.

Dental schools grant doctoral degrees in dentistry. Dental programs in the United States must earn accreditation from the ADA every seven years.

For More Information

The American Dental Education Association publishes the *ASDA Handbook*, which contains more useful information on requirements for application and admission to dental schools in the United States. Additionally, ADEA offers a predental membership to individuals interested in a dental career. For further details, write or contact:

American Student Dental Association
211 E. Chicago Ave., Suite 700
Chicago, IL 60611-2687
Toll-Free: 800-621-8099, ext. 2795
Phone: 312-440-2795
Fax: 312-440-2820
Website: www.asdanet.org

More information on a career in dentistry can also be found online at ADA.org. Be sure to ask your dentist about a career in dentistry.

Section 14.2

The Pediatric Dentist: Teaching Kids and Teens to Care for Their Teeth

"The Pediatric Dentist," © 2008 American Academy of Pediatric Dentistry (www.aapd.org). Reprinted with permission.

Pediatric dentistry is the specialty of dentistry that focuses on the oral health and unique needs of young people. After completing a four-year dental school curriculum, two to three additional years of rigorous training is required to become a pediatric dentist. This specialized program of study and hands-on experience prepares pediatric dentists to meet the unique needs of your infants, children and adolescents, including persons with special health care needs.

We are concerned about your child's total health care. Good oral health is an important part of total health. Establishing us as your child's "Dental Home" provides us the opportunity to implement preventive dental health habits that keep a child free from dental/oral disease. We focus on prevention, early detection, and treatment of dental diseases, and keep current on the latest advances in dentistry for children.

Pleasant visits to the dental office promote the establishment of trust and confidence in your child that will last a lifetime. Our goal, along with our staff, is to help all children feel good about visiting the dentist and teach them how to care for their teeth. From our special office designs, to our communication style, our main concern is what is best for your child.

Preventing Tooth Decay

Four things are necessary for cavities to form: 1) a tooth; 2) bacteria; 3) sugars or other carbohydrates; and 4) time. We can share with you how to make teeth strong, keep bacteria from organizing into harmful colonies, develop healthy eating habits, and understand the role that time plays. Remember, dental decay is an infection of the tooth. Visiting us early can help avoid unnecessary cavities and dental treatment.

The pediatric dental community is continually doing research to develop new techniques for preventing dental decay and other forms of oral disease. Studies show that children with poor oral health have decreased school performance, poor social relationships, and less success later in life. Children experiencing pain from decayed teeth are distracted and unable to concentrate on schoolwork.

Importance of Primary Teeth (Baby Teeth)

It is very important that primary teeth are kept in place until they are lost naturally. These teeth serve a number of critical functions. Primary teeth:

- maintain good nutrition by permitting your child to chew properly;

- are involved in speech development; and

- help the permanent teeth by saving space for them. A healthy smile can help children feel good about the way they look to others.

Infants and Children

Getting an early start in regular dental care is an important step on the road to teaching your child healthy lifetime habits. We want to share with you the latest available methods for keeping your child healthy and safe.

The first dental visit should occur shortly after the first tooth erupts and no later than the child's first birthday. Beginning tooth and mouth examinations early may lead to detection of early stages of tooth decay that can be easily treated. At the first visit we will present:

- a program of preventive home care including brushing, flossing, diet, and the importance of fluorides;

- a caries risk assessment;

- information about early childhood caries, which may be due to inappropriate nursing habits or inappropriate use of sippy cups;

- the latest facts about finger, thumb, and pacifier habits;

- what you need to know about preventing injuries to the mouth and teeth; and

- information on growth and development.

Adolescents

Adolescents have special needs. Appearance and self-image are very important to them. Decayed or poorly positioned teeth or jaws might make them more self-conscious. Teens also eat frequently, and unhealthy snack foods tend to become a major part of their regular diet. We provide a professional, sensitive, and caring approach to restoring and guiding teeth, and teaching preventive dental health care through the teen's high school years. When necessary, we will provide information on sealants, oral piercing, wisdom teeth, missing teeth, and tobacco use.

Young People with Special Needs

An integral part of our education is concerned with the medical and dental health of the special patient. People with significant medical, physical, or mental disabilities often present unique challenges to dentists. Our training allows us to address their special needs and provide the best care possible.

Team Approach to Total Health

Good oral health is an important part of total health. When helping children, we often work with pediatricians, other physicians, and dental specialists. All young people are served best through this team approach. We, the pediatric dentists, are an important part of your child's health team.

Section 14.3

Choosing a Dentist

Access to Dental Care

How can I find out about charitable or low-cost dental care for persons in need?

Assistance programs vary from state to state, so you may want to contact your state dental society to see if there are programs in your area.

Another possible source of lower-cost dental care is a dental school clinic. Generally, dental costs in school clinics are reduced and may include only partial payment for professional services covering the cost of materials and equipment. Your state dental society can tell you if there is a dental school clinic in your area, or you can search our list.

For more resources, please visit the National Institute of Health's website [http://www.nih.gov].

Where can people with special needs obtain dental care?

The ADA [American Dental Association] Council on Access, Prevention and Interprofessional Relations suggests the following tips:

- Inform the dentist about your special health or financial conditions.

- Ask if the dentist has training and/or experience in treating patients with your specific condition.

- Ask if the dentist has an interest in treating patients with your specific condition.

- Find out if the dentist participates in your dental benefit plan (dental insurance program).

- Ask if the dental facility is accessible to the disabled.

In addition, the Council suggests that patients with special needs:

- Call or write the dental director at your state department of public health.

- Contact the nearest dental school clinic or hospital dental department, especially if it is affiliated with a major university.

- Contact the Special Care Dentistry (Formerly Federation of Special Care Organizations in Dentistry), the Academy of General Dentistry, and the American Academy of Pediatric Dentistry for a referral.

- Also, the National Oral Health Information Clearinghouse may have useful information.

- Contact the National Foundation of Dentistry for the Handicapped (NFDH), a charitable affiliate of the American Dental Association since 1988. The NFDH, via several programs, facilitates the provision of comprehensive dental care for needy disabled, elderly, and medically compromised individuals.

- Dentists and dental institutions organizing or participating in voluntary projects that care for uninsured and underserved patients will find information, and grant opportunities through Volunteers in Health Care (VIH). VIH Program staff are available to assist you at the toll-free number 877-844-8442.

Choosing a Dentist

How do I find a dentist?

The American Dental Association offers these suggestions:

- Ask family, friends, neighbors, or co-workers for recommendations.

- Ask your family physician or local pharmacist.

- If you're moving, your current dentist may be able to make a recommendation.

- Call or write your local or state dental society. Your local and state dental societies also may be listed in the telephone directory under "dentists" or "associations."

- Use ADA.org's ADA Member Directory to search for dentists in your area.

You may want to call or visit more than one dentist before making your decision. Dental care is a very personalized service that requires a good relationship between the dentist and the patient.

What should I look for when choosing a dentist?

You may wish to consider several dentists before making your decision. During your first visit, you should be able to determine if this is the right dentist for you. Consider the following:

- Is the appointment schedule convenient for you?
- Is the office easy to get to from your home or job?
- Does the office appear to be clean, neat, and orderly?
- Was your medical and dental history recorded and placed in a permanent file?
- Does the dentist explain techniques that will help you prevent dental health problems? Is dental health instruction provided?
- Are special arrangements made for handling emergencies outside of office hours? (Most dentists make arrangements with a colleague or emergency referral service if they are unable to tend to emergencies.)
- Is information provided about fees and payment plans before treatment is scheduled?
- Is your dentist a member of the ADA? All ADA member dentists voluntarily agree to abide by the high ethical standards reflected in the ADA Principles of Ethics and Code of Professional Conduct as a condition of their membership.

You and your dentist are partners in maintaining your oral health. Take time to ask questions and take notes if that will help you remember your dentist's advice.

What is the difference between a DDS and a DMD?

The DDS (Doctor of Dental Surgery) and DMD (Doctor of Dental Medicine) are the same degrees. The difference is a matter of semantics.

The majority of dental schools award the DDS degree; however, some award a DMD degree. The education and degrees are the same.

Your Relationship with Your Dentist

What does this treatment recommendation mean?

If you don't understand any part of what your dentist recommends, don't be afraid to ask for more information.

Are other treatment options available?

You may want to ask your dentist the following:

- How do the options differ in cost?
- Which solution will last the longest?
- Do all the options solve the problem?

Among the dentist's recommendations, which treatments are absolutely necessary? Which are elective? Which are cosmetic? Which procedures are urgently needed, and which ones are less urgent?

Your dentist should be able to prioritize a treatment schedule to help you distinguish problems needing immediate attention from those that are less urgent. Often, treatment can be phased in over time. Be sure you understand the consequences of delaying treatment.

How much will this cost, and when and how are you expected to pay?

Does the dentist participate in your health plan? What method of payment does he or she expect? And when is payment due? Make sure you understand the fees, method, and schedule of payment before you agree to any treatment.

Should I comparison shop?

Feel free to call around the community to compare such factors as location, office hours, fees, and what arrangements will be made in case of emergency. If you are comparing fees, ask for estimates on full-mouth x-rays and a preventive dental visit that includes an oral exam and tooth cleaning.

If you have talked with your dentist and still are uncertain about what to do, get a second opinion. To find another dentist for a second opinion, call your local dental society, or ask a relative or friend for referrals. If there is a dental school in your area, you may be able to make an appointment at the school's clinic.

How do I resolve disputes or complaints?

Even in the best dentist-patient relationship, a problem may occur. First, discuss any concerns you have with your dentist. Many times this will help clear up the matter. If you are still not pleased, contact your state or local dental association.

Local dental societies have established a dispute resolution system called peer review to help resolve the occasional disagreement about dental treatment. Peer review provides an impartial and easily accessible means for resolving misunderstandings regarding the appropriateness or quality of care and, in certain instances, about the fees charged for dental treatment.

A peer review committee will attempt to mediate the problem. They may meet to discuss the case and may examine clinical records, talk to the dentist and patient and, when indicated, arrange for a clinical examination.

Can I get a copy of my dental records?

Talk with your dentist about getting a copy of your dental records. Dentists covered by the HIPAA [Health Insurance Portability and Accountability Act] privacy rule are required to provide patients with a copy of their records and state law may also apply.

The ADA Principles of Ethics and Code of Professional Conduct states: "A dentist has the ethical obligation on request of either the patient or the patient's new dentist to furnish, either gratuitously or for nominal cost, such dental records or copies or summaries of them, including dental x-rays or copies of them, as will be beneficial for the future treatment of that patient. This obligation exists whether or not the patient's account is paid in full."

What if I want a second opinion?

To find another dentist for a second opinion, call your local dental society, or ask a relative or friend for referrals. If there is a dental school in your area, you may be able to make an appointment at the school's clinic.

What happens if I miss a dental appointment?

Dental offices vary on their policies of missed appointments. Ask your dentist about his or her policy. Many dentists ask that you call to cancel an appointment at least 24 hours in advance. This will allow time for office staff to find someone else for your scheduled appointment. Those who don't call to cancel may be charged all or a portion of an office visit.

When should you cancel an appointment if you feel ill? If you feel up to the visit, keep it—unless you've got a fever, strep throat, can't breathe well, or are too uncomfortable to sit in the chair. Some dentists also request patients to cancel if they have an active herpes virus or a cold sore around the mouth. If in doubt, ask your dentist if the visit should be rescheduled.

Section 14.4

Dental Insurance: What You Need to Know

Excerpted from "Dental Benefit Coverage,"
© 2006 California Dental Association. Reprinted with permission.

To better understand the options available to employers in providing a dental benefit plan to their employees, it is important to understand the differences between dental and medical care. These differences drive the design of dental benefit plans, and create a distinction between approaches to dental and medical benefit coverage.

Unlike general medical disease, dental disease is not an insurable risk.

- There is near-universal incidence of dental disease—everyone has it, and hence, everyone needs and will utilize dental care.

- Apart from trauma and pain, the patient has complete control over when, or even if, treatment will be given. The nature and amount of that treatment has considerable effect on the outcome of treatment.

- Although the need for dental care varies between individuals, the dental needs of an employee group are highly predictable. Hence, a dental plan can often be self-funded and self-administered.

- Unlike general medical disease, dental disease is generally not acute or life-threatening; hence, the financial implications of dental treatment are not catastrophic.

Unlike many diseases, dental disease does not heal without therapeutic intervention; it is chronic, progressive, and destructive, becoming more severe over time.

Much of dental disease is preventable, at a minimum of cost and effort. Hence, dental coverage should always have a preventive orientation.

Dental disease generally progresses slowly. Hence dental treatment can be postponed and accumulated without symptoms for a considerable length of time.

The onset of dental disease occurs early in childhood. Hence, coverage extended to children is important in terms of a lifetime of satisfactory oral health.

The dental profession is organized differently than medicine:

- Eighty percent of dentists are general practitioners and primary dental care providers.

- The greatest percentage of dental care is rendered by one practitioner at a single site.

- Almost all dental care is done on an outpatient basis.

- There is a relatively small number of categories of dental auxiliary personnel [and probably a relatively small number of auxiliaries per dentist].

- There is no central facility, like a hospital, where dentists interact on a daily basis.

- Dentists own, equip, and operate their own "hospital," i.e., their dental office, without public subsidy.

"High-tech" advances in dental care generally are not very costly, add to the efficiency and capability of care, and have not resulted in severe inflation of dental costs.

Competition exists in the dental marketplace, since most dental care is not of an acute nature, enabling patients to seek out the best value in dental care.

The average annual amount of money spent per person for dental care in the United States is relatively small, even if restorative work is necessary. Dental care amounts to about 5% of annual healthcare expenditures in the United States.

Unlike the cost of medical care, the costs associated with dental care remain relatively stable; increases in the cost of dental care in the United States have been moderate.

In summary: There are significant differences between dentistry and medicine. These differences need to be taken into consideration when designing a dental benefit plan. A dental plan should not be designed as if it were a medical plan, and should not cover medical services. Ignoring the inherent differences between dentistry and medicine will result in costly mistakes in providing dental coverage to a group.

Types of Dental Benefit Plans

In many ways, the coverage of dental care mirrors the benefit plans used to cover medical care. Commercial benefit plans fall into two categories: managed care and fee-for-service.

Managed Care Plans

Preferred Provider Organization (PPO) programs are plans under which patients select a dentist from a network or list of providers who have agreed, by contract, to discount their fees. In PPOs that allow patients to receive treatment from a non-participating dentist, patients are penalized with higher deductibles and co-payments. PPOs can be fully insured or self-insured. They are usually less expensive than comparable indemnity plans and are regulated under the appropriate insurance statutes in the company's state of domicile and operation.

- **Type of Plan:** Group PPO/DPO [Dental Plan Organization] Plan

- **Benefits:** PPO plans are less expensive than indemnity plans. Employer may be able to customize plan's benefit levels and covered services. Similar to an indemnity plan, however, plan contracts with dentist to provide service for a reduced rate. PPO plan can limit the co-payment the dentist is allowed to charge, thus reduce employee's out-of-pocket expenses. Plans regulated by state laws. Private employer-sponsored plans protected under ERISA [Employee Retirement Income Security Act].

- **Limitations:** Limited to panel of participating dentists. Employee may be required to change dentists. This could discourage patients from seeking care. Reduced benefit if patient is seen by a non-participating dentist. Exclusive Provider Organization (EPO) does not cover any expenses when a patient is seen by a non-participating dentist. Annual calendar maximum.

Dental Health Maintenance Organization (DHMO)/Capitation Plan

Dental Health Maintenance Organizations or capitation plans pay contracted dentists a fixed amount (usually on a monthly basis) per enrolled family or individual, regardless of utilization. In return, participating dentists agree to provide specific types of treatment to the patient at no charge (for some treatments a co-payment may be required). Theoretically, the DHMO rewards dentists who keep patients in good health, thereby keeping costs low.

- **Type of Plan:** Group HMO/DHMO

- **Benefits:** Least expensive dental plan. Predictable co-payments or no co-payments. Preventative care generally provided at no cost to patient. Incentives for preventative treatment. Early diagnosis and preventative treatment keeps costs down. HMO plans are regulated by the Department of Managed Health Care. Plans are mandated by law to establish internal review processes for quality assurance.

- **Limitations:** Employee must select Primary Care Provider (PCP) from a list of participating dentists. Employee may be required to change dentists. This could discourage patients from seeking care. No benefit paid if patient does not seek treatment from PCP. Non-routine or major services require substantial patient co-payments, or may not be covered by plan. Dentist assumes financial risk. Dentist receives a monthly "capitation" fee (per head) for each patient assigned to practice, regardless of actual service performed. Treatment may be discouraged and quality of care could be compromised. Practice may limit number of patients seen each month, thus limit patient's access to care. Patient removed from actual cost of dental care; may not understand the value of the service provided. Annual calendar maximum.

Fee-for-Service Plan

An indemnity plan is a fully insured or self-insured plan where an assigned payment is provided to dentists for specific services, regardless of the actual charges made by the provider. Payment may be made to enrollees in the form of reimbursement payments, or directly to dentists.

- **Type of Plan:** Group Fully-Insured Indemnity Plan

- **Benefits:** Employee may see any dentist. Fixed premium for 6–12 months. Fee-For-Service; benefits paid off a UCR [Usual, Customary and Reasonable] schedule. Preventative services are usually paid at 100%, basic services at 80% and major services at 50%. Basic orthodontic coverage may be included. Plans regulated by state laws. Private employer-sponsored plan protected under ERISA.

- **Limitations:** Most expensive type of dental plan. Limit of calendar-year maximum of $1,000–$2,000 in expenses. Excluded coverage for esthetic dentistry, implants, treatment for TMJ [temporomandibular joint disorder]. Annual deductible of $50–$150. Patient is financially responsible for the balance remaining from the UCR fee to the actual fee charged. Waiting periods may apply.

- **Type of Plan:** Group Self-Funded Indemnity Plan

- **Benefits:** Employee may see any dentist. Fee-For-Service; benefits paid on a UCR schedule. Less expensive than a fully-insured indemnity plan. Claims usually paid directly to dentist. Private employer-sponsored plans protected under ERISA.

- **Limitations:** Employer bears sole financial responsibility; premiums are paid to a trust fund. Employer costs are not fixed, cost varies depending upon utilization. Employer responsible for selecting and paying for Third Party Administrator [TPA]. Check references of TPA. Self-funded plans are regulated by state law.

Direct Reimbursement (DR)

A self-funded dental benefits plan that reimburses patients according to dollars spent on dental care, not the type of treatment received.

It allows the patient complete freedom to choose any dentist. Instead of paying monthly insurance premiums employers pay a percentage of actual treatments received. Moreover, employers are removed from the potential responsibility of influencing treatment decisions due to plan selection or sponsorship.

- **Type of Plan:** Direct Reimbursement

- **Benefits:** Employees have freedom of choice to see their own dentist. No interference from insurance with patient-provider relationship. Employer determines benefit level. Employees have control of how they use their benefit dollars. Employees are directly involved in the payment process. Low administrative cost. Some employers may choose to self-administer or select a TPA. Almost all moneys go directly to dental benefits. Private employer-sponsored plan is regulated by ERISA.

- **Limitations:** Less predictable than a premium plan; costs vary month to month depending upon utilization. Plan is not regulated by state law. Employees may be required to pay dentist directly for services and are later reimbursed by the employer. This inconvenience can be avoided if employer establishes plan to directly pay dentist.

Chapter 15

Frequently Asked Questions about Teeth Cleanings and Dental Visits

Understanding Teeth Cleaning

When a dentist or dental hygienist cleans your teeth they remove soft (plaque) and hard (tartar, calculus, or stains) deposits from your teeth. The primary purpose of having your teeth cleaned is to prevent or delay the progression of periodontal diseases. Professional dental care alone, however, is inadequate to prevent periodontal diseases. Smoking has been implicated in approximately 50% of periodontal disease cases in adults. Abstaining from tobacco use, maintaining good oral hygiene, and having your teeth cleaned professionally are the most effective ways to prevent periodontal diseases.

How Often Should I Get My Teeth Cleaned?

As with routine dental examinations, the frequency of professional teeth cleaning will depend on the health of your teeth and gums. Healthy children and adults should have their teeth cleaned at least once every 12–24 months. If you are at risk of periodontal diseases because of age, tobacco use, rate of accumulation of deposits, personal oral hygiene practices, or medical conditions such as diabetes or HIV [human immunodeficiency virus] infection, your teeth may need to be cleaned more often. Your dentist or dental hygienist can help you determine how often you should have your teeth cleaned.

"Frequently Asked Questions: Teeth Cleaning," from the Centers for Disease Control and Prevention (CDC, www.cdc.gov), June 7, 2007.

Dental Visits

Routine dental visits aid in the prevention, early detection and treatment of tooth decay, oral soft tissue disease, and periodontal diseases. All information collected at the dental checkup should be kept in a dental record for future reference. If you change dentists, a copy of your dental record (including radiographs) should be given to your new dentist.

How Often Should I Visit the Dentist?

Although annual (or more frequent) dental examinations are often recommended, there is little scientific evidence that this frequency is necessary for the maintenance of oral health in healthy children or adults. The frequency of routine dental visits should be based on individual need—some people will need to see the dentist more often than others. More frequent visits may be necessary for persons at increased risk for oral diseases due to age, pregnancy, tobacco and alcohol use, periodontal diseases, oral hygiene, and health conditions (e.g., diabetes, dry mouth, HIV infection). Your dentist or dental hygienist can help you determine how often you should have your teeth cleaned.

What Should a Complete Dental Examination Include?

A complete dental examination should include the following: (1) a soft tissue examination, (2) a screening and examination for periodontal diseases, and (3) a detailed charting of cavities, existing restorations (fillings and crowns), and other tooth conditions.

The purpose of the soft tissue examination is to detect pathological changes in the tissues that line the inside of the mouth. While the vast majority of pathology in the mouth is benign, precancerous and cancerous changes in the oral tissues may be found. It is best if detected at an early stage when it can be successfully treated. Tobacco and heavy alcohol use are major risk factors for oral cancer. A thorough soft tissue examination should include a visual inspection and finger exploration of the tongue, floor of the mouth (under the tongue), palate (roof of the mouth), salivary glands, insides of the cheek, and the back of the throat. The tongue should be moved to allow for the inspection of its sides and base; the face, head, and neck should also be examined, and any enlarged lymph nodes identified.

In an examination for periodontal diseases, your dentist or hygienist should use a periodontal probe to measure the band of gum tissue that surrounds the tooth. The purpose of this examination is to detect gum disease at the early stages when prevention is most effective.

The third aspect of a complete dental examination is the inspection of every tooth surface for the presence of new decay and the status of existing restorations.

Dental radiographs (x-rays) may be part of your routine dental visit and will assist the dentist in locating disease that cannot be seen by the eye, such as cavities that develop between the teeth or bone loss that occurs beneath the gums.

When Should My Child First Visit the Dentist?

The American Academy of Pediatric Dentistry recommends an oral examination for all infants within 6 months of the eruption of the first tooth and no later than 12 months of age. An early examination will provide an opportunity for the parent or caregiver to receive anticipatory guidance regarding dental and oral development and oral health care. It will also help ensure that the infant's mouth is appropriately cleaned, that the infant has adequate fluoride exposure, and that the infant has no existing medical conditions or habits that could lead to oral disease.

Untreated Tooth Decay

Why is it important to fill decayed teeth, even baby teeth? For children, untreated decay can result in chronic pain and early tooth loss. These sequelae can lead to failure to thrive, inability to concentrate at or absence from school, reduced self-esteem, and psychosocial problems. Primary teeth should be retained until their permanent successor teeth emerge. Permanent teeth should be retained for life, if properly cared for. Decayed teeth should be repaired promptly so that fillings may be kept small and as much natural tooth structure as possible conserved. Typically, fillings have to be replaced several times during life; each time, additional tooth structure has to be removed, weakening the tooth. Of course, preventing the initial cavity is preferable to restoring the tooth after disease has occurred. Prevention is best accomplished with fluoride and dental sealants.

Chapter 16

Dealing with Dental Anxiety

Chapter Contents

Section 16.1—Calming the Anxious Child 180
Section 16.2—Tips on Easing Dental Anxiety for Adults 181

Section 16.1

Calming the Anxious Child

"Calming the Anxious Child," © 2008 American Academy of
Pediatric Dentistry (www.aapd.org). Reprinted with permission.

How does a pediatric dentist help with dental anxiety?

Pediatric dentists have special training in helping anxious children
feel secure during dental treatment. And, pediatric dental offices are
designed for children. Staff members choose to work in a pediatric
dental practice because they like kids. So, most children are calm,
comfortable, and confident in a pediatric dental office.

How will a pediatric dentist help my child feel comfortable?

Pediatric dentists are trained in many methods to help children
feel comfortable with dental treatment. For example, in the "Tell-
Show-Do" technique, a pediatric dentist might name a dental instrument, demonstrate the instrument by using it to count your child's
fingers, then apply the instrument in treatment.

The modeling technique pairs a timid child in dental treatment
with a cooperative child of similar age. Coaching, distraction, and
parent participation are other possibilities to give your child confidence in dentistry. But by far the most preferred technique is praise.
Every child does something right during a dental visit, and pediatric
dentists let children know that.

Should I accompany my child into treatment?

Infants and some young children may feel more confident when parents stay close during treatment. With older children, doctor-child communication is often enhanced if parents remain in the reception room.

What if a child misbehaves during treatment?

Occasionally a child's behavior during treatment requires assertive
management to protect him or her from possible injury. Voice control

(speaking calmly but firmly) usually takes care of it. Some children need gentle restraint of the arms or legs as well. Mild sedation, such as nitrous oxide/oxygen or a sedative, may benefit an anxious child. If a child is especially fearful or requires extensive treatment, other sedative techniques or general anesthesia may be recommended.

Section 16.2

Tips on Easing Dental Anxiety for Adults

From "Dental Treatment Anxiety," from the
U.S. Army Center for Health Promotion and Preventive Medicine
(http://chppm-www.apgea.army.mil/dhpw), 2006.

For many, going to the dentist's office can be a stressful experience associated with feelings of anxiety, nervousness, and even fear. Anxiety about dental visits shows up in a number of different ways.

• rapid heartbeat

• faster breathing

• sweaty palms

• feeling "keyed-up," edgy, or irritable

• foot tapping or fidgeting

• difficulty sleeping the night before a visit

• putting off making an appointment

• not showing up for your appointment

It's OK to have these feelings. Anxiety is a normal result of a built-in survival mechanism that is meant to help keep you out of danger. Several aspects of routine dental exams and procedures can be unpleasant and slightly painful making a person feel uncomfortable. Our minds and bodies relate these unpleasant sensations with any trip to the dentist. It causes us to be more anxious than we really need to be.

Use these methods to help ease some of these feelings:

- Schedule your appointment for a time when you will not feel rushed or under pressure.

- Get a good night's sleep—if you know that you have trouble sleeping, ask your dentist for a sedative.

- Eat a high protein meal or snack before your visit.

- Avoid caffeinated or sugary beverages or foods on the day of your visit.

- Wear loose-fitting, comfortable clothing.

- Distract yourself by listening to music. Bring a portable radio, tape, or CD player with headphones.

- Use relaxation techniques such as deep breathing exercises, progressive muscle relaxation exercises, or closing your eyes and visualizing restful or relaxing scenes.

- Make a list of any questions that you would like to ask and bring it with you.

- Do not drink alcohol the night before or the day of your visit to calm you. Alcohol causes the pain-numbing medicine to not work.

Talk with your dental provider about your fears. Your dentist may prescribe a small dose of a medication to be taken just before your appointment to help manage symptoms of pain and/or worry.

The bottom line is that anxiety associated with dental treatment is normal. Use the above simple and effective methods so worry doesn't keep you from taking care of your mouth.

Chapter 17

Holistic Dentistry:
Considerations and Cautions

A significant number of dentists have gone overboard in espousing pseudoscientific theories, particularly in the area of nutrition. Dentists who identify themselves as "holistic" or "biological" typically claim that disease can be prevented by maintaining "optimum" overall health or "wellness." In their offices, this typically involves inappropriate diagnostic tests, recommendations for expensive dietary supplements and/or homeopathic products; a plastic bite appliance; unnecessary replacement of amalgam fillings; and/or removal of root-canal-treated teeth. John E. Dodes, D.D.S., an expert on dental quackery, has remarked that "wellness" is "something for which quacks can get paid when there is nothing wrong with the patient."

Historical Perspective

Much of "holistic dentistry" is rooted in the activities of Weston A. Price, D.D.S. (1870–1948), a dentist who maintained that sugar causes not only tooth decay but physical, mental, moral, and social decay as well. Price made a whirlwind tour of primitive areas, examined the natives superficially, and jumped to simplistic conclusions. While extolling their health, he ignored their short life expectancy and high rates of infant mortality, endemic diseases, and malnutrition. While praising their diets for not producing cavities, he ignored the fact that malnourished people don't usually get many cavities.

"Stay Away from 'Holistic' and 'Biological' Dentists," by Stephen Barrett, M.D. © 2008 Quackwatch (www.quackwatch.com). Reprinted with permission.

Price knew that when primitive people were exposed to "modern" civilization they developed dental trouble and higher rates of various diseases, but he failed to realize why. Most were used to "feast or famine" eating. When large amounts of sweets were suddenly made available, they overindulged. Ignorant of the value of balancing their diets, they also ingested too much fatty and salty food. Their problems were not caused by eating "civilized" food but by abusing it. In addition to dietary excesses, the increased disease rates were due to: (a) exposure to unfamiliar germs, to which they were not resistant; (b) the drastic change in their way of life as they gave up strenuous physical activities such as hunting; and (c) alcohol abuse.

Price also performed poorly designed studies that led him to conclude that teeth treated with root canal therapy leaked bacteria or bacterial toxins into the body, causing arthritis and many other diseases. This "focal infection" theory led to needless extraction of millions of endodontically treated teeth until well-designed studies, conducted during the 1930s, demonstrated that the theory was not valid.[1,2]

Melvin Page, D.D.S. (1894–1983), one of Price's disciples, coined the phrase "balancing body chemistry" and considered tooth decay an "outstanding example of systemic chemical imbalances." Page ran afoul of the Federal Trade Commission by marketing a mineral supplement with false claims that widespread mineral deficiencies were an underlying cause of goiter, heart trouble, tuberculosis, diabetes, anemia, high and low blood pressure, hardening of the arteries, rheumatism, neuritis, arthritis, kidney and bladder trouble, frequent colds, nervousness, constipation, acidosis, pyorrhea, overweight, underweight, cataracts, and cancer. Page also claimed that milk was "unnatural" and was the underlying cause of colds, sinus infections, colitis, and cancer.

The human body contains many chemicals, ranging from water and simple charged particles (ions) to complex organic molecules. The amounts vary within limits. Some are in solution and others are not. Legitimate medical practitioners may refer to a specific chemical or a balance between a few chemicals that can be measured. But the idea that "body chemistry" goes in and out of balance is a quack concept.

Proponent Organizations

The Price-Pottenger Nutrition Foundation of La Mesa, California, was founded in 1952 as the Santa Barbara Medical Research Foundation, became the Weston Price Memorial Foundation in 1965, and adopted its current name in 1969. It has about 1,000 members. Its website describes it as "the source for quality information on the origins of health through nutrition and lifestyle." Its newsletter, book catalog, and information service promote food faddism, megavitamin therapy, homeopathy, chelation therapy, and many other dubious practices. It is also the repository for many of Price's manuscripts and photographs. In January 2008, its online membership directory listed 28 dentists as professional members.

The Weston A. Price Foundation, of Washington, D.C., is another membership organization founded to promote Price's principles. Founded in 1999, it advocates holistic dentistry, organic farming, raw (unpasteurized) milk, and many questionable dietary strategies. It also opposes fluoridation.

The Holistic Dental Association was founded in 1978 to provide a forum for developing and sharing of "health-promoting therapies that were not taught in dental schools." In March 2006, its online directory included 99 U.S. dentists.

The American Academy of Biological Dentistry was formed in 1985 and was renamed the International Academy of Biological Dentistry and Medicine (IABDM) in 2005. IABDM's founding mission statement says: "The IABDM supports dentists, physicians and allied practitioners committed to integrating body, mind, spirit and mouth, and caring for the whole person."[3] Its seminars have promoted "mercury-free dentistry," "detoxification, "cavitation surgery," electromagnetics, sound, light, acupuncture, homeopathy, herbal therapy, nutrition, and "an integrated approach to body, mind and spirit, with diagnosis and treatment of the whole person." In September 2005, its online directory included 55 dentists and 6 members from other professions. Fourteen of the dentists also belonged to the Holistic Dental Association.

Dubious Practices

"Holistic" and "biological" dentists use many approaches that are not only unsound but involve procedures and body areas that are outside of the legitimate scope of dentistry. Some practitioners use hair analysis, computerized dietary analysis, a blood chemistry screening test, or muscle-testing, as a basis for recommending supplements to "balance the body chemistry" of their patients. Hair analysis is not a reliable tool for measuring the body's nutritional state.[2] Computer analysis can be useful for determining the composition of a person's diet and can be a legitimate tool for dietary counseling. Dentists receive training in the nutritional aspects of dental health. However, few are qualified to perform general dietary counseling, and computerized "nutrient deficiency tests" are not legitimate. The blood chemistry tests, usually obtained from a reputable laboratory, are legitimate but misinterpreted. Instead of accepting the laboratory's range of "normal" values, "holistic dentists" use a much narrower range and tell patients that anything outside that range means they are out of balance and need treatment. Muscle-testing is a feature of applied kinesiology, a pseudoscientific system of diagnosis and treatment based on the notion every health problem can be related to a weak muscle and nutritional imbalances.[3] Variations used by dentists include behavioral kinesiology and autonomic response testing (ART).

Disorders of the TMJ [temporomandibular joint] (jaw joint) and facial muscles can cause facial pain and restrict opening of the mouth. Clicking alone is not considered a problem. Allegations that TMJ problems can affect scoliosis, premenstrual syndrome, or sexual problems are not supported by scientific evidence. Scientific studies show that 80% to 90% of patients with TMJ pain will get better within three months if treated with nonprescription analgesics, moist heat, and exercises.

Correction of a "bad bite" can involve irreversible treatments such as grinding down the teeth or building them up with dental restorations. The most widespread unscientific treatment involves placing a plastic appliance between the teeth. These devices, called mandibular orthopedic repositioning appliances (MORAs), typically cover only some of the teeth and are worn continuously for many months or even years. When worn too much, MORAs can cause the patient's teeth to move so far out of proper position that orthodontics or facial reconstructive surgery is needed to correct the deformity.

Proponents of "cranial osteopathy," "craniosacral therapy," "cranial therapy," and similar methods claim that the skull bones can be manipulated to relieve pain (especially TMJ pain) and remedy many other ailments. They also claim that a rhythm exists in the flow of the fluid that surrounds the brain and spinal cord and that diseases can be diagnosed by detecting aberrations in this rhythm and corrected by manipulating the skull. Proponents include dentists, physical therapists, osteopaths, and chiropractors. The theory underlying craniosacral therapy is erroneous because the bones of the skull are fused to each other, and cerebrospinal fluid does not have a palpable rhythm.[4] In one study, three physical therapists who examined the same 12 patients diagnosed significantly different "craniosacral rates."[5]

Homeopathy is a pseudoscience based on 200-year-old notions that (a) substances that produce symptoms in healthy people can cure ill people with similar symptoms and (b) infinitesimal doses can be highly potent.[6]

Some practitioners use procedures based on traditional Chinese medicine (TCM) theories that relate health and disease to alleged imbalances in the flow of "vital energy" ("chi") through imaginary channels called meridians. A few dentists use a quack "electrodiagnostic device" that supposedly detects these imbalances. These devices actually measure skin resistance to a low-voltage electric current, which the practitioners claim is related to "electromagnetic energy imbalance." The procedure is commonly referred to as electrodermal testing, galvanic testing, or electroacupuncture according to Voll (EAV). It typically leads to multiple false diagnoses, unnecessary tooth removal, and/or the sale of useless dietary supplements and/or homeopathic products.[7]

Some dentists who espouse TCM theories claim that areas of the body are "represented" by the tongue and the teeth, These claims have no anatomical basis and should be regarded as preposterous. I have also seen diagrams that relate each tooth to one or more of the body's internal organs.[8]

Auriculotherapy espouses the notion that the body and organs are represented on the surface of the ear. Proponents claim it is effective against facial pain and ailments throughout the body. Its practitioners twirl needles or administer small electrical currents at points on the ear that supposedly represent diseased organs. Courses on auriculotherapy are popular among "holistic" dentists. Complications from unsterile and broken needles have been reported. There is certainly no scientific evidence or logical reason to believe that fiddling with someone's ear can modify a disease process at a remote part of the body.[9]

A few hundred dentists claim that the mercury in amalgam fillings is toxic and causes a wide range of health problems, including multiple sclerosis, arthritis, headaches, Parkinson's disease, and emotional stress. They recommend that mercury fillings be replaced with either gold or plastic ones and that vitamin supplements be taken to prevent trouble during the process. However, scientific testing has shown that the amount of mercury absorbed from fillings is only a small fraction of the average daily intake from food and is insignificant. In 1992 an extensive review by the U.S. Public Health Service concluded that it was inappropriate to recommend restricting the use of dental amalgam.[10] The American Dental Association Council on Ethics, Bylaws, and Judicial Affairs considers the unnecessary removal of silver-amalgam fillings "improper and unethical."

The most outspoken advocate of mercury-amalgam toxicity has been Hal A. Huggins, D.D.S., of Colorado Springs, Colorado, who describes himself as one of Page's students. Huggins promoted "balancing body chemistry" so vigorously that in 1975 the American Dental Association Council on Dental Research denounced the diet that he recommended. Another Price follower is George A. Meinig, D.D.S., whose book *Root Canal Cover-up Exposed* was published in 1994.

In the mid-1980s the FDA forced Huggins to stop marketing mineral products with false claims that they would help the body rid itself of mercury. Huggins has also claimed that root canal therapy can make people susceptible to arthritis, multiple sclerosis, amyotrophic lateral sclerosis, and other autoimmune diseases. As with mercury-amalgam fillings, there is no objective evidence that teeth treated with root canal therapy have any adverse effect on the immune system or any other system or part of the body.[11] Huggins's dental license was revoked in 1996. During the revocation proceedings the administrative law judge concluded: (a) Huggins had diagnosed "mercury toxicity" in all patients who consulted him in his office, even some without mercury fillings; (b) he had also recommended extraction of all teeth that had had root canal therapy; and (c) Huggins's treatments were "a sham, illusory and without scientific basis."[12]

Huggins is among a small number of dentists who maintain that facial pain, heart disease, arthritis, and various other health problems are caused by "cavitations," within the jaw bones, that are not detectable on x-ray examination or treatable with antibiotics. Advocates now call this condition "neuralgia-inducing cavitational osteonecrosis (NICO)" and claim they can cure the patient by locating and scraping out the affected tissues. They may also remove all root-canal-treated teeth, most of the vital teeth close to the area where they say a problem exists, and even parts of the jawbone. Worse yet, the surgery may result in severe infections and a lifetime of pain.[13]

Huggins's website states that, "Cavitations are hard to find. They require lots of skill, years of experience, and most of all, a vivid imagination to spot them on an X-ray film." Vivid imagination may well be the basic requirement of holistic and biological dentistry.

The Bottom Line

My advice is simple. Steer clear of dentists who practice "holistic dentistry" or "biological dentistry" or who use or even recommend any of the dubious methods described in this text.

References

1. Easlick K. An evaluation of the effect of dental foci of infection on health. *Journal of the American Dental Association* 42:615–97, 1951.

2. Grossman L. Pulpless teeth and focal infection. *Journal of Endodontics* 8:S18–S24, 1982.

3. Founding mission statement. IABDM website, accessed Feb 3, 2008.

4. Barrett S. Commercial hair analysis: A cardinal sign of quackery. Quackwatch, April 20, 2006.

5. Barrett S. Applied kinesiology: Muscle-testing for "allergies" and "nutrient deficiencies." Quackwatch, Sept 26, 2004.

6. Barrett S. Why craniosacral therapy is silly. Quackwatch, Sept 21, 2004.

7. Hartman SE, Norton JM. Interexaminer reliability and cranial osteopathy. Scientific *Review of Alternative Medicine* 6(1):23–34, 2002.

8. Barrett S. Homeopathy: The ultimate fake. Quackwatch, Oct 4, 2007.

9. Barrett S. Quack "electrodiagnostic" devices. Quackwatch, Sept 5, 2007.

10. Barrett S. Bizarre tooth charts. Dental Watch, Nov 9, 2004.

11. Barrett S. Auriculotherapy: A skeptical look. Acupuncture Watch, Feb 2, 2008.

12. Benson JS and others. Dental Amalgam: A Scientific Review and Recommended Public Health Strategy for Research, Education and Regulation. Washington, D.C., 1993, US Public Health Service.

13. Barrett S. The "mercury toxicity" scam: How anti-amalgamists swindle people. Quackwatch.

14. Administrative Law Judge's conclusions about Hal A. Huggins, D.D.S (1999). Quackwatch, Dec 23, 1999.

15. Barrett S, Dodes J. A critical look at cavitational osteopathosis, NICO, and "biological dentistry." Aug 31, 2007.

Chapter 18

Avoiding Disease Transmission, Allergic Reactions, and Dangerous Exposures at the Dentist's Office

Chapter Contents

Section 18.1—Preventing Infectious Disease Transmission ... 192

Section 18.2—Preventing Contact Dermatitis and Latex
Allergy Reactions in Dental Settings 194

Section 18.3—Potential Risk for Lead Exposure in Dental
Offices 199

Section 18.1

Preventing Infectious Disease Transmission

"Protecting Against Disease Transmission,"
© American Dental Hygienists Association (www.adha.org).
Reprinted with permission. The date of this document is unknown.

Although experts agree it is extremely rare, it may be possible to get an infectious disease during a routine visit to the dental office.

Infected microorganisms live in blood and oral fluids, on contaminated instruments and countertops, and sometimes even in the air. Patients may be exposed to diseases such as hepatitis B and C, herpes simplex virus, HIV [human immunodeficiency virus], tuberculosis, staphylococci, and other viruses and bacteria that thrive in the oral cavity and respiratory tract. However, there has only been one report of possible HIV transmission in a dental setting and that was in 1991, and last transmission of hepatitis B was in 1987. There have been no documented cases of hepatitis C being transmitted in a dental setting.

But all of these diseases can be avoided if proper infection control is used in dental offices. Keep an eye out for improper infection control procedures and ask your dental hygienist about the procedures your dental office uses. Many offices post a list of the infection control procedures they follow in a reception area or elsewhere. If you don't see this information, ask about it.

In addition, the Centers for Disease Control and Prevention (CDC) recommends standard precautions that should be used in the care of all patients, regardless of their infection status. The precautions are intended to prevent or reduce the potential for disease transmission among patients and oral health care personnel.

Infection Control Patrol

Your oral health care provider should adhere to all of the following standard infection control procedures:

- Wear protective clothing and gear, including gloves, masks, gowns, or laboratory coats, and protective eyewear for all treatment procedures.

- Change gloves after each patient contact. Whenever possible, complete all work on one patient before regloving and performing procedures on another patient.

- Even though gloves are worn, wash hands thoroughly before and after each patient is treated. An alternative to hand washing between each patient is to hand wash before the first patient and then use an alcohol rub between patients. However, alcohol hand rubs have limitations. For instance, they are ineffective if there is visible dirt on hands, and they cannot be used for a sterile procedure. In the case of the latter, a surgical hand scrub is required. The rationale for using gloves despite the fact that hand washing and alcohol rubs are used is that gloves may become perforated, knowingly or unknowingly, during use. The perforations may allow fluids to pass through the gloves to contaminate hands. These fluids could contain infectious microorganisms.

- Use coverings to protect surfaces like light handles or x-ray unit heads that may be contaminated and are difficult or impossible to disinfect.

- Heat sterilize all non-disposable instruments and devices—heat-resistant needles, syringes, and other sharp instruments and devices—and disinfect surfaces and equipment after treatment of each patient.

- Discard disposable syringes and other sharp instruments in puncture-resistant containers. Needles must not be recapped, bent, or broken before disposal because this increases the risk of an unintentional needle stick injury.

- Place all potentially infectious waste in closable, leak-proof containers or bags that are color-coded, labeled, or tagged in accordance with applicable federal, state, and local regulations.

Many infection control precautions oral health care workers take to protect their patients and themselves are not easily apparent to patients, so feel free to ask your oral health care professionals to explain the policies and procedures in place in your office.

For more information on infection control, visit the CDC website at www.cdc.gov or the Organization for Safety and Asepsis Procedures at www.osap.org.

Section 18.2

Preventing Contact Dermatitis and Latex Allergy Reactions in Dental Settings

Excerpted from "Contact Dermatitis and Latex Allergy,"
by the Division of Oral Health, Centers for Disease Control and
Prevention (CDC, www.cdc.gov), August 7, 2007.

What is contact dermatitis?

Occupationally related contact dermatitis can develop from frequent and repeated use of hand hygiene products, exposure to chemicals, and glove use. Contact dermatitis is classified as either irritant or allergic. Irritant contact dermatitis is common, nonallergic, and develops as dry, itchy, irritated areas on the skin around the area of contact. By comparison, allergic contact dermatitis (type IV hypersensitivity) can result from exposure to accelerators and other chemicals used in the manufacture of rubber gloves as well as from exposure to other chemicals found in the dental practice setting. Allergic contact dermatitis often manifests as a rash beginning hours after contact and, like irritant dermatitis, is usually confined to the areas of contact.

What is latex allergy?

Latex allergy (type I hypersensitivity to latex proteins) can be a more serious systemic allergic reaction. It usually begins within minutes of exposure but can sometimes occur hours later. It produces varied symptoms, which commonly include runny nose, sneezing, itchy eyes, scratchy throat, hives, and itchy burning sensations. However, it can involve more severe symptoms including asthma marked by difficult breathing, coughing spells, and wheezing; cardiovascular and gastrointestinal ailments; and in rare cases, anaphylaxis and death.

What are some considerations if dental health care personnel are allergic to latex?

Dental health care personnel who are allergic to latex will need to take precautions at work and outside the workplace since latex is used in a variety of other common products in addition to gloves. The following recommendations are based on those issued by the National Institute for Occupational Health and Safety (NIOSH).

If definitively diagnosed with allergy to natural rubber latex (NRL) protein:

- Avoid, as far as feasible, subsequent exposure to the protein and only use nonlatex (e.g., nitrile or vinyl) gloves.
- Make sure that other staff members in the dental practice wear either nonlatex or reduced protein, powder-free latex gloves.
- Use only synthetic or powder-free rubber dams.

Dental personnel can further reduce occupational exposure to NRL protein by taking the following steps:

- Using reduced protein, powder-free latex gloves.
- Frequently changing ventilation filters and vacuum bags used in latex contaminated areas.
- Checking ventilation systems to ensure they provide adequate fresh or recirculating air.
- Frequently cleaning all work areas contaminated with latex dust.
- Educating dental staff on the signs and symptoms of latex allergies.

Why are powder-free gloves recommended?

Proteins responsible for latex allergies are attached to glove powder. When powdered gloves are worn, more latex protein reaches the skin. Also, when gloves are put on or removed, particles of latex protein powder become aerosolized and can be inhaled, contacting mucous membranes. As a result, allergic dental health care personnel and patients can experience symptoms related to cutaneous, respiratory, and conjunctival exposure. Dental health care personnel can become sensitized to latex proteins after repeated exposure. Work areas where only powder-free, low-allergen (i.e., reduced-protein) gloves are used show low or undetectable amounts of allergy-causing proteins.

What are some considerations for providing dental treatment to patients with latex allergy?

Patients with a latex allergy should not have direct contact with latex-containing materials and should be treated in a "latex safe"

Table 18.1. Categories of Glove-Associated Skin Reactions

	Irritant Contact Dermatitis	Allergic Contact Dermatitis (Type IV [delayed] Hypersensitivity)	Latex Allergy (Type I [immediate] Hypersensitivity or NRL* protein allergy)
Causative Agents	Toxic chemicals (e.g., biocides, detergents); excessive perspiration; irritating chemicals used in hand products and in glove manufacture	Accelerators and other chemicals used in glove manufacture; sterilants and disinfectants (e.g., glutaraldehyde); bonding agents (e.g., methacrylates); local anesthetics	Latex proteins from *Hevea brasiliensis* (rubber tree)
Reactions	Skin reactions usually confined to the area of contact	Skin reactions usually confined to the area of contact	Skin and systemic reactions can occur as soon as 2–3 minutes, or as long as several hours after skin or mucous membrane contact with the protein allergens
	Acute: Red, dry, itchy irritated areas	**Acute:** Itchy, red rash, small blisters	**Acute:** Hives, swelling, runny nose, nausea, abdominal cramps, dizziness, low blood pressure, bronchospasm, anaphylaxis (shock)
	Chronic: Dry, thickened skin, crusting, deep painful cracking, scabbing sores, peeling	**Chronic:** Dry thickened skin, crusting, scabbing sores, vesicles, peeling (appears 4–96 hours after exposure)	**Chronic:** As above, increased potential for extensive, more severe reaction
Diagnosis	By medical history, symptoms, and exclusion of Type IV and Type I hypersensitivity; Not an allergic reaction	By medical history, symptoms, and skin patch test	By medical history, symptoms, and skin-prick or blood test

Note: *NRL=natural rubber latex. American Dental Association, 1999. Dental health care personnel experiencing contact dermatitis or latex allergy symptoms should seek a definitive diagnosis by an experienced health care professional (e.g., dermatologist, allergist) to determine the specific etiology and appropriate treatment for their condition, as well as to determine what work restrictions or accommodations may be necessary.

environment. Such patients also may be allergic to the chemicals used in manufacturing natural rubber latex gloves, as well as to metals, plastics, or other materials used to provide dental care. By obtaining thorough patient health histories and preventing patients from having contact with potential allergens, dental health care professionals can minimize the possibility of patients having adverse reactions. Considerations in providing safe treatment for patients with possible or documented latex allergy include (but are not limited to) the following:

- Screen all patients for latex allergy (e.g., obtain their health history, provide medical consultation when latex allergy is suspected).

- Be aware of some common predisposing conditions (e.g., spina bifida, urogenital anomalies, or allergies to avocados, kiwis, nuts, or bananas).

- Be familiar with the different types of hypersensitivity—immediate and delayed—and the risks that these pose for patients and staff.

- Consider sources of latex other than gloves. Dental patients with a history of latex allergy may be at risk from a variety of dental products including, but not limited to, prophylaxis cups, rubber dams, and orthodontic elastics.

- Provide an alternative treatment area free of materials containing latex. Ensure a latex-safe environment or one in which no personnel use latex gloves and no patient contact occurs with other latex devices, materials, and products.

- Remove all latex-containing products from the patient's vicinity. Adequately cover/isolate any latex-containing devices that cannot be removed from the treatment environment.

- Be aware that latent allergens in the ambient air can cause respiratory and or anaphylactic symptoms in people with latex hypersensitivity. Therefore, to minimize inadvertent exposure to airborne latex particles among patients with latex allergy, try to give them the first appointments of the day.

- Frequently clean all working areas contaminated with latex powder/dust.

- Frequently change ventilation filters and vacuum bags used in latex-contaminated areas.

- Have latex-free kits (e.g., dental treatment and emergency kits) available at all times.

- Be aware that allergic reactions can be provoked from indirect contact as well as direct contact (e.g., being touched by someone who has worn latex gloves). Hand hygiene, therefore, is essential.

- Communicate latex allergy procedures (e.g., verbal instructions, written protocols, posted signs) to other personnel to prevent them from bringing latex-containing materials into the treatment area.

- If latex-related complications occur during or after the procedure, manage the reaction and seek emergency assistance as indicated. Follow current medical emergency response recommendations for management of anaphylaxis.

Section 18.3

Potential Risk for Lead Exposure in Dental Offices

From "Public Health Dispatch: Potential Risk for Lead Exposure in Dental Offices," from the Centers for Disease Control and Prevention (CDC, www.cdc.gov), *Morbidity and Mortality Weekly Report (MMWR)*, October 12, 2001. This document was reviewed by David A. Cooke, M.D., May 11, 2008.

In December 2000, the Washington State Health Department discovered white powder that was found to be lead oxide in boxes used to store dental intraoral radiograph film. The Washington State Health Department alerted state health departments throughout the United States. Subsequently, the Wisconsin Division of Public Health (WDPH) conducted an investigation of dental offices in the state. This report summarizes the investigation, which indicated that similar storage boxes are used in Wisconsin. The findings indicate that patients are at risk for exposure to a substantial amount of lead during a dental radiograph procedure if the office stores dental film in these boxes.

During January–March 2001, radiation safety inspectors in Wisconsin visited 240 (9%) of 2,748 dental offices with radiograph equipment. Of these, 43 (18%) stored radiograph film in table-top, lead-lined boxes. Of 11 dental offices in use for >20 years, four (36%) used this storage method.

The boxes were usually made of wood and shaped like a shoe box. All boxes contained a white powder residue. A bulk sample of the residue contained 77% lead identified as lead oxide. Visits to dental offices occurred before and after a mailing had been sent by WDPH to all dental offices with radiograph equipment warning about possible lead exposure and recommending that lead-lined storage boxes be discarded. Many offices discarded the boxes before the inspection. In one office, after receiving the warning, paper was placed in the bottom of the box and film was placed on top of the paper. In another office, dental instruments had been placed in the box. Other offices used a vertical wall-mounted, lead-lined film dispensing box. Some of these boxes and the film in them also contained lead.

199

A mock dental radiograph procedure was performed during which wipes were placed on the tips of a dental hygienist's fingers whenever a patient's mouth was touched. Analysis of these wipe samples found 3,378 mcg lead that could have been transferred from the hygienist's fingers to a patient's mouth. Lead also could have been introduced directly from the film. Wipe samples of eight film packets from two dental offices that used the lead-lined storage boxes identified average lead levels of 3,352 mcg (range: 262 mcg–34,000 mcg). During a typical radiographic procedure, usually conducted once per year, >4 separate views are taken. When children's teeth develop to the point where adjacent teeth touch (usually age 3 years), radiographs may be taken if the dentist suspects decay.

Because of the increased susceptibility of children and the developing fetus, lead exposure is particularly dangerous for children and for women who are or may soon become pregnant. The approximate half-life of lead in blood is 25 days; as a result, the window for identifying lead exposure following dental radiographs is a few months. Health-care providers who discover high blood lead levels of unexplained origin should consider this possible route of exposure.

Advances in dental radiograph technology have reduced scatter radiation—the reason for protective boxes—making lead-lined radiograph storage boxes unnecessary. Because lead oxide cannot be removed adequately, the film packets stored in lead-lined boxes and the film packets stored in them should be discarded.

Chapter 19

X-Rays for Diagnosing Dental Problems

Chapter Contents

Section 19.1—How Do Dental X-Rays Work? 202
Section 19.2—X-Ray Use and Safety in Children 203

Section 19.1

How Do Dental X-Rays Work?

"How Do X-rays work?," © Massachusetts Dental Society
(www.massdental.org). Reprinted with permission.
The date of this document is unknown.

When x-rays pass through your mouth during a dental exam, more x-rays are absorbed by the denser parts (such as teeth and bone) than by soft tissues (such as cheeks and gums) before striking the film. This creates an image called a radiograph. Teeth appear lighter because fewer x-rays penetrate to reach the film. Tooth decay, infections, and signs of gum disease, including changes in the bone and ligaments holding teeth in place, appear darker because of more x-ray penetration. Dental restorations (fillings, crowns) may appear lighter or darker, depending on the type of material used for the restoration. The interpretation of these radiographs allows the dentist to safely and accurately detect hidden abnormalities.

How often should radiographs be taken?

How often x-rays (radiographs) should be taken depends on the patient's individual health needs. It is important to recognize that just as each patient is different form the next, so should the scheduling of x-ray exams be individualized for each patient. Your dentist will review your history, examine your mouth, and then decide whether you need radiographs and what type. If you are a new patient, the dentist may recommend radiographs to determine the present status of the hidden areas of your mouth and to help analyze changes that may occur later. If you have had recent radiographs at your previous dentist, your new dentist may ask you to have the radiographs forwarded.

The schedule for needing radiographs at recall visits varies according to your age, risk for disease, and signs and symptoms. Recent films may be needed to detect new cavities, or to determine the status of gum disease or for evaluation of growth and development. Children may need x-rays more often than adults. This is because their teeth and jaws are still developing and because their teeth are more likely to be affected by tooth decay than those of adults.

If you have questions about receiving dental x-rays, be sure to speak to your dentist.

Section 19.2

X-Ray Use and Safety in Children

"X-Ray Use and Safety," © 2008 American Academy of Pediatric Dentistry (www.aapd.org). Reprinted with permission.

How often should a child have dental x-ray films?

Since every child is unique, the need for dental x-ray films varies from child to child. Films are taken only after a complete review of your child's health, and only when they are likely to yield information that a visual exam cannot.

In general, children need x-rays more often than adults. Their mouths grow and change rapidly. They are more susceptible to tooth decay than adults. The American Academy of Pediatric Dentistry recommends x-ray examinations every six months for children with a high risk of tooth decay. Children with a low risk of tooth decay require x-rays less frequently.

Why should x-ray films be taken if my child has never had a cavity?

X-ray films detect much more than cavities. For example, x-rays may be needed to survey erupting teeth, diagnose bone diseases, evaluate the results of an injury, or plan orthodontic treatment. X-rays allow dentists to diagnose and treat health conditions that cannot be detected during a clinical examination. If dental problems are found and treated early, dental care is more comfortable and affordable.

Will x-ray films be taken routinely?

No. X-ray films are recommended only when necessary to protect your child's dental health. The frequency of x-ray films is determined by your child's individual needs.

How safe are dental x-rays?

Pediatric dentists are particularly careful to minimize the exposure of child patients to radiation. With contemporary safeguards, the amount of radiation received in a dental x-ray examination is extremely small. The risk is negligible. In fact, dental x-rays represent a far smaller risk than an undetected and untreated dental problem.

How will my child be protected from x-ray exposure?

Lead body aprons and shields will protect your child. Today's equipment filters out unnecessary x-rays and restricts the x-ray beam to the area of interest. High-speed film and proper shielding assure that your child receives a minimal amount of radiation exposure.

Chapter 20

Managing Pain at the Dentist's Office

Chapter Contents

Section 20.1—Conscious Sedation for Adults 206

Section 20.2—Frequently Asked Questions about Dental
Anesthesia 209

Section 20.3—Air Abrasion: A Painless Drilling Technique.... 211

Section 20.4—Minimally Invasive Dentistry 213

Section 20.5—Lasers in Dentistry: How Do They Work? 215

Section 20.1

Conscious Sedation for Adults

From "Conscious (moderate) sedation for adults," by the National Institutes of Health Clinical Center (www.cc.nih.gov), August 2007.

This information explains moderate sedation. If you have questions after reading it, feel free to ask your nurse or doctor.

What is conscious (moderate) sedation?

During a procedure, conscious (moderate) sedation, lets you stay awake and aware, without feeling discomfort and without the stronger side effects and dangers of general anesthesia.

The doctor can speak with you and you will be able to respond.

Conscious sedation does not last long, but it may make you drowsy.

Let your doctor know if you have any allergies, especially to Fentanyl, Versed, or Ativan.

How will I receive sedation medications?

You will receive medications by vein (intravenously) or by injection into a muscle (intramuscularly). They can also be given by mouth.

Oral medications may take 30 to 60 minutes to take effect. The effects of intravenous medication may be felt immediately.

What are the side effects of sedation?

- Sedation may slow your breathing, and the nurse may need to give you oxygen to help you breathe.

- Your blood pressure may be affected, and you may get intravenous fluids to stabilize your blood pressure.

- Because sedation effects may linger, you may have a headache, nausea, and feel sleepy for several hours.

- Some people have a brief period of amnesia (not remembering what happened) after receiving conscious sedation.

How do I prepare for sedation?

One to 2 weeks before your procedure:

- Inform your doctor immediately if you take anti-inflammatory medications such as indomethacin, Daypro, Aleve, ibuprofen, aspirin, or even Pepto-Bismol. These medications contain salicylate. Your doctor will let you know if you can take them.

- Contact your doctor for specific instructions about your other medications. You may need to take some of these medications on the day of your procedure.

- If you smoke, you may be asked to stop the night before your procedure, and not restart until the day after (depending on the procedure).

- You may have restrictions on your diet; for example no solid foods for 8 to 12 hours before the procedure with sips of water or broth up to 4 hours before the procedure. Fasting means no eating or drinking, including water. Check with your doctor or nurse for your specific restrictions.

- Avoid drinking alcohol the night before and day of the procedure. Alcohol can interact with sedation and pain medications and cause problems for you.

The morning of your procedure:

- Your doctor will explain what to expect during the procedure, including its benefits, risks, and recovery period. You will have plenty of time to ask questions. If you agree to the procedure, you will be asked to sign a consent form.

- If you are an outpatient, you will be asked to bring a responsible adult to take you home. This person must be available when you are discharged from the procedure.

- You will have a physical examination that includes your vital signs (blood pressure, pulse, and respirations). We will also ask you about your medical, surgical, anesthetic and family histories, and current medications and allergies.

- The nurse will start an intravenous catheter (IV). This is a small plastic catheter placed in your vein to administer fluids and medications during the procedure.

207

- You may have blood drawn or be asked to provide a urine specimen.

- You may be asked to empty your bladder and change into hospital gown before the procedure.

What happens during the procedure?

- A nurse and doctor will stay with you at all times to check your level of drowsiness and your vital signs (pulse, blood pressure, and respiration).

- Your vital signs will be checked every 3 to 5 minutes.

- Your oxygen level (oxygen saturation) will be checked continuously with a device that clips onto one of your fingers.

- You will feel very relaxed and may even begin to sleep, but you will awaken easily and be able to talk with the doctors and nurses.

What happens immediately after the procedure?

- A nurse will watch you closely until you recover from the medications.

- Your oxygen level will continue to be measured with the device attached to your finger.

- A nurse will continue to closely monitor your blood pressure, breathing, and pulse at least every 15 minutes for 1 hour, or until they go back to what they were before the procedure.

- If you are an inpatient, you will be taken back to your room when your vital signs are stable.

When can I be discharged?

Expect to stay 1 to 2 hours after your procedure. The timing of your discharge depends on several things:

- You must be awake, alert, and know where you are.

- You must not be bleeding or vomiting.

- Your blood pressure, pulse, breathing, and oxygen saturation must be close to normal for you.

- You must be able to drink fluids.

- You must be able to urinate. Your intravenous line will be removed after you can drink and urinate.

- Your doctor must write an order for your discharge.

Should I do anything special after conscious sedation?

For your safety, a responsible adult must take you home. This person must be available when you are ready for discharge.

Do not take a bus, taxicab, or public transportation without a responsible adult to ride with you.

Do not drive, drink alcohol, use machinery, or sign legal documents for 24 hours after receiving conscious sedation.

Section 20.2

Frequently Asked Questions about Dental Anesthesia

"Patient Information," © American Dental Society of
Anesthesiology (www.adsahome.org). Reprinted with permission.
The date of this document is unknown.

It is common for many patients to feel nervous or anxious about their dental procedures. Your dentist has advanced training in ways to help with your anxiety which may include other medications to make you feel more comfortable. By having a more relaxed patient your dentist may be able to complete more of your dentistry in one appointment. In other cases, a more relaxed patient may be safer for them as well as being more relaxed.

This text will address the most commonly asked questions regarding anesthesia. The decisions of which type of sedation/anesthesia will be determined by you in consultation with your doctor.

What is sedation and anesthesia?

During dental and oral surgical procedures local anesthesia (Novocain) is administered to block sensations. However, the anxiety that some people have can be controlled by administering sedative drugs, such as Valium-type medications. A sedated patient may remember the procedures, but will be more relaxed. Additional medications such as agents similar to pentothal are sometimes used to cause anesthesia, which places the patient more deeply asleep.

How is the medication administered?

The sedative and anesthetic medications are typically given intravenously (IV). Since the effects are so rapid by this means of administration, your doctor can precisely give the correct amounts of the medications to make you relaxed and comfortable. Also, if more medications are needed during the procedure, the IV allows easy administration of additional medications.

How am I monitored during the procedure?

Depending on the depth of the sedation and anesthetic being used, as well as your own medical condition, various monitors are used. These vary from automatic blood pressure cuffs, to the use of pulse oximeters which through a light sensor measure the oxygen concentration in your blood. Sometimes an EKG [electrocardiogram] may be used as well.

The doctor along with at least one trained member of the staff will always be with you and closely observing you throughout your treatment.

Is anesthesia safe?

The use of sedation and anesthesia in dentistry has a commendable record of safety. This is due to the advanced training your doctor has and his/her commitment to your overall health. It is important to advise your doctor of all medications that you take as well as any changes in your health since your last visit.

In most states a special permit is required to administer intravenous medications. In order to qualify your doctor had to provide evidence of advanced training in anesthesia and often a site visit is required. The ability to handle emergency situations as well as having specific emergency medications and equipment is also mandatory.

What is the ADSA?

The American Dental Society of Anesthesiology is a group of dentists who are committed to the task of making dental care more pleasant through a variety of advanced pain and anxiety control techniques. Membership in this organization is evidence of his/her concern for your comfort and health.

Section 20.3

Air Abrasion: A Painless Drilling Technique

"What is Air Abrasion?" © 2007 Academy of General Dentistry (www.agd.org). Reprinted with permission.

Air abrasion, also called microabrasion and kinetic cavity preparation, is a method of tooth-structure removal considered to be an effective alternative to the standard dental drill.

Air abrasion technology functions much like the sandblasting technique used to clear graffiti from walls. An air abrasion handpiece blows a powerful air stream of tiny aluminum oxide particles out of its tip onto the tooth structure. As particles bounce off the tooth, they blast the decay away.

It most commonly is used to prepare various types of cavities to be restored with composites, or "white fillings." Air abrasion also can be effectively used to repair cracks and discolorations and prepare tooth surfaces for bonding procedures or sealants.

What are its advantages?

Air abrasion procedures are virtually painless, which, in most cases, eliminates the need for an anesthetic injection. Air abrasion systems produce no vibration and no heat from friction. The technology can't harm soft mouth tissue and operates very quietly. Because air abrasion cuts tooth surfaces with the utmost precision, it removes less tooth than the drill and it reduces the risk of enamel micro-fracturing. In other words, the advantages are more of your tooth is preserved, there is little or no discomfort, no anesthetic numbness is needed and treatment time is usually shorter.

211

Will I feel anything during the procedure?

Air abrasion procedures can leave an accumulation of harmless, dusty particle debris in the patient's mouth, resulting in a gritty feeling that is eradicated by rinsing. Your dentist may require you to wear protective glasses during the procedure, and a rubber dam may be applied inside your mouth and around the tooth area being treated to serve as a particle barrier. To reduce dust build-up, the dentist or dental assistant may use a vacuum hose or a water spray technique while administering air abrasion.

If you have a deep cavity, you may experience some sensitivity. Your dentist will make every effort to make you comfortable and may administer local anesthesia, depending on the depth of your cavity.

Is air abrasion suitable for everyone?

Yes. It is an especially good option for children who may be afraid of the needle and the noise and vibration of a regular dental drill. However, there are some treatments, like crown and bridge preparation and "silver fillings," or amalgam, that still require the use of a dental drill. Air abrasion can't be used as an alternative in every procedure.

Who will provide my air abrasion treatment?

Your general dentist, who has been trained in restorative dentistry techniques, will perform any procedures that use air-abrasion technology. Ask your dentist if he or she uses air-abrasion equipment and if this technique is right for you.

Section 20.4

Minimally Invasive Dentistry

"Minimally Invasive Dentistry," © 2008 Academy of General Dentistry
(www.agd.org). Reprinted with permission.

What is minimally invasive dentistry and how is it different from regular dentistry?

The goal of minimally invasive dentistry, or microdentistry, is to conserve healthy tooth structure. It focuses on prevention, remineralization, and minimal dentist intervention. Using scientific advances, minimally invasive dentistry allows dentists to perform the least amount of dentistry needed while never removing more of the tooth structure than is required to restore teeth to their normal condition. In addition, in minimally invasive dentistry, dentists use long-lasting dental materials that conserve the maximum tooth structure so the need for future repairs is reduced.

How does it work?

First your dentist will evaluate your risk for tooth decay. The presence of bacteria, quality and quantity of saliva, and your diet are all contributors to decay. Your dentist will then use strategies to prevent or reduce your risk for tooth decay. For instance, if you have a high level of oral bacteria, you might be advised to use mouthwash daily, limit the intake of certain carbohydrates, and practice good oral hygiene.

Which techniques are used?

Minimally invasive dentistry techniques include:

- **Remineralization:** Remineralization is the process of restoring minerals. Remineralization can repair the damage created by the demineralization process. Fluoride plays a very important role in remineralization.

- **Air abrasion:** When a tooth cannot be remineralized and decay is present, your dentist may use air abrasion to remove the decay.

Air abrasion is used instead of a traditional drill and may not require anesthesia. It resembles microscopic sand blasting and uses a stream of air combined with a super-fine abrasive powder.

• **Sealants:** Usually made of plastic resin, dental sealants protect teeth from bacteria that cause decay. Sealants fit into the grooves and depressions of the tooth and act as a barrier, protecting against acid and plaque. Sealants do not require any cutting of the tooth and can be placed on teeth that might be susceptible for decay at any time.

• **Inlays and onlays:** Usually dentists use crowns to restore a tooth, but inlays and onlays do not require them to remove as much of the tooth structure. Inlays are similar to fillings except that they are custom-made to fit the cavity in your tooth and are typically the same color as the tooth or gold colored. Onlays are used for more substantial reconstruction and also do not require your dentist to remove as much of the tooth as would a crown.

• **Bite splints:** Many people grind their teeth at night. Grinding, or bruxism, may cause serious damage to the teeth, and may require you to need crowns. Grinding, which often begins in your teenage years or early 20s, can be detected and corrected before much damage has been done. Dentists can create bite splints for you to wear at night or during stressful times when most teeth-grinding occurs.

Where can I find a dentist who practices minimally invasive dentistry?

Most dentists use minimally invasive dentistry techniques in their everyday practice. Ask your dentist if he or she uses these techniques.

Section 20.5

Lasers in Dentistry: How Do They Work?

What is a laser and how does it work?

A laser is an instrument that produces a very narrow, intense beam of light energy. When laser light comes in contact with tissue, it causes a reaction. The light produced by the laser can remove, vaporize, or shape tissue.

Are lasers used in dentistry?

Yes, lasers have been used in dentistry since 1990. The U.S. Food and Drug Administration has determined that lasers can be used as a safe and effective treatment for a wide range of dental procedures. Lasers are often used in conjunction with other dental instruments.

How are lasers used in dentistry?

Dental lasers can be used to:

- correct speech problems caused by a tongue-tie, which prevents normal tongue movement.
- uncover partially erupted wisdom teeth.
- remove decay from a cavity and prepare the tooth for a new filling.
- remove muscle pulls, as seen in orthodontic patients.
- manage gum tissue during impressions for crowns.
- remove swollen tissues caused by medications.
- perform biopsy procedures.
- remove inflamed gum tissues and reduce the amount of bacteria within a periodontal pocket.

- remove or reshape excess gum and bone tissues during crown lengthening procedures.

- treat abscessed gums and infections in root canals.

- reduce the discomfort of canker and cold sores.

- activate whitening chemicals that are used to lighten teeth.

What are the benefits of using dental lasers?

There are several advantages. Dentists may not need to use a drill or administer anesthesia, allowing the patient to enjoy a more relaxed dental experience. Laser procedures can be more precise. Also, lasers can reduce symptoms and healing times associated with traditional therapies; reduce the amount of bacteria in both diseased gum tissue and in tooth cavities; and control bleeding during surgery.

Are dental lasers safe?

If the dental laser is used according to accepted practices by a trained practitioner, then it is at least as safe as other dental instruments. However, just as you wear sunglasses to protect your eyes from prolonged exposure to the sun, when your dentist performs a laser procedure, you will be asked to wear special eyeglasses to protect your eyes from the laser.

How can I be sure my dentist is properly trained to use a laser?

Ask your dentist questions about the extent of his or her laser education and training. Make sure that your dentist has participated in educational courses and received training by the manufacturer.

Many dental schools, dental associations, and the Academy of Laser Dentistry (ALD) offer dental laser education. The ALD is the profession's independent source for current dental laser education and credentialing.

How will I know if treatment with a dental laser is an option for me?

Ask your dentist. Although the laser is a very useful dental instrument, it is not appropriate for every dental procedure.

Part Four

Treating Common
Dental Concerns

Chapter 21

Plaque and Tooth Decay

Chapter Contents

Section 21.1—Understanding Plaque 220
Section 21.2—What Is a Cavity? 221

Section 21.1

Understanding Plaque

Excerpted from "Plaque," by the National Institute for Dental and Cranio-facial Research (NIDCR, www.nidcr.nih.gov), part of the National Institutes of Health, July 1999. This document was reviewed by David A. Cooke, M.D., May 11, 2008.

People used to think that as you got older you naturally lost your teeth. We now know that's not true. By following easy steps for keeping your teeth and gums healthy plus seeing your dentist regularly, you can have your teeth for a lifetime!

Plaque: What Is It?

Plaque is made up of invisible masses of harmful germs that live in the mouth and stick to the teeth.

- Some types of plaque cause tooth decay.
- Other types of plaque cause gum disease.

Red, puffy, or bleeding gums can be the first signs of gum disease. If gum disease is not treated, the tissues holding the teeth in place are destroyed and the teeth are eventually lost.

Dental plaque is difficult to see unless it's stained. You can stain plaque by chewing red "disclosing tablets," found at grocery stores and drug stores, or by using a cotton swab to smear green food coloring on your teeth. The red or green color left on the teeth will show you where there is still plaque—and where you have to brush again to remove it. Stain and examine your teeth regularly to make sure you are removing all plaque. Ask your dentist or dental hygienist if your plaque removal techniques are OK.

Step One: Floss

Use floss to remove germs and particles between teeth. Rinse.

Note: Ease the floss into place gently. Do not snap it into place—this could harm your gums.

Another way of removing plaque between teeth is to use a dental pick—a thin plastic or wooden stick. These picks can be purchased at drug stores and grocery stores.

Step Two: Brush Teeth

Use any tooth brushing method that is comfortable, but do not scrub hard back and forth. Small circular motions and short back and forth motions work well. Rinse.

To prevent decay, it's what's on the toothbrush that counts. Use fluoride toothpaste. Fluoride is what protects teeth from decay.

Brush the tongue for a fresh feeling. Rinse again.

Remember: Food residues, especially sweets, provide nutrients for the germs that cause tooth decay, as well as those that cause gum disease. That's why it is important to remove all food residues, as well as plaque, from teeth. Remove plaque at least once a day—twice a day is better. If you brush and floss once daily, do it before going to bed.

Section 21.2

What Is a Cavity?

Reprinted with permission from "Open Wide: Oral Health Training for Health Professionals," © 2006 National Maternal & Child Oral Health Resource Center (www.mchoralhealth.org).

What Is Tooth Decay?

Tooth decay is an active process of tooth destruction resulting from interactions between teeth, food, and bacteria.

Bacteria, transmitted via saliva, adhere to tooth surfaces in a sticky film, called dental plaque. When foods containing carbohydrates are consumed, bacteria are able to break down carbohydrates in the mouth, producing acids that attack the enamel of the teeth and that cause mineral loss from teeth. Each time such foods are consumed, the acids attack the enamel of the teeth. After repeated acid attacks, tooth decay may occur, and the acids may create a cavity in the tooth. Cavities occur when the attack is prolonged and exceeds an individual's resistance and the ability of the teeth to heal. Resistance and healing ability are determined partly by an individual's physiology and partly by health behaviors.

At first, while the decay is limited to the subsurface of the enamel, the tooth can restore itself. But if the decay progresses and the tooth is not restored, the cavity continues to grow, extending deeper into the hard structures of the tooth and finally into the living pulp tissues within the tooth. The bacterial infection can then spread through the tissue spaces and blood vessels to other parts of the face and body.

What Is Streptococcus Mutans?

The bacterium *S. mutans* is the main contributor to tooth decay. *S. mutans* can grow under conditions that would kill other bacteria.

S. mutans is found mostly on tooth surfaces. One tooth may have a large number of these bacteria, while the tooth next to it may have only a small number. The bacteria are most concentrated in the crevices, pits, and fissures that are a normal part of the teeth and surrounding structures.

Can a Parent Infect an Infant or Child with Streptococcus Mutans?

Adults may have a high concentration of *S. mutans* in their mouths. Bacteria can be transmitted from a parent or another intimate caregiver to an infant or child via saliva, for example, by allowing infants or children to put their fingers in the parent's mouth and then into their own mouths, testing the temperature of a bottle with the mouth, sharing forks and spoons, and "cleaning" a pacifier or a bottle nipple that has fallen by sucking on it before giving it back to the infant or child.

Even if an infant or child is already infected with *S. mutans*, transmission can increase the concentration of bacteria in the infant's or child's mouth, increasing the likelihood of tooth decay or resulting in more severe decay. Therefore, it is important that parents and other intimate caregivers practice good oral hygiene and avoid behaviors that could transmit *S. mutans* to an infant or child.

Food Interactions with Streptococcus Mutans

Foods containing fermentable carbohydrates, which include all sugars and cooked starches, interact with *S. mutans*, producing acids that can cause mineral loss from teeth.

- **Sucrose**, which is highly concentrated in candy, cookies, cake, and sweetened beverages (for example, fruit drinks and soda), is a major contributor to tooth decay.

- **Fructose**, the naturally occurring sugar contained in fruit, contributes to tooth decay, although fruit is more nutritious than candy, cookies, and cake.

- **Lactose**, the sugar contained in milk, contributes to tooth decay, although milk is more nutritious than candy, cookies, and cake.

- **Starch**, contained in processed foods such as bread, crackers, pasta, potato chips, pretzels, sweetened cereal, and french fries breaks down into simpler sugars. Processed foods containing starch produce as much acid in plaque as sucrose alone, but at a slower rate.

Frequent consumption of foods high in sugar (for example, candy, cookies, cake, sweetened beverages, and fruit juice) increases the risk for tooth decay. Even very small amounts of these foods consumed frequently over the course of a day will create an acid environment lasting many hours.

Even though they contain sugar (fermentable carbohydrates), healthy foods like fruit, vegetables, grain products (especially whole grain), and dairy products should not be avoided. Snacking is important for infants and children; because their stomachs are small, they need to eat small amounts frequently to meet their nutritional requirements. However, it is important to limit snacking on foods high in sugar, to offer snacks only at regular times between meals, and to develop good oral hygiene habits.

Can Tooth Decay Lead to Other Problems?

Tooth decay can spread and be extremely painful. It may lead to:

- destruction of teeth;

- difficulty chewing, which can result in undernutrition and, in turn, to impaired physical development;

- speech problems;

- inability to concentrate, difficulty with learning, absence from child development programs (such as Head Start) and school, difficulty completing schoolwork, and impaired performance in school;

- psychological problems such as low self-esteem and poor social interaction; and

- severe infections that can even result in death on rare occasions.

The primary teeth are important to a child's overall development. Permanent teeth will eventually replace them, but this does not make primary teeth less important. Tooth decay in primary teeth most often means that there will be tooth decay in permanent teeth.

Healthy primary teeth are important for:

- proper chewing, which helps ensure proper nutrition;

- proper speech development;

- holding the space in the dental arch until the permanent teeth; and

- development of the facial structure.

Don't assume that tooth decay will occur no matter what. Even if everyone in a family has tooth decay, this doesn't mean that tooth decay cannot be prevented or reduced. Any effort to save teeth, including primary teeth, will help promote healthy development and reduce or eliminate the pain associated with tooth decay.

Chapter 22

Sealants: Questions and Answers

What are dental sealants?

Sealants are thin, plastic coatings painted on the chewing surfaces of the back teeth.

Sealants are put on in dentists' offices, clinics, and sometimes in schools. Getting sealants put on is simple and painless. Sealants are painted on as a liquid and quickly harden to form a shield over the tooth.

Why get sealants?

The most important reason for getting sealants is to avoid tooth decay.

Fluoride in toothpaste and in drinking water protects the smooth surfaces of teeth but back teeth need extra protection. Sealants cover the chewing surfaces of the back teeth and keep out germs and food.

Having sealants put on teeth before they decay will also save time and money in the long run by avoiding fillings, crowns, or caps used to fix decayed teeth.

What causes tooth decay?

Germs in the mouth use the sugar in food to make acids. Over time, the acids can make a cavity in the tooth.

"Seal Out Tooth Decay" is from the National Institute of Dental and Craniofacial Research (NIDCR, www.nidcr.nih.gov), part of the National Institutes of Health, November 9, 2007.

Of course a healthy tooth is the best tooth. So it is important to prevent decay. That's why sealants are so important.

Why do back teeth decay so easily?

The chewing surfaces of back teeth are rough and uneven because they have small pits and grooves. Food and germs can get stuck in the pits and grooves and stay there a long time because toothbrush bristles cannot brush them away.

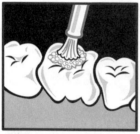 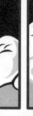 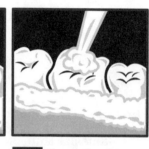

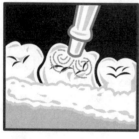 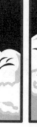 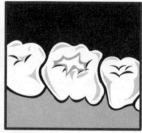

1 The tooth is cleaned.

2 The tooth is dried, and cotton is put around the tooth so it stays dry.

3 A solution is put on the tooth that makes the surface a little rough. (It is easier for the sealant to stick to a slightly rough surface.)

4 The tooth is rinsed and dried. Then new cotton is put around the tooth so it stays dry.

5 The sealant is applied in liquid form and hardens in a few seconds.

6 The sealant is in place.

Figure 22.1. *How sealants are put on.*

Who should get sealants?

Children should get sealants on their permanent molars as soon as the teeth come in—before decay attacks the teeth.

The first permanent molars—called "6 year molars"—come in between the ages of 5 and 7.

The second permanent molars—"12 year molars"—come in when a child is between 11 and 14 years old.

Other teeth with pits and grooves also might need to be sealed.

Teenagers and young adults who are prone to decay may also need sealants.

Should sealants be put on baby teeth?

Your dentist might think it is a good idea, especially if your child's baby teeth have deep pits and grooves.

Baby teeth save space for permanent teeth. It is important to keep baby teeth healthy so they don't fall out early.

Does insurance pay for sealants?

Some health insurance programs pay for sealants. Check with your state Medicaid program or your insurance company for details.

How long do sealants last?

Sealants can last up to 10 years. But they need to be checked at regular dental checkups to make sure they are not chipped or worn away. The dentist or dental hygienist can repair sealants by adding more sealant material.

What if a small cavity is accidentally covered by a sealant?

The decay will not spread, because it is sealed off from its food and germ supply.

Are sealants new?

No, sealants have been around since the 1960s. Studies by the National Institute of Dental and Craniofacial Research and others led to the development of dental sealants and showed that they are safe and effective.

But many people still do not know about sealants. About one third of children in the United States have sealants on their teeth.

227

Besides sealants, are there other ways to prevent tooth decay?

Yes. Using fluoride toothpaste and drinking fluoridated water can help protect teeth from decay.

Water is fluoridated in about two thirds of cities and towns in the United States. If your water is not fluoridated or if your children's teeth need more fluoride to stay healthy, a dentist can prescribe it in the form of a gel, mouth rinse, or tablet.

Fluoride is the best defense against tooth decay. Fluoride:

- makes teeth more resistant to decay;
- repairs tiny areas of decay before they become big cavities; and
- makes germs in the mouth less able to cause decay.

Fluoride helps the smooth surfaces of the teeth the most. It is less effective on the chewing surfaces of the back teeth. Regular brushing—with fluoride toothpaste—also helps prevent tooth decay.

Sealants and fluoride together can prevent almost all tooth decay.

How can I get dental sealants for my children?

Talk to your dentist, state or local dental society, or health department. Sometimes sealants are put on at school. Check with your school about whether it has a sealant program.

Chapter 23

Dental Erosion and Tooth Sensitivity

Chapter Contents

Section 23.1—What Is Dental Erosion? 230
Section 23.2—What Are Sensitive Teeth? 231

Section 23.1

What Is Dental Erosion?

From "Are You at Risk for Dental Erosion?," from the
U.S. Army Center for Health Promotion and Preventive Medicine
(http://chppm-www.apgea.army.mil/dhpw), 2006.

Dental erosion is the process where the hard outer tooth structure (the enamel) gradually dissolves through repeated exposure to stomach acid or acidic foods and drinks. Over time, this erosion leaves the inner tooth structure (the dentin) exposed, weakened, and sensitive. Back teeth can even become worn and shortened, causing changes in your bite (the way your upper and lower teeth come together).

Stomach Acid

Teeth are exposed to stomach acid in three ways:

- severe acid reflux (heartburn) or gastroesophageal reflux disease (GERD);
- vomiting from illness or morning sickness; or
- bulimia.

Stomach acids irritate the gum tissues and soften the outer layers of tooth enamel, allowing them to be removed easily, often by simply brushing your teeth. If this happens repeatedly, the enamel will become thinned and your teeth will become more sensitive.

- Never brush your teeth immediately after your mouth is exposed to stomach acid.
- Rinse with a solution of water that contains baking soda to neutralize the acid.
- If baking soda is not available, liquid antacid or plain water may be used.
- Wait at least an hour after rinsing before brushing your teeth. This allows your saliva to remineralize (harden) your tooth surfaces.

If your teeth are exposed to stomach acids repeatedly on a daily basis, talk to your dentist. You may need a fluoride mouth rinse or prescription fluoride gel that can be used at home to prevent dental erosion.

Acidic Food or Drink

Many foods and drinks are very acidic. Sodas, even diet sodas, contain strong acids that soften the outer layers of enamel. Damage usually occurs to the teeth along the gumline, and is often followed by decay. Here are some examples of foods and beverages that are acidic:

- tomatoes;
- pickles;
- citrus;
- tea;

- coffee;
- apple juice;
- orange juice;
- lemon juice;

- soft drink (soda or pop);
- sports drink; and
- white wine.

Drink water or eat cheddar cheese after eating acidic foods or drinks to dilute the acids.

Wait at least 30 minutes, preferably an hour, before brushing after eating or drinking acidic foods. This will allow your saliva to remineralize (harden) your tooth surfaces as much as possible.

Section 23.2

What Are Sensitive Teeth?

"Don't Be So Sensitive," © 2006 Massachusetts Dental Society (www.massdental.org). Reprinted with permission.

If you've ever taken a lick of an ice cream cone or a sip of hot tea only to be met with an excruciatingly sharp pain in your tooth, or if brushing or flossing causes you to flinch, you may be suffering from sensitive teeth. But just what causes this condition, and how you stop being so "sensitive"?

Sensitive teeth may be caused by many things, including cavities, a cracked tooth, worn tooth enamel, worn fillings, and exposed tooth roots, according to the American Dental Association (ADA). If a cavity, filling, or cracked tooth is behind this hypersensitivity, your dentist can rectify the situation by filling the cavity, replacing the filling, or fixing the fractured tooth. However, if your dentist determines that cavities and fractured teeth are not the source of the problem, then the cause could be either worn tooth enamel or an exposed tooth root.

All healthy teeth are composed of three layers of substances: enamel, cementum, and dentin. Enamel, the strongest substance in the body, protects the tooth's crown, making up the top layer. Cementum, the middle layer, protects the tooth root under the gum line. Dentin, which can be found under the enamel and cementum, is the least dense part of the tooth. When the dentin loses its protective covering, hot and cold foods, as well as acidic or sticky foods, stimulate the nerves and cells inside the tooth, leading to hypersensitivity and discomfort.

Dentin can also be exposed when gums recede, leading to sensitivity near the gum line. Good oral hygiene is the best way to prevent gums from receding and causing hypersensitivity. Flossing regularly and brushing correctly—using a soft-bristled brush and not brushing too roughly, which can injure the gums and expose tooth roots—can help keep your gums healthy and prevent them from receding.

In the interim, desensitizing toothpastes may help reduce your discomfort. These toothpastes contain compounds that help block transmission of sensation from the tooth surface to the nerve. However, you should note that several applications are required before sensitivity is reduced.

Additionally, if desensitizing toothpastes do not offer you relief, your dentist may be able to treat you using in-office techniques, such as applying a fluoride gel that strengthens the tooth enamel and reduces the transmission of sensation. If you suffer from receding gums, your dentist may be able to "seal" the sensitive teeth by using agents, composed of plastic material, that bond to the tooth root.

Regardless of the severity of your sensitivity and discomfort, and even if desensitizing toothpastes temporarily alleviate the pain, you should visit your dentist to determine the cause of the sensitivity. Doing this will not only allow you to enjoy that ice cream cone pain-free, but it will help head off any conditions, such as exposed roots, that if left untreated could eventually require further treatment, such as a root canal.

Chapter 24

Tooth Pain

Chapter Contents

Section 24.1—Toothaches 234
Section 24.2—Abscessed Teeth 236

Section 24.1

Toothaches

"The truth about toothaches," by Dennis R. Horanic, D.M.D.,
January 2007. © 2007 *Lake Mary Life Magazine*. Reprinted with permission.

Approximately five million people visit their dentist with tooth-aches every year. A common problem that can be prevented with good oral hygiene, toothaches occur because the pulp of the tooth is exposed, disturbed, or infected. The pulp is the inner layer of the tooth that is engulfed in a layer of dentin and then by the hard layer that we see called the enamel, which is packed full of minerals. Toothaches can also occur if just the outer enamel layer is damaged exposing only the dentin. The most common dental causes of toothaches:

- **Tooth root sensitivities:** Oversensitivity when consuming hot or cold, sweet or sour food, and beverages. Tooth root sensitivities occur when bacterial toxins get to work and dissolve the bone around the root of the tooth. The gum and bone recede exposing the root of the tooth, causing the sensitivity and toothache. Treatment: Visit your dentist. Fluoride gel and sensitivity toothpastes that contain fluoride will both help the root to become stronger and in turn reduce the toothache. If the root sensitivity causes the pulp to die, a root canal procedure or tooth extraction will need to be carried out to stop the toothache.

- **Tooth decay:** Also known as tooth 'cavities' or tooth 'caries.' Tooth decay occurs when the minerals of the enamel are dissolved by acid created by bacteria in our mouths (a buildup of this bacteria is known as plaque). This demineralization of the enamel forms a hole in the tooth exposing the dentin, causing the toothache. If the toothache is severe, then the hole has most likely exposed the pulp as well. The obvious prevention for tooth decay is to eat as little sugar as possible because the acid that causes the enamel to decay is created by the bacteria eating the sugar and starch left in our mouths. So brush your teeth with fluoride toothpaste, preferably after every meal or snack. Flossing will also help a lot. Being thorough with your brushing and flossing will stop any buildup of plaque forming. Treatment: Your dentist will in most cases remove the decay and place a filling in the tooth, although large cavities may need a crown. If the cavity damages the pulp, then a root canal procedure or extraction of the tooth may be necessary to stop the toothache.

- **Tooth abscess:** A complication of tooth decay or nerve injury. Tooth abscesses occur when a dental cavity has been left untreated. The bacteria has infected the tooth from the pulp all the way up to the bone tissue at the end of the root, causing a severe toothache. Treatment: Your dentist will have to carry out a root canal procedure where the pulp of the tooth is removed and then filled and sealed with an inert material. If this is unsuccessful, then the tooth will have to be removed.

- **Gum disease:** Also known as gingivitis and in severe cases, periodontal disease. Gum disease occurs when the soft tissue in our mouths becomes infected due to a build up of plaque or tartar along the gum line. It is highly likely that your toothache will be accompanied with bleeding gums if you have gum disease. Treatment: In mild cases of gum disease, your dentist will help you become more informed in order to improve your oral hygiene. Root planing, the removal of plaque and tartar from the exposed roots, may be necessary. In more severe cases, the surface of the inflamed gum tissue will have to be removed. This is known as subgingival curettage.

- **Jaw disease:** Also known as TMJ (temporomandibular joint) dysfunction. Jaw disease usually occurs when there has been an impact or injury to the head such as whiplash. Bruxism (grinding of the teeth) often leads to TMJ as well as arthritis and having an overbite. Jaw disease is often characterized by pain in the muscles around the jaw joint and limitations in jaw movement. Treatment: Your dentist will fit a special intraoral splint for you to wear. If your bite needs to be fixed, then crowns and orthodontic treatment are likely, as well as medication to relieve the toothache.

- **A cracked tooth:** This can occur for many reasons including an injury to the mouth, bruxism, chewing on hard objects, or extreme changes in temperature on your teeth (such as eating hot food immediately followed by an iced drink). The toothache may occur when the crack closes after releasing the pressure of a bite. The toothache gets worse over time if left untreated as the pulp can become infected. If you have a visible crack in your tooth that is not accompanied by a toothache, then it is known as a "craze line" and is considered to be part of the natural anatomy of the tooth. These "craze lines" usually occur as we age. Treatment: Your dentist will evaluate the treatment needed depending on the severity of the crack. This can involve bonding for a small crack or root canal treatment for a large crack where the inner pulp of the tooth has been damaged. In severe cases the tooth may need to be removed to stop the toothache.

Whatever the cause of your toothache, you should see a dentist who will determine the cause and apply the appropriate treatment. While waiting for a dental appointment, try to soothe the pain by applying a cold compress to the area of the cheek where the toothache is. Rinsing your mouth with warm salt water and taking aspirin will also help.

Dennis R. Horanic, D.M.D., is the sole practitioner of his private practice, Lake Forest Family Dentistry. He is a member of the American Dental Association, Florida Dental Association, and Dental Society of Greater Orlando.

Section 24.2

Abscessed Teeth

© 2008 A.D.A.M., Inc. Reprinted with permission.

Definition

A tooth abscess is a collection of infected material (pus) resulting from bacterial infection of the center of a tooth.

Causes

A tooth abscess is a complication of tooth decay. It may also result from trauma to the tooth, such as when a tooth is broken or chipped. Openings in the tooth enamel allow bacteria to infect the center of the tooth (the pulp). Infection may spread out from the root of the tooth and to the bones supporting the tooth.

Infection results in a collection of pus (dead tissue, live and dead bacteria, white blood cells) and swelling of the tissues within the tooth. This causes a painful toothache. If the root of the tooth dies, the toothache may stop, unless an abscess develops. This is especially true if the infection remains active and continues to spread and destroy tissue.

Symptoms

- Toothache
- Severe, continuous pain
- Gnawing or throbbing pain
- Sharp or shooting pain
- Pain when chewing
- Sensitivity of the teeth to hot or cold
- Bitter taste in the mouth
- Breath odor
- Possible fever
- Swollen glands of the neck
- General discomfort, uneasiness, or ill feeling
- Swollen area of the upper or lower jaw—a very serious symptom

Exams and Tests

The patient will feel pain when the dentist taps the tooth. Biting or closing the mouth tightly also increases the pain. The gums may be swollen and red and may drain thick material.

Treatment

The goals of treatment are elimination of the infection, preservation of the tooth, and prevention of complications. Antibiotics may be given to fight the infection. Warm salt-water rinses may be soothing. Over-the-counter pain relievers may relieve the toothache and fever. Do not place aspirin directly over the tooth or gums because this increases irritation of the tissues and can result in mouth ulcers.

Root canal therapy may be recommended in an attempt to preserve the tooth. The center of the tooth, including the nerve and vascular tissue (pulp), is removed along with decayed portions of the tooth. The root and surface of the tooth remain in place. The cavity that is created in the core is filled and repaired, and a crown may be placed over the tooth.

Surgical drainage of the abscess or extraction of the affected tooth may be necessary.

Outlook (Prognosis)

The infection of tooth abscess is usually curable with treatment. Preservation of the tooth is possible in many cases.

Possible Complications

- Loss of the tooth
- Spread of infection to soft tissue (facial cellulitis, Ludwig angina)
- Spread of infection to the jaw bone (osteomyelitis of the mandible or maxilla)
- Spread of infection to other areas of the body resulting in brain abscess, endocarditis, pneumonia, or other disorders

When to Contact a Medical Professional

Call your dentist if persistent, throbbing toothache or other symptoms of tooth abscess occurs.

Prevention

Prompt treatment of dental caries reduces the risk of tooth abscess. Traumatized teeth should be examined promptly by the dentist.

Chapter 25

Cracked Teeth

With their more sophisticated procedures, dentists are helping people keep their teeth longer. Because people are living longer and more stressful lives, they are exposing their teeth to many more years of crack-inducing habits, such as clenching, grinding, and chewing on hard objects. These habits make our teeth more susceptible to cracks.

How do I know if my tooth is cracked?

Cracked teeth show a variety of symptoms, including erratic pain when chewing, possibly with release of biting pressure, or pain when your tooth is exposed to temperature extremes. In many cases, the pain may come and go, and your dentist may have difficulty locating which tooth is causing the discomfort.

Why does a cracked tooth hurt?

To understand why a cracked tooth hurts, it helps to know something about the anatomy of the tooth. Inside the tooth, under the white enamel and a hard layer called the dentin, is the inner soft tissue called the pulp. The loose pulp is a connective tissue that contains cells, blood vessels, and nerves.

When the outer hard tissues of the tooth are cracked, chewing can cause movement of the pieces, and the pulp can become irritated. When biting pressure is released, the crack can close quickly, resulting in a momentary, sharp pain. Irritation of the dental pulp can be repeated many times by chewing. Eventually, the pulp will become damaged to the point that it can no longer heal itself. The tooth will not only hurt when chewing but may also become sensitive to temperature extremes. In time, a cracked tooth may begin to hurt all by itself. Extensive cracks can lead to infection of the pulp tissue, which can spread to the bone and gum tissue surrounding the tooth.

How will my cracked tooth be treated?

There are many different types of cracked teeth. The treatment and outcome for your tooth depends on the type, location, and extent of the crack.

- **Craze Lines:** Craze lines are tiny cracks that affect only the outer enamel. These cracks are extremely common in adult teeth. Craze lines are very shallow, cause no pain, and are of no concern beyond appearances.

- **Fractured Cusp:** When a cusp (the pointed part of the chewing surface) becomes weakened, a fracture sometimes results. The weakened cusp may break off by itself or may have to be removed by the dentist. When this happens, the pain will usually be relieved. A fractured cusp rarely damages the pulp, so root canal treatment is seldom needed. Your tooth will usually be restored with a full crown by your dentist.

- **Cracked Tooth:** This crack extends from the chewing surface of the tooth vertically towards the root. A cracked tooth is not completely separated into two distinct segments. Because of the position of the crack, damage to the pulp is common. Root canal treatment is frequently needed to treat the injured pulp. Your dentist will then restore your tooth with a crown to hold the pieces together and protect the cracked tooth. At times, the crack may extend below the gingival tissue line, requiring extraction. Early diagnosis is important. Even with high magnification and special lighting, it is sometimes difficult to determine the extent of a crack. A cracked tooth that is not treated will progressively worsen, eventually resulting in the loss of the tooth. Early diagnosis and treatment are essential in saving these teeth.

- **Split Tooth:** A split tooth is often the result of the long term progression of a cracked tooth. The split tooth is identified by a crack with distinct segments that can be separated. A split tooth cannot be saved intact. The position and extent of the crack, however, will determine whether any portion of the tooth can be saved. In rare instances, endodontic treatment and a crown or other restoration by your dentist may be used to save a portion of the tooth.

- **Vertical Root Fracture:** Vertical root fractures are cracks that begin in the root of the tooth and extend toward the chewing surface. They often show minimal signs and symptoms and may therefore go unnoticed for some time. Vertical root fractures are often discovered when the surrounding bone and gum become infected. Treatment may involve extraction of the tooth. However, endodontic surgery is sometimes appropriate if a portion of the tooth can be saved by removal of the fractured root.

After treatment for a cracked tooth, will my tooth completely heal?

Unlike a broken bone, the fracture in a cracked tooth will not heal. In spite of treatment, some cracks may continue to progress and separate, resulting in loss of the tooth. Placement of a crown on a cracked tooth provides maximum protection but does not guarantee success in all cases.

The treatment you receive for your cracked tooth is important because it will relieve pain and reduce the likelihood that the crack will worsen. Once treated, most cracked teeth continue to function and provide years of comfortable chewing. Talk to your endodontist about your particular diagnosis and treatment recommendations. S/he will advise you on how to keep your natural teeth and achieve optimum dental health.

What can I do to prevent my teeth from cracking?

While cracked teeth are not completely preventable, you can take some steps to make your teeth less susceptible to cracks.

- Don't chew on hard objects such as ice, unpopped popcorn kernels, or pens.

- Don't clench or grind your teeth.

241

- If you clench or grind your teeth while you sleep, talk to your dentist about getting a retainer or other mouth guard to protect your teeth.

- Wear a mouth guard or protective mask when playing contact sports.

Chapter 26

Fillings

Chapter Contents

Section 26.1—Overview of Dental Filling Options 244

Section 26.2—Tooth-Colored Fillings 254

Section 26.3—Questions and Answers on Dental Amalgam ... 255

Section 26.4—Studies Evaluate Health Effects of Dental
Amalgam Fillings in Children 257

Section 26.5—Mercury Exposure and Dental Fillings 260

Section 26.1

Overview of Dental Filling Options

"Dental Filling Facts," © American Dental Association.
Reprinted with permission. 2005.

Preventing Fillings—What You Can Do

You can avoid the need for fillings by preventing tooth decay in the first place. Brushing, flossing, eating a balanced diet, and seeing your dentist regularly are important factors in staying healthy. Because of improvement in disease prevention and the availability of new materials, most people need far fewer fillings than they did in the past and many filling materials are more esthetically pleasing. Knowing what dental filling materials are available and the benefits and drawbacks of each of those is important. This text is designed to help you understand your filling choices and provide you with information on how to prevent tooth decay and avoid the need for any fillings.

About Cavities and Dental Decay

A cavity (caused by a disease called caries) happens when bacteria in the mouth produce acids that attack your teeth. In time, this acid can dissolve away the enamel on your teeth and cause a hole, which is known as a cavity. Unlike some other diseases or injuries, a cavity will not heal by itself, but if the early signs of dental decay are promptly treated before a cavity forms, it can be stopped and even reversed by your dentist.

Without treatment by your dentist, dental decay may continue to advance. Extreme decay can result in the loss of the affected tooth or teeth, potentially preceded by great discomfort, infection, and other health problems.

Preventing Dental Decay

Over the past 60 years many successful preventive measures have helped to reduce dental disease. Preventing decay is the best way to protect your oral health. If you keep decay from starting, you won't need fillings and you'll save money.

Follow these basic steps to prevent dental disease:

- brush twice a day with a fluoride toothpaste;
- floss or use an interdental cleaner once a day;
- eat a balanced diet;
- limit eating and drinking between meals. Give preference to nutritious foods for snacks;
- visit your dentist regularly;
- ask your dentist whether supplemental fluoride would be appropriate to strengthen tooth enamel and prevent decay; and
- ask your dentist about dental sealants.

Talking with Your Dentist

Because of the wide variety of potential dental procedures any patient may need, it is important to talk openly with your dentist. Therefore, during your appointment, let your dentist know of any changes to your health since your last visit. This information will help your dentist to recommend the best treatment options for you. Examples of the type of information you should tell your dentist include:

- Are you pregnant or nursing?
- Do you have any allergies?
- Do you plan to have braces soon?
- What medications are you taking? For what conditions? Any over-the-counter medications or supplements?
- Do you have any other health conditions or specific health concerns?

By knowing facts like these your dentist will be better able to help you make the best treatment choice.

If you need to have a tooth restored (filled), your options may include several different materials. Your dentist will discuss with you which material is best for you and the tooth that needs to be filled. Each material has advantages and disadvantages and you should know what these are so you can make an informed choice that is best for you.

If you have any questions or concerns about the types of fillings you already have, read this text and talk with your dentist about those questions or concerns.

What choice you make will depend on your needs and the best way to repair the cavity in your tooth. Many factors may affect your choice of filling material and the recommendations made by your dentist. These factors include: your oral and general health; esthetics; the location of the filling; the biting force in the affected area of the mouth; the length and number of visits needed to place the filling; the durability required; and the cost.

For many years the only available choices were metals. These are 1) gold alloy or 2) a mixture or "amalgam" of mercury, silver, and other metals. In the past few decades, other materials have been developed for restoring teeth. They are "tooth colored" rather than silver-colored or gold. They include composite resin, glass ionomer, and porcelain materials.

Dental fillings fall into two categories based on the method used to place them: They are: direct restorations and indirect restorations.

Direct restorations are fillings placed immediately into a prepared cavity in a single visit. They include dental amalgam, glass ionomers, resin ionomers, and most composite (resin) fillings. The dentist prepares the tooth, places the filling, and adjusts it during one appointment.

Indirect restorations may require two or more visits. They include inlays, onlays, veneers, crowns, and bridges fabricated with gold, ceramics, or composites. During the first visit, the dentist prepares the tooth and makes an impression of the area to be treated. The impression is sent to a dental laboratory, which creates the dental restoration (filling). At the next appointment, the dentist cements the restoration to the prepared tooth and adjusts it as needed.

This text outlines the alternatives available and will help you decide on the right choice for you. The final choice is between you and your dentist.

Direct Restorations

Amalgam

The word "amalgam" when referring to dental fillings means a mixture of two or more metals in which mercury is a component. Dental amalgam is a mix of approximately 43 percent to 54 percent mercury with other metals, including silver, copper, and tin. Dental amalgams have commonly been called "silver fillings" because of their silver color when they are first placed. Today, amalgam is used most commonly in the back teeth. It is one of the oldest filling materials and has been used (and improved) for more than 150 years. Dental amalgam is the most thoroughly researched and tested filling material.

Advantages

- Strong, durable, and stands up to biting force;

- can be placed in one visit;

- normally the least expensive filling material;

- self-sealing with minimal-to-no shrinkage and it resists leakage (leakage occurs when a filling does not completely seal, permitting food and bacteria to "leak in" and promote new decay behind or beneath the filling);

- resistance to further decay is high;

- frequency of repair and replacement is low; and

- amalgam is the only material that can be used in a wet environment, especially important when treating small children or special needs patients.

Disadvantages

- While agencies like the U.S. Food and Drug Administration (FDA), the U.S. Centers for Disease Control (CDC), and the World Health Organization (WHO) have not found evidence of harm from dental amalgam, there are some individuals and groups who have raised concerns about the very low levels of mercury vapor released by amalgam. These concerns are discussed later in this text;

- amalgam scrap (waste left over after repairing a cavity) contains mercury and requires special handling to protect the environment;

- amalgam can darken over time as it corrodes. This does not affect the function of the filling, but many people find it less attractive than tooth-colored materials;

- placement of amalgam requires removal of some healthy tooth; and

- in rare cases, a localized, allergic reaction such as inflammation or rash may occur.

Composite (Resin)

Composite is a mixture of acrylic resin and powdered glass-like particles that produce a tooth-colored filling. This type of material may be self-hardening or may be hardened by exposure to blue light. Composite is used for fillings, inlays, and veneers. Sometimes it is used to replace a portion of a broken or chipped tooth.

Advantages

- Color and shading can be matched to the existing tooth;
- composite is a relatively strong material, providing good durability in small to mid sized restorations that need to withstand moderate chewing pressure;
- composite may generally be used on either front or back teeth;
- fillings are usually completed in a single visit (with exceptions noted below);
- moderately resistant to breakage;
- often permits preservation of as much of the tooth as possible;
- low risk of leakage if bonded only to enamel;
- does not corrode;
- generally holds up well to biting force (dependent on the material used);
- moderately resistant to further decay, new decay is easy to find; and
- frequency of repair or replacement is low to moderate.

Disadvantages

- This type of filling can break and wear out more easily than metal fillings, especially in areas of heavy biting force. Therefore, composite fillings may need to be replaced more often than metal fillings;
- compared to other fillings, composites are sometimes difficult and time-consuming to place. They can not be used in all situations;
- composite generally is more expensive than amalgam;

- may require more than one visit for inlays, veneers, and crowns;
- may wear faster than natural dental enamel;
- may leak over time when bonded beneath the layer of enamel; and
- in rare cases, a localized, allergic reaction such as inflammation or rash may occur.

Glass Ionomer

Glass ionomers are tooth-colored materials made of a mixture of acrylic acids with fine glass powders that are used to fill cavities, particularly those on the root surfaces of teeth. They are primarily used for small fillings in areas that need not withstand heavy chewing pressure. Glass ionomers also are used to cement dental crowns.

Advantages

- Tooth-colored so the filling looks more natural;
- can contain fluoride that may help prevent further decay;
- minimal amount of tooth structure removed;
- low incidence of localized allergic reaction; and
- usually completed in a single visit.

Disadvantages

- Low resistance to fracture. Use is limited to small areas of decay on non-biting surfaces of teeth;
- moderate cost, similar to composite (costs more than amalgam);
- as it ages, this material may become rough and plaque can build up increasing the risk of gum (periodontal) disease;
- can be dislodged; and
- in rare cases, a localized allergic reaction such as inflammation or rash may occur.

Resin Ionomer

Resin ionomers are also made from glass filler with acrylic acids and acrylic resin. They harden with exposure to blue light. Resin ionomers are most commonly used in fillings on non-chewing surfaces and fillings in primary (baby) teeth.

Advantages

- Tooth-colored, more translucent than glass ionomer;
- can contain fluoride that may help prevent further decay;
- minimal amount of tooth structure removed to place it;
- low incidence of localized allergic reaction;
- may be used for short-term fillings in primary (baby) teeth;
- may last longer than glass ionomer but is not as durable as composite; and
- usually completed in a single visit.

Disadvantages

- Limited use because it is not recommended for biting surfaces in adult teeth;
- moderate cost, similar to composite (more than amalgam);
- wears faster than composite and amalgam; and
- in rare cases, a localized allergic reaction such as inflammation or rash may occur.

Indirect Restorations

Porcelain (ceramic)

All-porcelain (ceramic) materials include porcelain, ceramic, or glass-like fillings and crowns. They are used in inlays, onlays, crowns, and cosmetic veneers. Porcelain fused to metal is another application for this material and has similar properties as described below with the notable exceptions of increased durability due to the metal substructure, the necessity for more tooth removal for that substructure and, in rare cases, a localized, allergic reaction may occur.

Advantages

- Tooth-colored with excellent translucency; the color looks similar to natural tooth enamel;

- very little tooth is removed when used as a veneer, more tooth is removed for a crown;
- good resistance to further decay if it fits well;
- is resistant to surface wear but can cause some wear on opposing teeth;
- resists leakage because of precise shaping and fitting; and
- does not cause allergic reaction.

Disadvantages

- Material is brittle and is prone to cracking under biting force;
- may not be recommended for molars;
- generally, requires a minimum of two appointments to complete; and
- high cost, similar to gold.

Gold Alloys

Gold alloys contain gold, copper, and other metals that result in a strong, effective filling, crown, or bridge. They are primarily used for inlays, onlays, crowns, and fixed bridges.

Advantages

- Excellent durability, does not crack under stress;
- good resistance to decay if it fits well;
- minimal amount of tooth structure needs to be removed;
- wears well, does not cause excessive wear to opposing teeth;
- resistant to corrosion and tarnishing; and
- resists leakage because it can be shaped and fit very accurately.

Disadvantages

- Gold is normally the highest cost material;
- a minimum of two appointments is required to complete the restoration;
- not tooth colored; and

- in rare cases, a localized allergic reaction such as inflammation or rash may occur.

Allergic Reactions to Dental Materials

Just like any other material we come in contact with during our daily lives, substances in dental fillings may trigger a localized allergic reaction. For all dental filling materials the risk of this type of reaction is extremely low, but they do exist. Normally, an allergy is revealed as a rash and is easily reversed when the affected area is not in contact with the material causing the allergy (known as an "allergen").

No matter which material is used, a filling is not a natural tooth. Filling materials are man-made and as such are foreign materials to your body. Whenever something foreign is put into your body, there is a chance of side effects. Dental materials may cause a localized allergic reaction in a very small number of individuals. This is why your dentist needs to know about your allergies.

If you have or may be prone to allergies, tell your dentist before a filling material is chosen. It may be an important part of determining what the right material is for you.

Dental Amalgam and Mercury

Health

Dental amalgam fillings are created by mixing elemental mercury (between 43 percent and 54 percent) and an alloy powder composed mainly of silver, tin, and copper. In its elemental form, mercury can be toxic, although this form is far less toxic than organic mercury, such as the methylmercury found in some seafood such as tuna and swordfish. This has generated discussion about the potential risks and toxicity of the mercury in dental amalgam. When mixed as an alloy the vast majority of the mercury in the dental amalgam becomes stable, however a miniscule amount is released as vapor. How much vapor is emitted depends on the number of fillings you have. It also depends on how much time you spend chewing, grinding your teeth, and drinking hot liquids. Miniscule amounts of this vapor can be inhaled and enter the bloodstream where it may then be taken throughout the body. The amounts absorbed are well below safety limits set by the federal government and are harmlessly excreted from the body. Should you swallow a bit of an amalgam filling, the mercury within it is very poorly absorbed and typically does not enter the bloodstream and is excreted.

Scientific research continues on the safety of dental amalgam. Many public and private agencies reconsider this issue on an ongoing basis. The U.S. Food and Drug Administration (FDA) and other public health organizations have investigated the safety of dental amalgams and concluded that "no valid scientific evidence has shown that amalgams cause harm to patients with dental restorations, except in rare cases of allergy."[1] The World Health Organization (WHO) reached a similar conclusion,[2] and the U.S. Centers for Disease Control (CDC) maintains that "At present, there is scant evidence that the health of the vast majority of people with amalgam is compromised, nor that removing amalgam fillings has a beneficial effect on health."[3] While questions have been raised concerning the safety of amalgam fillings, no public agency has found evidence to support discontinuation of the material and the FDA places no restrictions on their use.

Environment

When new fillings are placed in teeth or when old fillings are removed, there is a certain amount of leftover material that needs to be discarded. Because dental amalgam contains mercury, that means dental amalgam waste also contains mercury. While this waste does not represent a major environmental concern as compared to other sources of mercury, your dentist employs best management practices to ensure that the vast majority of any waste amalgam is captured before it enters the environment.

In addition to using premeasured amalgam capsules, dentists also use traps and filters to remove amalgam before it enters the sewer system. Most recently, some dentists have installed amalgam separators, devices that remove almost all of the remaining amalgam waste beyond that removed by the traps and filters. While the mercury used in dental amalgams is not a major contributor to the pollution that results in fish consumption warnings, these actions strive to ensure that any potential environmental impact is negligible.

1. U.S. Food and Drug Administration (FDA), Consumer Update: Dental Amalgams, December 31, 2002.

2. World Health Organization (WHO), WHO Consensus Statement on Dental Amalgam, September, 1997.

3. U.S. Centers for Disease Control (CDC), Fact Sheet: Dental Amalgam Uses and Benefits, Updated February 2, 2005.

Section 26.2

Tooth-Colored Fillings

What are tooth-colored fillings?

Tooth-colored fillings are made from durable plastics called composite resins. Similar in color and texture to natural teeth, the fillings are less noticeable, and much more attractive, than other types of fillings.

What are the advantages of tooth-colored fillings?

Because composite resins are tooth-colored, they look more natural than other filling materials. Your child can smile, talk, and eat with confidence. In addition, tooth-colored fillings are compatible with dental sealants. A tooth can be filled and sealed at the same time to prevent further decay.

What are the disadvantages?

First, tooth-colored fillings are not for every tooth. They work best in small restorations and low-stress areas. For example, your pediatric dentist may not recommend a tooth-colored filling for a large cavity or for the chewing surface of a back tooth. Second, tooth-colored fillings may cost a bit more than silver fillings because they take longer to place.

How do I decide if tooth-colored fillings are right for my child?

Talk to your pediatric dentist. Together you will decide what type of filling is best for your child.

How do I care for a tooth-colored filling?

Take care of a tooth-colored filling the same way you take care of a silver filling: Brush, floss, and visit your dentist. Any filling will last longer with good oral hygiene. Your pediatric dentist will regularly check the fillings for color change, leakage, or unusual wear and inform you of the need for repair or replacement.

Section 26.3

Questions and Answers on Dental Amalgam

Excerpted from "Questions and Answers on Dental Amalgam," by the Center for Devices and Radiological Health (CDRH, www.fda.gov/cdrh), U.S. Food and Drug Administration (FDA), October 31, 2006.

What is dental amalgam?

Dental amalgam is the silver-colored material used to fill (restore) teeth that have cavities. Dental amalgam is made of two nearly equal parts: liquid mercury and a powder containing silver, tin, copper, zinc, and other metals. Mercury concentration in dental amalgams is generally about 50% by weight, while the silver concentration ranges from 20–35%.

What is FDA's role in dental amalgam?

Dental amalgams are medical devices and are regulated by FDA's Center for Devices and Radiological Health (CDRH). CDRH is responsible for ensuring that medical devices are reasonably safe and effective and that the labeling has adequate directions for use and any appropriate warnings.

What are the safety concerns about dental amalgam?

Dental amalgams contain mercury, which may have neurotoxic effects on the nervous systems of developing children and fetuses. When amalgam fillings are placed in teeth or removed from teeth, they release mercury vapor. Mercury vapor is also released during chewing.

Since the 1990s, FDA and other government agencies (CDC, NIH) have reviewed the scientific literature looking for links between dental amalgams and health problems. In September 2006, an advisory

255

panel to the FDA reviewed FDA's research and heard presentations from the public about the benefits and risks of mercury and amalgam.

You can read the summary of the panel meeting at: http://www.fda .gov/cdrh/meetings/090606-summary.html. In addition, a complete transcript is available at: http://www.fda.gov/ohrms/dockets/ac/cdrh06.html #dentalproductspanel

Are there other dental filling materials that can be used instead of amalgam?

Yes, there are several other types of dental fillings.

Resin composites are tooth-colored materials made from powdered glass and resin compounds. When composites were initially introduced, they were not very strong and were used primarily in the front teeth. Newer composites are stronger, although they still tend to wear more than metal-based materials and generally need earlier replacement.

Glass ionomer cement is also a tooth-colored material. It is not usually used for long-term fillings because it breaks easily.

Porcelain, gold, and other metals are also used as filling materials. Gold and porcelain are used for inlays, veneers, crowns, and bridges. These fillings are made outside the mouth and cemented into place after they are formed.

Should I have my amalgam fillings removed and replaced with these other materials? If I have a cavity, should I choose to get amalgam fillings?

FDA does not recommend that you have your amalgam fillings removed. FDA is engaged in a rulemaking that may lead to revised labeling. It is also reviewing evidence about safe use, particularly in sensitive subpopulations.

If you are concerned about the possible health effects of amalgam fillings, you should talk with your qualified health care practitioner.

Dental amalgam fillings are very strong and durable, they last longer than most other types of fillings, and they are relatively inexpensive. You may want to weigh these advantages against the possibility that dental amalgam could pose a health risk.

Should pregnant women and young children use or avoid amalgam fillings?

The recent advisory panel believed that there was not enough information to answer this question.

Some other countries follow a "precautionary principle" and avoid the use of dental amalgam in pregnant women.

Pregnant women and persons who may have a health condition that makes them more sensitive to mercury exposure, including individuals with existing high levels of mercury bioburden, should not avoid seeking dental care, but should discuss options with their health practitioner.

Section 26.4

Studies Evaluate Health Effects of Dental Amalgam Fillings in Children

From the National Institute of Dental and Craniofacial Research (NIDCR, www.nidcr.nih.gov), part of the National Institutes of Health, April 18, 2006.

Scientists supported by the National Institute of Dental and Craniofacial Research (NIDCR), part of the National Institutes of Health, report in the *Journal of the American Medical Association* the results of the first-ever randomized clinical trials to evaluate the safety of placing amalgam fillings, which contain mercury, in the teeth of children.

Both studies—one conducted in Europe, the other in the United States—independently reached the conclusion: Children whose cavities were filled with dental amalgam had no adverse health effects. The findings included no detectable loss of intelligence, memory, coordination, concentration, nerve conduction, or kidney function during the 5–7 years the children were followed. The researchers looked for measurable signs of damage to the brain and kidneys because previous studies with adults indicated these organs might be especially sensitive to mercury.

The authors noted that children in both studies who received amalgam, informally known as "silver fillings," had slightly elevated levels of mercury in their urine. But after several years of analysis, they determined the mercury levels remained low and did not correlate with any symptoms of mercury poisoning.

"What's particularly impressive is the strength of the evidence," said NIDCR director Dr. Lawrence Tabak. "The studies evaluated mercury exposure in two large, geographically distinct groups of children and reached similar conclusions about the safety of amalgam."

Dentists have used silver-colored amalgam to fill cavities for more than 150 years. The material is made from an alloy powder of silver, copper, zinc, and other metals held together like glue by mercury. The mercury comprises about half the total weight of a filling.

For decades, it was believed that a person's direct exposure to the mercury in amalgam was brief, occurring only while the dentist packed the filling into the tooth. But with the arrival of more sensitive laboratory tools in the late 1970s and into the 1980s, scientists showed that dental amalgam continuously releases a mercury vapor into the mouth, which is inhaled and absorbed by the body.

The discovery raised concerns about the possible toxicity of chronic low-level exposure to mercury from dental amalgam. The toxicity of mercury at higher levels, such as from industrial exposures, is well established. Possible symptoms of mercury poisoning include irritability, memory loss, tremors, poor physical coordination, insomnia, kidney failure, and anorexia.

To help fill gaps in knowledge about the potential risks of dental amalgam, the NIDCR began supporting in 1996 the first two safety trials of amalgam in children. The decision to support the trials stemmed in part from the fact that millions of children receive amalgam fillings each year. But nearly all of the available safety data on mercury exposure involved adults, typically those who worked in environments where the element is present in relatively large doses, such as dental offices.

"It was clear that we needed to determine whether the potential risks of dental amalgam in any way outweigh its benefits, and we needed to make the determination first in children, who may be more sensitive to any adverse effects of mercury," said Tabak.

The two studies, whose results are reported in *JAMA,* are: the New England study, which was undertaken in the urban Boston, Massachusetts area and rural Farmington, Maine, and the Portuguese study, conducted in Lisbon, Portugal. Each study enrolled over 500 children who had existing untreated decay in permanent posterior, or back, teeth but no previously placed dental amalgam fillings. Each child was randomly assigned to receive either amalgam or composite resin (tooth-colored) fillings while participating in the research studies. All were evaluated for several years thereafter to determine if any health changes occurred, with emphases on IQ changes in the New England study and memory, concentration, coordination, and nerve conduction measures in the Portuguese study.

"The children received free comprehensive dental care while they participated in both studies," said Dr. Tim DeRouen, the principal investigator of the Portuguese study and a scientist at the University of Washington in Seattle. "These treatments represent the standard of care for kids with cavities throughout most of the world."

In the Portuguese study, which enrolled children ages eight through 10, DeRouen and colleagues found no differences over seven years between the 253 participants who received amalgam fillings and the 254 volunteers who were treated with composites. This conclusion was reached following annual standardized tests of memory, attention, physical coordination, and velocity of nerve conduction. Neither did the scientists detect a pattern of decline in the test scores of individual children who received amalgam fillings.

DeRouen noted that children who received amalgam fillings had slightly elevated levels of mercury in their urine, measuring on average 1.5 micrograms per liter of urine for the first two years and leveling off to 1.0 micrograms per liter or less thereafter. However, these numbers fall within the so-called "background" level (0-4 micrograms per liter) that is typical for an average person not exposed to industrial or other known sources of mercury. A microgram equals one millionth of a gram.

The scientists noted that children in both groups were in great need of dental care. Among those in the amalgam group, children had on average 10.1 tooth surfaces treated upon entry into the study. By year seven of the study, they had received on average a total of 18.7 surface restorations. Each tooth has either four or five defined surface areas, totaling 128 surfaces in our 32 permanent teeth.

In the New England study, which enrolled children ages six through 10, the scientists also found after five years no significant differences in the well being of the 267 participants who randomly received amalgam and their 267 counterparts who received composite fillings. "We took great pains to design our study in a way that our tests would be sensitive enough to detect as little as a three-point drop in IQ," said Dr. Sonja McKinlay, the principal investigator of the American study and a scientist at New England Research Institutes in Watertown, Mass. "What we found over the course of the study is the amalgam fillings had no adverse effects on the IQ of these children as well as on a range of other neuropsychological measures and kidney function."

The New England scientists also found that children with amalgam fillings had very slightly increased mercury in their urine. On average, these children had mercury levels of 1.0 micrograms per liter of urine compared to an average measure of 0.5 in those who received composite fillings. Both averages remained within the range of background exposure and were not related to IQ, other tests of brain function, or kidney function.

The New England study participants also had fairly extensive tooth decay, with 9.5 decayed tooth surfaces at the start of the study, of which 1.7 were in permanent teeth. By the end of the study, the children had on average 15 tooth surfaces restored. In the United States, children between the age of 6 and 10 have on average only 1.6 decayed surfaces among both their primary and permanent teeth.

"Given the rigorous nature of the study designs and that both clinical trials confirmed the other's results, I think these findings should be reassuring for parents, children, and dental professionals," said McKinlay.

Section 26.5

Mercury Exposure and Dental Fillings

Excerpted from "Mercury Exposure," from the National Toxicology Program, Center for the Evaluation of Risks to Human Reproduction (cerhr.niehs.nih.gov), National Institute of Environmental Health Sciences, part of the National Institutes of Health, April 28, 2004.

Mercury is a metal found in various forms. Metallic mercury is the silver colored liquid used in thermometers. Mercury combined with carbon is called organic mercury; methylmercury is a common example of an organic mercury. Mercury compounds which contain non-carbon substances such as chlorine, oxygen, or sulfur are called inorganic mercurials. Mercury occurs naturally in the environment, and the levels are increased by certain human activities such as the burning of coal by power plants. Burning coal increases the amount of airborne mercury, which eventually falls back to earth into bodies of water. Mercury in water accumulates in fish. Common ways in which people are exposed to mercury include breathing contaminated air, eating contaminated fish, and through the use of mercury-based amalgams (fillings) in dental treatments. Mercury can also enter the body through direct skin contact, and exposures to mercury may occur by contact with broken household items such as thermometers.

The effects of mercury on unborn children have been documented in cases of accidental poisonings and in scientific studies. During the 1950s, large amounts of organic mercury were dumped into Minamata Bay in Japan, and mercury-contaminated fish were eaten by many pregnant women. Many of the children born to those women had severe nervous system damage, which was later referred to as Fetal Minamata Disease. In Iraq, studies showed that children born to mothers who ate grain contaminated with organic mercury may have learned to walk at a later age than non-exposed children. In the Faroe Islands, where mercury exposure occurs by eating contaminated whale meat, children born to mothers with higher body levels of mercury scored lower on brain function tests than children born to mothers with lower body levels of mercury. In contrast, no adverse effects were seen in children of the Seychelles Islands, where residents are routinely exposed to mercury by eating fish 12 times a week.

The Food and Drug Administration (FDA) and Environmental Protection Agency (EPA) recommend that young children and women who are pregnant, could become pregnant, or are nursing reduce their exposure to mercury by not eating fish containing high levels of mercury such as swordfish, shark, king mackerel, and tilefish. The FDA and EPA state that women and children can eat up to 12 ounces (2 average meals) per week of fish containing lower levels of mercury, such as shrimp, canned light tuna, salmon, Pollock, and catfish. Because albacore tuna contains higher levels of mercury, it is recommended that not more than 6 ounces be eaten per week.

Another possible source of mercury exposure to unborn children is the use of dental amalgams (mercury-based fillings) in pregnant women. Some special interest groups in the United States have attempted to place limits on the use of these amalgams. However, the U.S. Public Health Service and the FDA have taken the position that there is no scientific evidence to support limiting the use of mercury-based amalgams at this time. Similar conclusions were also reached by the World Health Organization and the government of New Zealand. German and Canadian governments concluded there was no evidence indicating that amalgams in pregnant women are harmful to unborn children, but suggested avoiding the use of, or even removing amalgams in pregnant women as a safety measure.

The EPA is proposing national standards for hazardous air pollutants and intends to require lower emissions of mercury and other pollutants from coal and oil-fired utility plants.

Some individuals may also be exposed to mercury through religious practices. According to a health alert issued by the Agency of Toxic Substances and Disease Registry (ATSDR), mercury may be sprinkled around homes or cars by practitioners of religions such as Esperitismo, Santeria, or Voodoo. Broken thermometers may also be a source of mercury exposure in homes. Household exposures to mercury can be minimized by properly cleaning spills from items such as broken thermometers. Skin contact should be avoided and the spilled mercury should be placed into a vial which should then be tightly capped and properly disposed of.

The California Environmental Protection Agency (Cal/EPA) has classified mercury, methylmercury, and mercury compounds as developmental toxicants, which means there is evidence that these compounds can be harmful to unborn children. Acceptable levels of mercury have been established by other regulatory agencies. A limit of 2 parts mercury per billion parts of drinking water (2 ppb) has been established by the EPA. In addition, the EPA requires the reporting of spills or releases of 1 pound or more of mercury. The FDA has set a limit of 1 part per million (ppm) of mercury in seafood. The FDA also regulates the use of mercury in medical treatments such as dental amalgams. The Occupational Safety and Health Administration (OSHA) limits the level of mercury in workplaces to 1 milligram per 10 cubic meters of air (1 mg/10 m^3).

Mercury in Dental Amalgams (Fillings)

Dental amalgams contain about 50% mercury and there are concerns that unborn children can be exposed to mercury vapors given off by the amalgams in mothers. Some special interest groups have tried to ban or limit the use of mercury based amalgams. In order to investigate this issue, the U.S. Public Health Service (PHS) assembled a group of scientists from various governmental agencies. The following excerpts, taken directly from the report generated in 1993, summarize some of the primary conclusions reached by the scientists:

"Dental amalgam, an inter-metallic compound, contains elemental mercury that is emitted in minute amounts as vapor. Because vapor emitting from amalgam restorations can be absorbed by the patient through inhalation, ingestion, or other means, concerns have been raised about possible toxicity. At present, there is scant evidence that the health of the vast majority of people with amalgam is compromised, nor that removing amalgam fillings has a beneficial effect on health. It also is recognized that a total conversion from dental amalgam to alternative materials would cause a significant increase in U.S. health care costs. Nonetheless, the possibility that this material, as well as currently available alternatives, could pose health risks cannot be totally ruled out because of the paucity of definitive human studies.

Given the limitations of existing scientific data, a research program should be designed and implemented to fill as many gaps as possible in current knowledge about the potential long-term biological effects of dental amalgam and alternative restorative materials. The PHS should be a leader in this effort.

The PHS should also educate dental personnel and consumers about the risks and benefits of dental amalgam. An educational program should include information on all restorative materials to help dentists and their patients make informed dental treatment decisions, and encourage dental care providers to report adverse reactions. Such a program should promote the use of preventive measures such as fluoride and dental sealants to prevent caries and thus further reduce the need for dental restorations.

The U.S. Public Health Service believes it is inappropriate at this time to recommend any restrictions on the use of dental amalgam, for several reasons. First, current scientific evidence does not show that exposure to mercury from amalgam restorations poses a serious health risk in humans, except for an exceedingly small number of allergic reactions. Second, there is insufficient evidence to assure the public that components of alternative restorative materials have fewer potential health effects than dental amalgam, including allergic-type reactions. Third, there are significant efforts underway in the United States to reduce the amount of mercury in the environment. And finally, as stated previously, amalgam use is declining due to a lessening of the incidence of dental caries and the increasing use of alternative materials."

The U.S. Public Health Service reassembled the group in 1997 to discuss new information published since the original report in 1993. According to the 1997 report, "In 1997, with input from a broad cross-section of scientists and dental professionals within USPHS, the FDA completed a review of nearly 60 studies that were published in peer reviewed scientific literature and were cited by citizen groups that petitioned the agency for stringent regulatory actions against dental amalgam. The analysis of the cited studies indicated that the current body of data does not support claims that individuals with dental amalgam restorations will experience adverse effects, including neurologic, renal or developmental effects, except for rare allergic or hypersensitivity reactions." The FDA concluded that "the agency does not believe there is scientific justification for discontinuing or curtailing amalgam use."

The 1997 U.S. Public Health Service Report also discussed opinions of foreign governments regarding the use of mercury amalgams. According to the report U.S. Department of Health and Human Services Public Health Service, October 1997, "The governments of Sweden and Denmark have recommended against the use of mercury-containing materials as part of national environmental protection initiatives provided that suitable non-amalgam materials are available. The German government has recommended against the placement of dental amalgam and dental restorative materials in general in patients with demonstrated allergy to such materials, as well as patients with severe renal dysfunction. Germany has also advised against the placement of dental amalgam and the removal of amalgam fillings in pregnant women as a precautionary measure while at the same time acknowledging the lack of evidence that exposure of the unborn to mercury released from the mother's amalgam fillings causes any health damage to the child. The European Commission, the governments of Canada, Quebec, and New Zealand, and the World Health Organization have independently evaluated the current body of science relating to dental amalgam safety and universally concluded that the vast majority of people treated with dental amalgam are not at risk. Notwithstanding this conclusion, Canada and its province of Quebec have recommended prudence in dental intervention therapies for certain patient subpopulations such as pregnant women."

Research to address health concerns of dental amalgams continues.

Chapter 27

Periodontal (Gum) Disease and Its Impact on Health

Chapter Contents

Section 27.1—Facts and Fallacies about Periodontal
Disease 266
Section 27.2—Frequently Asked Questions about Gum
Disease and General Health 269

Section 27.1

Facts and Fallacies about Periodontal Disease

Fallacy: Tooth loss is a natural part of aging.

Fact: With good oral hygiene and regular professional care, your teeth are meant to last a lifetime. However, if left untreated, periodontal (gum) disease can lead to tooth loss. It is the primary cause of tooth loss in adults 35 and over.

Fallacy: People who have gum disease are "dirty" and don't brush their teeth.

Fact: Research proves that up to 30% of the population may be genetically susceptible to gum disease. Despite aggressive oral care habits, these people may be six times more likely to develop periodontal disease. Identifying these people with a genetic test before they even show signs of the disease and getting them into early interventive treatment may help them keep their teeth for a lifetime.

Fallacy: Gum disease doesn't affect overall health.

Fact: Emerging research links periodontal disease to other health problems including heart and respiratory diseases; preterm, low birth weight babies; stroke; osteoporosis; and diabetes.

Fallacy: Gum disease is a minor infection.

Fact: The mass of tissue in the oral cavity is equivalent to the skin on your arm that extends from the wrist to the elbow. If this area was red, swollen, and infected, you would visit the doctor. Gum disease is not a small infection. Its result, tooth loss, leads to a very different lifestyle—dentures. The changes in your appearance, breath, and ability to chew food are dramatic.

Fallacy: *Bleeding gums are normal.*

Fact: Bleeding gums are one of nine warning signs of gum disease. Think of gum tissue as the skin on your hand. If your hands bled every time you washed them, you would know something is wrong. Other signs of gum disease include: red, swollen or tender gums; sores in your mouth; gums that have pulled away from the teeth; persistent bad breath; pus between the teeth and gums (leaving bad breath); loose or separating teeth; a change in the way the teeth fit together; and a change in the fit of partial dentures.

Fallacy: *Treatment for gum disease is painful.*

Fact: New periodontal procedures including local anesthesia and over-the-counter medications, have made patients' treatment experiences pleasant and comfortable. Many patients find they are back to normal routines on the same day or by the next day.

Fallacy: *Gum disease is easy to identify, even in its early stages, so my dentist would tell me if I had it.*

Fact: Millions of people don't know they have this serious infection that can lead to tooth loss if not treated. You should always get involved in your dental care, so that problems are detected in the early stages. You should inform your dentist if any signs of gum disease are present; or if any changes in your overall health or medications occurred in between visits. Most importantly, you should ask your dentist about your periodontal health and what method was used to evaluate its condition. This level of participation enables you to work in a team approach with your dentist to identify subtle changes that may occur in the oral cavity.

Fallacy: *Once teeth are lost, the only treatment options are crowns, bridges, or dentures.*

Fact: Dental implants are a permanent tooth-replacement option for teeth lost to trauma, injury, or periodontal disease. Dental implants are so natural-looking and feeling that many patients forget they ever lost a tooth.

Fallacy: *Cavities are the number-one cause of tooth loss.*

Fact: Periodontal disease is the number-one cause of tooth loss. According to the 1996 American Dental Association/Colgate survey,

U.S. dentists say gum disease is a more pressing oral health concern than tooth decay by a 2-to-1 margin.

Fallacy: *Because gum disease is a bacterial infection, antibiotics can be used to treat it.*

Fact: Research demonstrates that antibiotics can be a helpful adjunct to treating periodontal disease. However, medical and dental communities are concerned about the overuse of these medications in treating infections because of the possibility of the development of antibiotic resistant strains of bacteria. This overuse would be detrimental to patients if they develop a life-threatening illness for which antibiotics would no longer be helpful.

Fallacy: *Pregnant women should skip professional dental checkups.*

Fact: Teeth and gums are affected during pregnancy like other tissues in the body. In order to decrease the risk of damaging the gums and tissues surrounding the teeth, pregnant women should schedule an appointment for a periodontal evaluation.

Section 27.2

Frequently Asked Questions about Gum Disease and General Health

What is the relationship between periodontal disease and respiratory disease?

More research is needed to confirm how periodontal disease may put people at increased risk for respiratory disease. What we do know is that mouth infections like periodontal disease are associated with increased risk of respiratory infection. An analysis of research has revealed that periodontal (gum) disease may be a far more serious threat to your health than previously realized.

How does periodontal disease increase my risk for heart disease?

Several theories exist to explain the link between periodontal disease and heart disease. One theory is that oral bacteria can affect the heart when they enter the bloodstream, attaching to fatty plaques in the coronary arteries (heart blood vessels) and contributing to clot formation. Coronary artery disease is characterized by a thickening of the walls of the coronary arteries due to the buildup of fatty proteins. Blood clots can obstruct normal blood flow, restricting the amount of nutrients and oxygen required for the heart to function properly. This may lead to heart attacks. Researchers have found that people with periodontal disease are almost twice as likely to suffer from coronary artery disease as those without periodontal disease.

Can periodontal disease increase my risk for having a premature baby?

Pregnant women who have periodontal disease may be seven times more likely to have a baby that is born too early and too small. More research is needed to confirm how periodontal disease may affect pregnancy outcomes. What we do know is that periodontal disease is an infection and all infections are cause for concern during pregnancy because they pose a risk to the health of the baby. If you are thinking about becoming pregnant, be sure to include an evaluation with a periodontist as part of your prenatal care.

What is the relationship between periodontal disease and diabetes?

For years we've known that people with diabetes are more likely to have periodontal disease than people without diabetes. Recently, research has emerged suggesting that the relationship goes both ways—periodontal disease may make it more difficult for people who have diabetes to control their blood sugar. Though more research is needed, what we do know is that severe periodontal disease can increase blood sugar, putting diabetics at increased risk for complications. If you are among the 16 million Americans who live with diabetes or are at risk for diabetes or periodontal disease, see a periodontist for an evaluation.

What can I do to reduce the health risks associated with periodontal disease?

Sometimes the only way to detect periodontal disease is through a periodontal evaluation. If you value your oral health as well as your overall health, a periodontal evaluation is a good idea—especially if you notice any symptoms of periodontal disease; have heart disease, diabetes, respiratory disease, or osteoporosis; are thinking of becoming pregnant; have a family member with periodontal disease; or have a sore or irritation in your mouth that does not get better within two weeks.

Chapter 28

Causes, Symptoms, and Treatments for Gum Disease

Chapter Contents

Section 28.1—Understanding Gum Disease and Its
    Causes 272

Section 28.2—Fighting Gum Disease: How to Keep
    Your Teeth 278

Section 28.3—Oral Rinse Fights Gum Disease 287

Section 28.1

Understanding Gum Disease and Its Causes

From "Periodontal (Gum) Disease: Causes, Symptoms, and Treatments," a brochure by the National Institute of Dental and Craniofacial Research (NIDCR, www.nidcr.nih.gov), part of the National Institutes of Health, November 19, 2007.

If you have been told you have periodontal (gum) disease, you're not alone. An estimated 80 percent of American adults currently have some form of the disease.

Periodontal diseases range from simple gum inflammation to serious disease that results in major damage to the soft tissue and bone that support the teeth. In the worst cases, teeth are lost.

Gum disease is a threat to your oral health. Research is also pointing to possible health effects of periodontal diseases that go well beyond your mouth (more about this later). Whether it is stopped, slowed, or gets worse depends a great deal on how well you care for your teeth and gums every day, from this point forward.

What Causes Periodontal Disease?

Our mouths are full of bacteria. These bacteria, along with mucus and other particles, constantly form a sticky, colorless "plaque" on teeth. Brushing and flossing help get rid of plaque. Plaque that is not removed can harden and form bacteria-harboring tartar that brushing doesn't clean. Only a professional cleaning by a dentist or dental hygienist can remove tartar.

Gingivitis

The longer plaque and tartar are on teeth, the more harmful they become. The bacteria cause inflammation of the gums that is called gingivitis. In gingivitis, the gums become red, swollen, and can bleed easily. Gingivitis is a mild form of gum disease that can usually be reversed with daily brushing and flossing and regular cleaning by a dentist or dental hygienist. This form of gum disease does not include any loss of bone and tissue that hold teeth in place.

Periodontitis

When gingivitis is not treated, it can advance to periodontitis (which means inflammation around the tooth.) In periodontitis, gums pull away from the teeth and form pockets that are infected. The body's immune system fights the bacteria as the plaque spreads and grows below the gum line. Bacterial toxins and the body's enzymes fighting the infection actually start to break down the bone and connective tissue that hold teeth in place. If not treated, the bones, gums, and connective tissue that support the teeth are destroyed. The teeth may eventually become loose and have to be removed.

Risk Factors

- **Smoking:** Need another reason to quit smoking? Smoking is one of the most significant risk factors associated with the development of periodontitis. Additionally, smoking can lower the chances of success of some treatments.

- **Hormonal changes in girls/women:** These changes can make gums more sensitive and make it easier for gingivitis to develop.

- **Diabetes:** People with diabetes are at higher risk for developing infections, including periodontal disease.

- **Stress:** Research shows that stress can make it more difficult for our bodies to fight infection, including periodontal disease.

- **Medications:** Some drugs, such as antidepressants and some heart medicines, can affect oral health because they lessen the flow of saliva. (Saliva has a protective effect on teeth and gums.)

- **Illnesses:** Diseases like cancer or AIDS [acquired immunodeficiency syndrome] and their treatments can also affect the health of gums.

- **Genetic susceptibility:** Some people are more prone to severe periodontal disease than others.

Who Gets Periodontal Disease?

People usually don't show signs of gum disease until they are in their 30s or 40s. Men are more likely to have periodontal disease than women. Although teenagers rarely develop periodontitis, they can develop gingivitis, the milder form of gum disease. Most commonly, gum disease develops when plaque is allowed to build up along and under the gum line.

What Can I Do to Prevent Gum Disease?

Here are some things you can do to prevent periodontal diseases:

- Brush your teeth twice a day (with a fluoride toothpaste).
- Floss every day.
- Visit the dentist routinely for a check-up and professional cleaning.
- Eat a well balanced diet.
- Don't use tobacco products.

How Do I Know If I Have Periodontal Disease?

Symptoms are often not noticeable until the disease is advanced. They include:

- bad breath that won't go away;
- red or swollen gums;
- tender or bleeding gums;
- painful chewing;
- loose teeth; and
- sensitive teeth.

Any of these symptoms may signal a serious problem, which should be checked by a dentist. At your dental visit:

- The dentist will ask about your medical history to identify underlying conditions or risk factors (such as smoking) that may contribute to periodontal disease.
- The dentist or hygienist will examine your gums and note any signs of inflammation.
- The dentist or hygienist will use a tiny ruler called a probe to check for periodontal pockets and to measure any pockets. In a healthy mouth, the depth of these pockets is usually between 1 and 3 millimeters.

- The dentist or hygienist may take an x-ray to see whether there is any bone loss.

- The dentist may refer you to a periodontist, a specialist who treats gum diseases.

How Is Periodontal Disease Treated?

The main goal of treatment is to control the infection. The number and types of treatment will vary, depending on the extent of the gum disease. Any type of treatment requires that the patient keep up good daily care at home. Additionally, modifying certain behaviors, such as quitting tobacco use, might also be suggested as a way to improve treatment outcome.

Deep Cleaning (Scaling and Root Planing)

The dentist, periodontist, or dental hygienist removes the plaque through a deep-cleaning method called scaling and root planing. Scaling means scraping off the tartar from above and below the gum line. Root planing gets rid of rough spots on the tooth root where the germs gather, and helps remove bacteria that contribute to the disease.

Medications

Medications may be used with treatment that includes scaling and root planing, but they cannot always take the place of surgery. Depending on the severity of gum disease, the dentist or periodontist may still suggest surgical treatment. Long-term studies will be needed to determine whether using medications reduces the need for surgery and whether they are effective over a long period of time.

Table 28.1 lists some medications that are currently used.

Surgery

Flap Surgery: Surgery might be necessary if inflammation and deep pockets remain following treatment with deep cleaning and medications. A periodontist may perform flap surgery to remove tartar deposits in deep pockets or to reduce the periodontal pocket and make it easier for the patient, dentist, and hygienist to keep the area clean. This common surgery involves lifting back the gums and removing the tartar. The gums are then sutured back in place so that the tissue fits snugly around the tooth again.

275

Table 28.1. Medications Used to Treat Gum Disease

Medications	What is it?	Why is it used?	How is it used?
Prescription anti-microbial mouthrinse	A prescription mouthrinse containing an antimicrobial called chlorhexidine	To control bacteria when treating gingivitis and after gum surgery	It's used like a regular mouthwash.
Antiseptic "chip"	A tiny piece of gelatin filled with the medicine chlorhexidine	To control bacteria and reduce the size of periodontal pockets	After root planing, it's placed in the pockets where the medicine is slowly released over time.
Antibiotic gel	A gel that contains the antibiotic doxycycline	To control bacteria and reduce the size of periodontal pockets	The periodontist puts it in the pockets after scaling and root planing. The antibiotic is released slowly over a period of about seven days.
Antibiotic micro-spheres	Tiny, round particles that contain the antibiotic minocycline	To control bacteria and reduce the size of periodontal pockets	The periodontist puts the micro-spheres into the pockets after scaling and root planing. The particles release minocycline slowly over time.
Enzyme suppressant	A low dose of the medication doxycycline that keeps destructive enzymes in check	To hold back the body's enzyme response—If not controlled, certain enzymes can break down gum tissue	This medication is in pill form. It is used in combination with scaling and root planing.

Bone and Tissue Grafts: In addition to flap surgery, your periodontist may suggest bone or tissue grafts. Grafting is a way to replace or encourage new growth of bone or gum tissue destroyed by periodontitis. A technique that can be used with bone grafting is called guided tissue regeneration, in which a small piece of mesh-like fabric is inserted between the bone and gum tissue. This keeps the gum tissue from growing into the area where the bone should be, allowing the bone and connective tissue to regrow.

Since each case is different, it is not possible to predict with certainty which grafts will be successful over the long term. Treatment results depend on many things, including severity of the disease, ability to maintain oral hygiene at home, and certain risk factors, such as smoking, which may lower the chances of success. Ask your periodontist what the level of success might be in your particular case.

Getting a Second Opinion about Treatment

When considering any extensive dental or medical treatment options, you should think about getting a second opinion. To find a dentist or periodontist for a second opinion, call your local dental society. They can provide you with names of practitioners in your area. Additionally, dental schools may sometimes be able to offer a second opinion. Call the dental school in your area to find out whether it offers this service.

Can Periodontal Disease Cause Health Problems beyond the Mouth?

Maybe. But so far the research is inconclusive. Studies are ongoing to try to determine whether there is a cause-and-effect relationship between periodontal disease and:

- an increased risk of heart attack or stroke;
- an increased risk of delivering preterm, low birth weight babies; and
- difficulty controlling blood sugar levels in people with diabetes.

In the meantime, it's a fact that controlling periodontal disease can save your teeth—a very good reason to take care of your teeth and gums.

Clinical Trials

Clinical trials are research studies of new and promising ways to prevent, diagnose, or treat disease. If you want to take part in a clinical

277

trial about periodontal disease, visit www.clinicaltrials.gov. In the box under "Search Clinical Trials," type in: periodontal diseases. This will give you a list of clinical trials on gum disease for which you might be eligible.

Section 28.2

Fighting Gum Disease: How to Keep Your Teeth

From "Fighting Gum Disease: How to Keep Your Teeth," by Carol Lewis, *FDA Consumer* magazine, U.S. Food and Drug Administration, May-June 2002. This document was reviewed by David A. Cooke, M.D., May 11, 2008.

More than 75 percent of Americans over 35 have some form of gum disease. In its earliest stage, your gums might swell and bleed easily. At its worst, you might lose your teeth. The bottom line? If you want to keep your teeth, you must take care of your gums.

The mouth is a busy place, with millions of bacteria constantly on the move. While some bacteria are harmless, others can attack the teeth and gums. Harmful bacteria are contained in a colorless sticky film called plaque, the cause of gum disease. If not removed, plaque builds up on the teeth and ultimately irritates the gums and causes bleeding. Left unchecked, bone and connective tissue are destroyed, and teeth often become loose and may have to be removed.

A recent poll of 1,000 people over 35 done by Harris Interactive Inc. found that 60 percent of adults surveyed knew little, if anything, about gum disease, the symptoms, available treatments, and—most importantly—the consequences. And 39 percent do not visit a dentist regularly. Yet, gum disease is the leading cause of adult tooth loss. Moreover, a Surgeon General's report issued in May 2000 labeled Americans' bad oral health a "silent epidemic" and called for a national effort to improve oral health among all Americans.

The good news is that in most people gum disease is preventable. Attention to everyday oral hygiene (brushing and flossing), coupled with professional cleanings twice a year, could be all that's needed to prevent gum disease—and actually reverse the early stage—and help you keep your teeth for a lifetime.

In addition, several products have been approved by the Food and Drug Administration specifically to diagnose and treat gum disease, and even regenerate lost bone. These products may help improve the effectiveness of the professional care you receive.

What Is Gum Disease?

In the broadest sense, the term gum disease—or periodontal disease—describes bacterial growth and production of factors that gradually destroy the tissue surrounding and supporting the teeth. "Periodontal" means "around the tooth."

Gum disease begins with plaque, which is always forming on your teeth, without you even knowing it. When it accumulates to excessive levels, it can harden into a substance called tartar (calculus) in as little as 24 hours. Tartar is so tightly bound to teeth that it can be removed only during a professional cleaning.

Gingivitis and periodontitis are the two main stages of gum disease. Each stage is characterized by what a dentist sees and feels in your mouth, and by what's happening under your gumline. Although gingivitis usually precedes periodontitis, it's important to know that not all gingivitis progresses to periodontitis.

In the early stage of gingivitis, the gums can become red and swollen and bleed easily, often during toothbrushing. Bleeding, although not always a symptom of gingivitis, is a signal that your mouth is unhealthy and needs attention. The gums may be irritated, but the teeth are still firmly planted in their sockets. No bone or other tissue damage has occurred at this stage. Although dental disease in America remains a serious public health concern, recent developments indicate that the situation is far from hopeless.

Frederick N. Hyman, D.D.S., a dental officer in the FDA's dermatologic and dental drug products division, says that because people seem to be paying more attention to oral hygiene as part of personal grooming, the payoff is "a decline in gingivitis over recent years." Hyman adds that "gingivitis can be reversed in nearly all cases when proper plaque control is practiced," consisting, in part, of daily brushing and flossing.

When gingivitis is left untreated, it can advance to periodontitis. At this point, the inner layer of the gum and bone pull away from the teeth (recede) and form pockets. These small spaces between teeth and gums may collect debris and can become infected. The body's immune system fights the bacteria as the plaque spreads and grows below the gumline. Bacterial toxins and the body's enzymes fighting the infection actually start to break down the bone and connective tissue that hold teeth in place. As the disease progresses, the pockets deepen and more gum tissue and bone are destroyed.

At this point, because there is no longer an anchor for the teeth, they become progressively looser, and the ultimate outcome is tooth loss.

Signs and Symptoms

Periodontal disease may progress painlessly, producing few obvious signs, even in the late stages of the disease. Then one day, on a visit to your dentist, you might be told that you have chronic gum disease and that you may be at increased risk of losing your teeth.

Although the symptoms of periodontal disease often are subtle, the condition is not entirely without warning signs. Certain symptoms may point to some form of the disease. They include:

- gums that bleed during and after toothbrushing;
- red, swollen, or tender gums;
- persistent bad breath or bad taste in the mouth;
- receding gums;
- formation of deep pockets between teeth and gums;
- loose or shifting teeth; and
- changes in the way teeth fit together on biting, or in the fit of partial dentures.

Even if you don't notice any symptoms, you may still have some degree of gum disease. Some people have gum disease only around certain teeth, such as those in the back of the mouth, which they cannot see. Only a dentist or a periodontist—a dentist who specializes in gum disease—can recognize and determine the progression of gum disease.

The American Academy of Periodontology (AAP) says that up to 30 percent of the U.S. population may be genetically susceptible to gum disease. And, despite aggressive oral care habits, people who are genetically predisposed may be up to six times more likely to develop some form of gum disease. Genetic testing to identify these people can help by encouraging early treatment that may help them keep their teeth for a lifetime.

Diagnosis

During a periodontal exam, your gums are checked for bleeding, swelling, and firmness. The teeth are checked for movement and sensitivity. Your bite is assessed. Full-mouth x-rays can help detect breakdown of bone surrounding your teeth.

Periodontal probing determines how severe your disease is. A probe is like a tiny ruler that is gently inserted into pockets around teeth. The deeper the pocket, the more severe the disease.

In healthy gums, the pockets measure less than 3 millimeters—about one-eighth of an inch—and no bone loss appears on x-rays. Gums are tight against the teeth and have pink tips. Pockets that measure 3 millimeters to 5 millimeters indicate signs of disease. Tartar may be progressing below the gumline and some bone loss could be evident. Pockets that are 5 millimeters or deeper indicate a serious condition that usually includes receding gums and a greater degree of bone loss.

Following the evaluation, your dentist or periodontist will recommend treatment options. Methods used to treat gum disease vary and are based on the stage of the disease.

Treatment

The goal of periodontal treatment is to control any infection that exists and to halt progression of the disease. Treatment options involve home care that includes healthy eating and proper brushing and flossing, non-surgical therapy that controls the growth of harmful bacteria and, in more advanced cases of disease, surgery to restore supportive tissues.

Although brushing and flossing are equally important, brushing eliminates only the plaque from the surfaces of the teeth that the brush can reach. Flossing, on the other hand, removes plaque from in between the teeth and under the gumline. Both should be used as part of a regular at-home, self-care treatment plan. Some dentists also recommend specialized toothbrushes, such as those that are motorized and have smaller heads, which may be a more effective method of removing plaque than a standard toothbrush.

John J. Golski, D.D.S., a Frederick, Maryland, periodontist, says that the rationale behind flossing is not "just to get the food out." From the periodontal standpoint, Golski says, "You're flossing to remove plaque—the real culprit behind gum disease," adding that proper brushing and flossing techniques are critical.

During a typical checkup your dentist or dental hygienist will remove the plaque and tartar from above and below the gumline of all your teeth. If you have some signs of gingivitis, your dentist may recommend that you return for future cleanings more often than twice a year. Your dentist may also recommend that you use a toothpaste or mouth rinse that is FDA-approved for fighting gingivitis.

In addition to containing fluoride to fight cavities, Colgate Total—the only toothpaste approved by the FDA for helping to prevent gingivitis—also contains triclosan, a mild antimicrobial that has been clinically proven to reduce plaque and gingivitis if used regularly. A chlorhexidine-containing rinse, also approved to fight plaque and gingivitis, is available only with a prescription.

If your dentist determines that you have some bone loss or that the gums have receded from the teeth, the standard treatment is an intensive deep-cleaning, nonsurgical method called scaling and root planing (SRP). Scaling scrapes the plaque and tartar from above and below the gumline. Root planing smoothes rough spots on the tooth root where germs collect and helps remove bacteria that can contribute to the disease. This smooth, clean surface helps allow the gums to reattach to the teeth.

A relatively new drug in the arsenal against serious gum disease called Periostat (doxycycline hyclate) was approved by the FDA in 1998 to be used in combination with SRP. While SRP primarily eliminates bacteria, Periostat, which is taken orally, suppresses the action of collagenase, an enzyme that causes destruction of the teeth and gums.

Periodontal procedures such as SRP, and even surgery, are most often done in the office. The time spent, the degree of discomfort, and healing times vary. All depend on the type and extent of the procedure and the person's overall health. Local anesthesia to numb the treatment area usually is given before some treatments. If necessary, medication is given to help you relax. Incisions may be closed with stitches designed to dissolve and may be covered with a protective dressing.

Susan Runner, D.D.S., chief of the Dental Devices Branch in the FDA's Center for Devices and Radiological Health, says that devices have been approved both for diagnosing gum diseases and promoting regeneration of periodontal tissue.

"Periodontal membranes, along with bone-filling material, are used in treatment of the condition to help repair damage resulting from periodontal disease," Runner says. "Tissue engineering devices mimic the biological characteristics of the wound-healing process, and may help stimulate bone cells to grow."

Opinions about which treatment methods to use vary in the periodontal field. For some people, certain procedures may be safer, more effective, and more comfortable than others may be. Which treatment your dentist or periodontist chooses will most likely depend on how far your disease has progressed, how you may have responded to earlier treatments, or your overall health.

"Generally, we all have the same goals, but the methods for getting to them may be different," says Golski. "One size doesn't fit all." Professional treatment can promote reattachment of healthy gums to teeth, reduce swelling, the depth of pockets, and the risk of infection, and stop further damage.

"But in the end," Golski says, "nothing will work without a compliant patient."

Antibiotic Treatments

Antibiotic treatments can be used either in combination with surgery and other therapies, or alone, to reduce or temporarily eliminate the bacteria associated with periodontal disease.

However, doctors, dentists, and public health officials are becoming more concerned that overuse of these antibiotics can increase the risk of bacterial resistance to these drugs. When germs become resistant to antibiotics, the drugs lose the ability to fight infection.

"The resistance we're worried about," explains Robert Genco, D.D.S., Ph.D., chairman of the oral biology department at The State University of New York at Buffalo, "is in association with antibiotics in the traditional use; those at higher levels in the blood that kill bacteria."

Jerry Gordon, D.M.D., of Bensalem, Pennsylvania, shares Genco's concerns. "There is a role for antibiotics in periodontal disease," Gordon says, "but you have to be very selective in your use."

Each time a person takes penicillin or another antibiotic for a bacterial infection, the drug may kill most of the bacteria. But a few germs may survive by mutating or acquiring resistance genes from other bacteria. These surviving genes can multiply quickly, creating drug-resistant strains. The presence of these strains may mean that the person's next infection will not respond to another dose of the same antibiotic. And this overuse would be detrimental to people if they develop a life-threatening illness for which antibiotics would no longer be helpful.

John V. Kelsey, D.D.S., dental team leader in the FDA's dermatologic and dental drug products division, says, "The widespread use of systemic antibiotics is generating resistant organisms, and that's a problem." And that fact, he says, "has prompted the industry to develop new strategies that would reduce the risk of resistance developing."

For example, three relatively new drugs—Atridox (doxycycline hyclate), PerioChip (chlorhexidine gluconate), and Arestin (minocycline)—are antibiotics that were approved in sustained-release doses to be applied into the periodontal pocket. Local application of antibiotics to the gum surface may not affect the entire body, as do oral antibiotics.

Oral Health and Overall Health

According to the Centers for Disease Control and Prevention (CDC), researchers have uncovered potential links between periodontal disease and other serious health conditions. In people with healthy immune systems, the influx of oral bacteria into the bloodstream is usually harmless. But under certain circumstances, the CDC says, the microorganisms that live in the human mouth can cause problems elsewhere in the body "if normal protective barriers in the mouth are breached."

If you have diabetes, for example, you are at higher risk of developing infections such as periodontal disease. These infections can impair the body's ability to process or use insulin, which may cause your diabetes to be more difficult to manage. Diabetes is not only a risk factor for periodontal disease, but periodontal disease may make diabetes worse.

However, the CDC cautions that there is not enough evidence to conclude that oral infections actually cause or contribute to cardiovascular disease, diabetes, and other serious health problems. More research is underway to determine whether the associations are causal or coincidental.

Other Common Measures for Treating Gum Disease

- **Curettage:** a scraping away of the diseased gum tissue in the infected pocket, which permits the infected area to heal.

- **Flap surgery:** involves lifting back the gums and removing the tartar. The gums are then sewn back in place so that the tissue fits snugly around the tooth. This method also reduces the pocket and areas where bacteria grow.

- **Bone grafts:** used to replace bone destroyed by periodontitis. Tiny fragments of your own bone, synthetic bone, or donated bone are placed where bone was lost. These grafts serve as a platform for the regrowth of bone, which restores stability to teeth.

- **Soft tissue grafts:** reinforce thin gums or fill in places where gums have receded. Grafted tissue, most often taken from the roof of the mouth, is stitched in place over the affected area.

- **Guided tissue regeneration:** stimulates bone and gum tissue growth. Done in combination with flap surgery, a small piece of mesh-like fabric is inserted between the bone and gum tissue. This keeps the gum tissue from growing into the area where the bone should be, allowing the bone and connective tissue to regrow to better support the teeth.

- **Bone (osseous) surgery:** smoothes shallow craters in the bone due to moderate and advanced bone loss. Following flap surgery, the bone around the tooth is reshaped to decrease the craters. This makes it harder for bacteria to collect and grow.

- **Medications:** in pill form are used to help kill the germs that cause periodontitis or suppress the destruction of the tooth's attachment to the bone. There are also antibiotic gels, fibers, or chips applied directly to the infected pocket. In some cases, a dentist will prescribe a special anti-germ mouth rinse containing a chemical called chlorhexidine to help control plaque and gingivitis. These are the only mouth rinses approved for treating periodontal disease.

Other Potential Factors That Contribute to Gum Disease

While plaque is the primary cause of periodontal disease, the American Academy of Periodontology (AAP) says that other factors are thought to increase the risk, severity, and speed of gum disease development. These can include:

- **Tobacco use:** one of the most significant risk factors associated with the development of periodontitis. People who smoke are seven times more likely to get periodontitis than nonsmokers, and smoking can lower the chances of success of some treatments.

- **Hormonal changes:** may make gums more sensitive and make it easier for gingivitis to develop.

- **Stress:** may make it difficult for the body's immune system to fight off infection.

Table 28.2. FDA-Approved Products for Gum Disease

Name	What It Is	Why It's Used	How It's Used
Colgate Total triclosan and fluoride toothpaste	Over-the-counter toothpaste containing the antibacterial triclosan	The antibacterial ingredient reduces plaque and resulting gingivitis. The fluoride protects against cavities.	Used like a regular toothpaste.
Peridex or generic chlorhexidine mouth rinse	Prescription mouth rinse containing an anti-microbial called chlorhexidine	To control bacteria, resulting in less plaque and gingivitis	Used like a regular mouthwash.
PerioChip	A tiny piece of gelatin filled with chlorhexidine	To control bacteria and reduce the size of periodontal pockets	Chip is placed in the pockets after root planing, where the medicine is slowly released over time.
Atridox	A gel that contains the antibiotic doxycycline	To control bacteria and reduce the size of periodontal pockets	Placed in pockets after scaling and root planing. Antibiotic is released slowly over a period of about 7 days.
Actisite	Thread-like fiber that contains the antibiotic tetracycline	To control bacteria and reduce the size of periodontal pockets	These fibers are placed in the pockets. The medicine is released slowly over 10 days. The fibers are then removed.
Arestin microspheres	Tiny round particles that contain the antibiotic minocycline	To control bacteria and reduce the size of periodontal pockets	Microspheres placed into pockets after scaling and root planing. Particles release minocycline slowly over time.
Periostat	A low dose of the medication doxycycline that keeps destructive enzymes in check	To hold back the body's enzyme response—if not controlled, certain enzymes can break down bone and connective tissue.	This medication is in pill form. It is used in combination with scaling and root planing.

- **Medications:** can affect oral health because they lessen the flow of saliva, which has a protective effect on teeth and gums. Some drugs, such as the anticonvulsant medication diphenylhydantoin and the anti-angina drug nifedipine, can cause abnormal growth of gum tissue.

- **Poor nutrition:** may make it difficult for the immune system to fight off infection, especially if the diet is low in important nutrients. Additionally, the bacteria that cause periodontal disease thrive in acidic environments. Eating sugars and other foods that increase the acidity in the mouth increases bacterial counts.

- **Illnesses:** may affect the condition of your gums. This includes diseases such as cancer or AIDS that interfere with the immune system.

- **Clenching and grinding teeth:** may put excess force on the supporting tissues of the teeth and could speed up the rate at which these tissues are destroyed.

Section 28.3

Oral Rinse Fights Gum Disease

From "FDA Approves New Oral Rinse to Help Treat Gingivitis," by the U.S. Food and Drug Administration (FDA, www.fda.gov), April 18, 2005.

The Food and Drug Administration (FDA) has approved a prescription treatment for gingivitis, a common gum disease that affects most adults at some point in their lives. The Decapinol Oral Rinse treats gingivitis by reducing the number of bacteria that attach to tooth surfaces and cause dental plaque. Decapinol is approved for use in persons 12 years of age or older when routine oral hygiene is not adequate to prevent gingivitis. Decapinol is not recommended for use by pregnant women.

"This new dental rinse helps treat gingivitis when tooth brushing and flossing are not enough," said Dr. Daniel Schultz, Director of FDA's

Center for Devices and Radiological Health. "This product can lead to a substantial reduction in gingivitis."

Gingivitis is an inflammation of the gums that often appears as swollen, red, or bleeding gums. Scientists believe plaque-forming bacteria that live in the mouth and on tooth surfaces are a cause of gingivitis. Substances released by the bacteria cause the gum inflammation. Reduction of plaque bacteria can decrease the inflammatory substances and cause a reduction in gingivitis.

Clinical studies were conducted in adults with mild to severe gingivitis. In these studies, Decapinol was compared either to "no treatment" or to an antimicrobial rinse. The studies showed that Decapinol decreases gingivitis up to 60%—compared to no treatment and when used as instructed with recommended brushing and flossing.

Decapinol Oral Rinse is being regulated as a medical device and not as a drug because its primary mode of action is to create a physical barrier, rather than to act chemically. Decapinol contains a substance called a surfactant that acts as a physical barrier, making it harder for bacteria to stick to tooth surfaces. FDA also has approved a number of other antigingivitis oral rinses, but since these products act chemically to kill bacteria that live in the mouth, they are regulated as antimicrobial drugs rather than as devices.

Decapinol Oral Rinse is manufactured by Sinclair Pharmaceuticals Limited, based in the United Kingdom.

Chapter 29

Tooth Injuries and Other Dental Emergencies

Chapter Contents

Section 29.1—Tips on Dealing with Dental Emergencies 290

Section 29.2—What to Do If a Tooth Is Knocked Out 291

Section 29.3—Facial Trauma 292

Section 29.4—Many Facial Sports Injuries Are
              Preventable 295

Section 29.5—Mouth Guards Protect More Than Teeth 298

Section 29.1

Tips on Dealing with Dental Emergencies

Knocked-Out Tooth

It's important to retrieve the tooth, hold it by the crown, and rinse off the root of the tooth if it's dirty. Do not scrub it or remove any attached tissue fragments. If possible, put the tooth back in its socket. If that isn't possible, put it in a container with milk or water and then get to the dentist as soon as possible.

Broken Tooth

Rinse your mouth with warm water to keep the area clean. Use cold compresses on the area to keep the swelling down and get to your dentist's office quickly.

Bitten Tongue or Lip

Clean the area gently with a cloth and then apply cold compresses to reduce the swelling. If the bleeding doesn't stop, go to a hospital emergency room immediately.

Objects Caught between the Teeth

Try to gently remove the object with dental floss and avoid cutting the gums. Do not use a sharp instrument. If you're not successful in removing the object, go to the dentist.

Toothache

Rinse the mouth with warm water to clean it out. Make sure food or foreign objects aren't lodged around the tooth by using dental floss. Don't ever put aspirin or any painkiller on the gums or around the aching tooth. It can cause a burn on the mouth and do more harm than good.

Knowing how to handle a dental emergency can mean the difference between saving or losing a tooth. Time is important in saving teeth. If your tooth or your child's tooth has been fractured, or especially if the tooth has been knocked out, you need to get to a dental office or emergency room as quickly as possible.

Section 29.2

What to Do If a Tooth Is Knocked Out

"Knocked-out Tooth Instruction Sheet," June 2007, reprinted with permission from www.kidshealth.org. Copyright © 2007 The Nemours Foundation. This information was provided by KidsHealth, one of the largest resources online for medically reviewed health information written for parents, kids, and teens. For more articles like this one, visit www.KidsHealth.org, or www.TeensHealth.org. This information was reviewed by Larissa Hirsch, M.D.

A knocked-out permanent tooth is a dental emergency. Baby teeth do not need to be put back in, but quickly putting a permanent tooth back in its socket is key to preserving the tooth.

Watch the clock. Every minute a tooth is out of its socket means the less chance it will survive. A tooth has the best chance of survival if replaced within 30 minutes.

What to Do

1. Find the knocked-out permanent tooth. If you're not sure whether it's a baby or permanent tooth (a baby tooth has a smooth edge), call a dentist or doctor or go to your local emergency room immediately.

2. Handle the tooth only by its crown (the top part), never by the root.

3. Gently rinse (don't scrub) the tooth immediately with saline solution or milk. (Tap water should only be used as a last resort; it contains chlorine, which may damage the root.)

4. Keep the tooth from drying out until you see the dentist by:

   - inserting the tooth back into its socket in the child's mouth if he or she is old enough to hold it in place

   - storing the tooth in milk (not water), or

   - placing the tooth between your cheek and lower gum.

5. See the child's dentist or go to your local emergency room right away.

Think Prevention

Children often lose teeth from playing contact sports such as football or ice hockey, from riding bikes, or from being in a motor vehicle crash. Children should wear mouth guards and protective gear when playing a contact sport. They should also always be buckled up in an age-appropriate car seat, booster seat, or seatbelt when in a motor vehicle.

Section 29.3

Facial Trauma

© 2008 A.D.A.M., Inc. Reprinted with permission.

Definition

Facial trauma is any injury of the face and upper jaw bone.

Causes

Blunt or penetrating trauma can cause injury to the midface region, which includes the upper jaw (maxilla). Common causes of facial injury include:

- Automobile accidents
- Violence
- Penetrating injuries

Symptoms

- Difficulty breathing through the nose due to swelling and bleeding
- Changes in sensation and feeling over the face
- Swelling around the eyes may cause vision problems
- Double vision
- Missing teeth

Exams and Tests

The doctor will perform a physical exam, which may show:

- Lacerations (breaks in the skin)
- Bruising around the eyes or widening of the distance between the eyes, which may mean injury to the bones between the eye sockets

The following may suggest bone fractures:

- An upper jaw that moves when the head is still
- Abnormal sensations on the cheek and irregularities that can be felt

A CT scan of the head may be done.

Treatment

Surgery is needed if the person can not function normally or if a substantial deformity is present.

The goal of treatment is to:

- Create a clear airway
- Control bleeding
- Treat the fracture
- Rule out other injuries
- Fix broken bone segments with titanium plates and screws
- Leave the fewest amount of scars possible

Treatment should be immediate, as long as the patient is stable and there are no neck fractures or life-threatening injuries.

Outlook (Prognosis)

Patients generally do very well with proper treatment. The patient should gently be told that they will probably look different than they did before their injury, and that additional surgeries may be needed 6–12 months later.

Possible Complications

General complications include, but are not limited to:

- Bleeding
- Infection
- Neurologic complications
- Facial asymmetry

When to Contact a Medical Professional

Go to the emergency room or call the local emergency number (such as 911) if you have a severe injury to your face.

Prevention

Wear seat belts and use protective head gear when appropriate. Avoid triggering potentially violent confrontations with other people.

Section 29.4

Many Facial Sports Injuries Are Preventable

From "Sports Injuries: In Your Face," by Ruth Levy Guyer, Ph.D.,
National Institutes of Health Office of Science Policy, 1997. This document was reviewed by David A. Cooke, M.D., May 29, 2008.

What do kissing, playing baseball and field hockey without a mouth
guard, and chugging soda from a glass bottle have in common?

They can all leave you with a chipped front tooth or, worse, no front
tooth at all.

Drinking soda through a mouth guard can be rough going, and a
face guard makes it next to impossible to enjoy kisses from the one
you love. But it simply makes good sense to shield your face and head
with protective gear when you play contact sports and sports where
balls, bats, pucks, and other missiles fly in your face.

"Sports and recreational injuries are easily prevented," says Ruth
Nowjack-Raymer, coauthor of a 1996 report on the use of protective
head gear—mouth guards and helmets—in organized sports.[1] The
strongest proof of this, she says, comes from the example of football.
In the 1950s, a faculty member in the dental school at Ohio State
University wrote a series of articles about mouth guards and their
cushioning effects.

Not only could a mouth guard protect the teeth and jaw but the
custom-made style molded by dentists could even prevent a concus-
sion, a form of brain injury. In the early 1960s, before rules and regulations governed the use of football gear, 50% of all injuries to high
school football players involved their faces and heads. Then, guidelines were established for shielding those parts of the body, and football players suited up with helmets and mouth guards. Today, only
1.4% of all football injuries involve the head and face.

It is strange that the example set by football players has not been
adopted by athletes who participate in other potentially dangerous
sports. Fans and athletes alike readily accept and even admire the
armored appearance of football players. Football players are, in fact,
among the most popular athletes in high schools and colleges in the
United States: the annual homecoming dance is always associated

295

with a fall football game, the school's band and cheerleaders perform more often at football games than at other sporting events, and graduates typically return to their schools to see football games. There is no stigma attached to helmets, mouth guards, and padding in this sport.

But, for some reason, there is great resistance among athletes in other sports to wearing protective gear. Nine million students in the United States play baseball and softball (three million play football). But it is rare to see baseball and softball players sporting protective head gear in the field and not even all at-bat players wear helmets. Nowjack-Raymer found that only 35% of kids wear helmets most or all of the time when they play baseball and softball and only 7% wear mouth guards. In Little League ball games, 86% of injuries involve athletes in the field, and most of the injuries affect heads and faces.[2]

As students get older, says Nowjack-Raymer, they are more likely to wear protective gear. This may, in part, reflect their growing understanding of the physical risks they face. It may also have something to do with who sponsors and pays for a sport. Organized sports programs for little children are often run by community centers, parents chip in money to support them, and the organization is relatively low key. As kids grow, she says, more of the programs are coordinated by schools and governed by "rules and regs." The survey documented some disturbing gender differences. "Girls are injured in sports too," notes Nowjack-Raymer, "and the injuries can be expensive and painful and cause problems that last a lifetime." But girls and women are much less likely to wear protective gear than are boys and men. Is this because they rarely see famous women athletes wearing mouth guards and helmets?

Nowjack-Raymer points to an example in her own family. Her sister, she says, is still dealing with problems that started years ago when she fractured her front teeth during a field hockey game. Field hockey, she notes, is a sport in which the disparity in safety practices between female and male athletes is striking. Male field hockey players at all levels wear head gear. Female hockey players typically do not, and whether they should is the subject of a raging debate. One group has been lobbying strongly for equal protection for female athletes. Another group is strongly opposed, arguing that, if girls and women wear protective gear, the nature and culture of the game will change toward more aggressive, violent play.

The data that Nowjack-Raymer analyzed were collected in a national health survey that was conducted in 1991. Nearly 10,000 parents and guardians of children in the 7 to 17 year old age range answered questions about the use of head gear and mouth guards in a number of organized sports. Nowjack-Raymer and her colleagues—epidemiologists, social scientists, health educators, behavioral scientists and others—are now beginning to look at the research that has already been done to address the problems that exist and define what research should be conducted next. They are trying to determine what coalitions of students, parents, coaches, trainers, organizations, and others could actually establish educational programs and binding rules that will support the use of protective gear. They are assessing what approaches work best to get student athletes to protect themselves. They are considering looking at the design of protective gear—is it comfortable, well made, effective?—and what makes a product acceptable.

In the United States, says Nowjack-Raymer, the strategies that have proved most effective are those based on establishment of and compliance with regulations, and often these have been instituted at local levels. This country has "no overarching authority" that makes rules, as is true in other countries. In Australia, for example, public health agencies provide information about injuries and also develop rules and guidelines for enhancing the safety of sports.

Will head gear ever become stylish? It hasn't yet, notes Nowjack-Raymer, but it has come a long way. "When a new sport comes along," she says, "it is important to think about what gear really makes sense." For example, in-line skating is a relatively new sport in which both beginners and more experienced skaters routinely wear lots of protective gear. Why this has occurred is unclear; perhaps it stems from good training from the beginning, the ready availability of colorful gear, a general acceptance of protective equipment, or some combination of these.

Accidents happen not only during official games but also during informal play, so, warns Nowjack-Raymer, it is important for athletes to wear their gear even when they are just practicing at home. Over 14 million children and teens in the United States participate in at least one organized sport, and injuries are on the rise. Teeth are knocked out in basketball games by the elbows of other players; eye injuries are common for badminton and squash players not wearing protective goggles;[3] 144,000 children in the United States suffer annually from head injuries in bicycle accidents, and 85% of these injuries would not have occurred had the child worn a helmet.[4] Getting athletes to readily don their helmets and mouth guards may involve major changes in the "cultures" of some sports.

And yet, some cultures have really valued helmets and other protective gear, which have been around as long as people have participated in sports and engaged in battles. Some 5,000 years ago, a prince of Ur named Meskalamdug apparently valued his gold and silver helmet so fully that he was buried in it. He also was buried with his bodyguards, all of whom were wearing helmets of copper.[5]

References

1. *Public Health Reports* 1996, 111:82–86.

2. *Pediatrics,* 1996, 98(3):445–448.

3. *J. R. Coll Surg,* Edinb, 1993 38(3):127–133.

4. *Public Health Reports* 1995, 110(3):251–259.

5. Aust. N.Z. *J. Surg.* 1996, 66:314–324.

Section 29.5

Mouth Guards Protect More Than Teeth

Upon heading back to school this fall, young athletes of all ages and skill levels will be joining their friends on basketball courts, soccer fields, baseball diamonds, and hockey rinks. Remember to add a mouth guard for each child to your list of school supplies. Protecting your child's head, jaw, and teeth, even for seemingly non-contact sports, is very important.

"Mouth guards not only protect the teeth," states Dr. Ian McConnachie, President of the Ontario Dental Association and a pediatric dentist. "They may also prevent concussions and other serious injuries by helping to avoid situations where the lower jaw and teeth are forced up against the upper teeth and jaw."

Sports Canada reports that overall, 69 percent of Canadian youth participate in organized sport. In any sport, whether it's full-contact hockey or a friendly game of racquetball, a little preparation can prevent costly and sometimes painful mistakes later on.

Who Should Wear a Mouth Guard?

All athletes. All ages. Any sport with a strong chance for contact with other participants or hard surfaces requires mouth protection. Players who participate in basketball, baseball, soccer, wrestling, squash, racquetball, lacrosse, rugby, in-line skating. and martial arts, or even recreational sports such as skateboarding and bicycling, should wear mouth guards when practicing or competing.

What Are the Factors That Affect the Fit of a Mouth Guard?

"A dentist will consider a number of factors when fitting a patient for a mouth guard," says Dr. McConnachie. "Size of mouth, bite, type of sport played, and whether or not the patient wears braces or other appliances are all important considerations. Each patient's very specific needs must be addressed for maximum comfort and protection."

Many athletes resist wearing a mouth guard because of bulkiness and poor fit. Custom-made mouth guards are the most comfortable, non-bulky, and form-fitting. This leads to increased use and fewer injuries.

Are There Different Types of Mouth Guards?

There are three basic types of mouth guards.

Table 29.1. Types of Mouth Guards

Type	Description
Custom-made	The dentist takes an impression of the patient's mouth and the mouth guard is fabricated from a cast model of the patient's teeth. This method provides the best fit, protection, and comfort. The custom-made mouth guard is most durable, can be modified for specific sports and patient need, and does not interfere with speech or breathing.
Boil and bite or mouth-formed	This type of mouth guard requires heating in warm water and then the user bites into the warm plastic. Because it is not vacuum-fitted onto a model of the patient's teeth, the fit is not as precise. The heating process will also reduce the longevity of the mouth guard. Discuss this option with your dentist.
Stock or ready-made	Made of rubber or polyvinyl, the ready-made mouth guard is a generic fit with limited comfort, protection, and durability. It is often bulky and loose-fitting and may interfere with breathing and speech.

Care for Your Mouth Guard So It Cares for You

Caring for your mouth guard will help it take care of your teeth longer. Take a few moments to:

- Rinse your mouth guard under cold water after each use and air-dry.

- Occasionally clean it with mild soap and water or mouthwash.

- Store your mouth guard in a plastic container when not in use to avoid damage due to excessive heat and cold.

- Wear your mouth guard properly. Do not cut or alter it and do not chew on it.

- Check your mouth guard regularly and let your dentist know if it shows any signs of wear, or has any tears or cracks that may weaken it. If the bite has changed and the mouth guard no longer fits well, it can sometimes be adjusted by the dentist.

Dos and Don'ts of Tooth Injuries

Prevention isn't always fool-proof, so if you play any sports, learn what to do in case of a mouth injury. Here are some dos and don'ts:

- **Do** make sure you receive prompt medical treatment in the case of injury sustained to the jaw where there was a loss of consciousness, no matter how brief the loss of consciousness was.

- **Do** make sure that you go to the dentist as quickly as possible after an injury to the teeth and/or jaw has occurred. Time is critical to the chances of saving the tooth/teeth.

- **Don't** place the lost or broken tooth/teeth in tissue paper or gauze while on the way to the dentist.

- **Do** store the dislodged tooth/teeth in cold milk or in sterile saline solution on your way to the dentist. Ideally, ask your dentist about commercially available tooth injury kits.

- **Don't** assume that noncontact sports can't cause mouth injuries.

Part Five

Surgical, Orthodontic, and Cosmetic Dental Procedures

Chapter 30

Oral and Maxillofacial Surgery

Chapter Contents

Section 30.1—Types of Oral and Maxillofacial Surgeries 304
Section 30.2—Home Care after Oral and Maxillofacial
    Surgery 307

303

Section 30.1

Types of Oral and Maxillofacial Surgeries

What is oral and maxillofacial surgery?

Oral and maxillofacial surgery is the specialty of dentistry which
includes the diagnosis, surgical and adjunctive treatment of disease,
injuries, and defects involving both the functional and esthetic aspects
of the hard and soft tissues of the oral and maxillofacial region.

What does it mean to be board certified in oral and maxillofacial surgery?

Education: Your board certified oral and maxillofacial surgeon
has graduated from an accredited dental school and is licensed in the
state in which he/she practices. In addition, this individual has completed an oral and maxillofacial surgery residency program approved
by the American Dental Association's Commission on Dental Accreditation.

The American Board of Oral and Maxillofacial Surgery is recognized by the American Dental Association as the specialty board for
oral and maxillofacial surgery. The Board is responsible for reviewing all applicants for board certification as well as administering the
examinations involved in the certification process.

During his/her oral and maxillofacial surgery residency, your board
certified oral and maxillofacial surgeon received graduate training in
other disciplines such as general surgery, plastic surgery, medicine,
anesthesia, and pathology. Oral and maxillofacial surgeons are trained
to treat patients in the hospital, outpatient facilities, surgery centers,
and in private offices.

Certification: In order to become board certified, an individual
must complete an intensive application and examination process. Applicants for board certification in oral and maxillofacial surgery must

provide verified written evidence of their educational and training qualifications. In addition, these individuals must provide evidence of their experience in all aspects of oral and maxillofacial surgery. Letters of recommendation from board certified oral and maxillofacial surgeons attesting to an applicant's acceptable ethical and moral standing in the profession and community are also required as part of the certification procedure. The applications of all candidates for board certification are reviewed by the Board's Credentials Committee.

Continued Competence: Finally, your board certified oral and maxillofacial surgeon was required to pass both a thorough written qualifying examination and a rigorous oral certifying examination to be certified as a Diplomate of the American Board of Oral and Maxillofacial Surgery. Diplomates are encouraged to maintain current competence by ongoing continuing education.

Diplomates are recertified in current competency every 10 years by a comprehensive written examination.

Continuing professional education is an important tool keeping oral and maxillofacial surgeons current on new developments in the field. This is accomplished through national meetings, seminars, lectures, special courses, panels, symposia, and self study. The board certified oral and maxillofacial surgeon has demonstrated a commitment to continued professional development. The American Board of Oral and Maxillofacial Surgery encourages its Diplomates to continue their professional development through various educational experiences.

What services do board certified oral and maxillofacial surgeons provide?

Removal of diseased and impacted teeth and anesthesia: Oral and maxillofacial surgeons remove impacted, damaged, and non-restorable teeth. They also provide sophisticated, safe, and effective anesthesia services in their office including intravenous (IV) sedation and general anesthesia.

Dental implants: Oral and maxillofacial surgeons, in close collaboration with restorative dentists, help plan and then place implants used to replace missing teeth. They can also reconstruct bone in places needing bone for implant placement and modify gingival (gum) tissue surrounding implants when necessary to make teeth placed on implants look even more natural.

Facial trauma: Oral and maxillofacial surgeons care for facial injuries by repairing routine and complex facial skin lacerations (cuts), setting fractured jaw and facial bones, reconnecting severed nerves and ducts, and treating other injuries. These procedures include care of oral tissues, the jaws, cheek and nasal bones, the forehead, and eye sockets.

Pathologic conditions: Oral and maxillofacial surgeons manage patients with benign and malignant cysts and tumors of the oral and facial regions. Severe infections of the oral cavity, salivary glands, jaws, and neck are also treated.

Reconstructive and cosmetic surgery: Oral and maxillofacial surgeons correct jaw, facial bone, and facial soft tissue problems left as the result of previous trauma or removal of pathology. This surgery to restore form and function often includes moving skin, bone, nerves, and other tissues from other parts of the body to reconstruct the jaws and face. These same skills are also used when oral and maxillofacial surgeons perform cosmetic procedures for improvement of problems due to unwanted facial features or aging.

Facial pain including temporomandibular joint disorders: Oral and maxillofacial surgeons possess skills in the diagnosis and treatment of facial pain disorders including those due to temporomandibular joint (TMJ) problems.

Correction of dentofacial (bite) deformities and birth defects: Oral and maxillofacial surgeons, usually in conjunction with an orthodontist, surgically reconstruct and realign the upper and lower jaws into proper dental and facial relationships to provide improved biting function and facial appearance. They also surgically correct birth defects of the face and skull including cleft lip and palate.

Section 30.2

Home Care after Oral and Maxillofacial Surgery

You have had oral or maxillofacial surgery. You may have had a
routine tooth extraction, removal of wisdom teeth, surgery for bone
reshaping or dental implants, or an intraoral biopsy. Below are instructions to follow at home after your surgery.

- Bite with light, steady pressure for 1 hour on the gauze placed
  in your mouth at the clinic.

- Mild bleeding after oral surgery is normal. If you still have
  bleeding after 3 to 4 hours, raise your head higher than the rest
  of your body. Then bite with firm, steady pressure on a moist
  gauze pad or a wet tea bag for 20 minutes. If the bleeding does
  not stop, call your nurse or doctor.

- Prop your head with several pillows when lying down or sleeping. This will help to reduce swelling and bleeding.

- Swelling after surgery is common. Hold an ice pack on the outside of your face for 20 minutes, then remove it for 10 minutes.
  Repeat this procedure while awake for the first 24 hours. After
  24 hours, stop using ice.

- If you had a routine extraction of one or several teeth with very
  little bone smoothing, you may eat and drink. Eat as much solid
  food as you comfortably can. Avoid crunchy foods.

- If you had more than 20 teeth removed or a lot of bone removal,
  follow a full liquid diet or a very soft diet for 5 to 7 days.

- If you had surgery to remove wisdom teeth, or if you have been
  sedated, take only clear liquids at first, and then soft foods, for

the first 24 hours. After 24 hours, you may return to your normal diet as soon as you comfortably can.

- If you had surgery for bone reshaping or dental implants or had an intraoral biopsy, follow a full liquid diet or a very soft diet for 5 to 7 days.

- After 24 hours, begin to rinse your mouth frequently with salt water. Rinse four to five times a day, especially after eating. Mix 1/4 teaspoon of salt in a tall glass of warm tap water. Rinse with salt water for 3 days. Do not swallow the salt water.

- Brush your teeth as you normally do. Be careful when brushing in the area where you had surgery.

- Take your medication exactly as your doctor prescribes.

- Do not smoke. It will take longer to heal if you do. Do not use chewing tobacco.

- Do not use a straw. Sucking may cause bleeding.

- Return for your postoperative visit as instructed by your doctor to have your stitches or dressings removed.

If you have any questions about these instructions or any concerns not listed here, call your nurse or doctor.

Chapter 31

Impacted Teeth

Chapter Contents

Section 31.1—Impacted Teeth and Their Removal 310
Section 31.2—Removing Wisdom Teeth during Adolescence
Prevents Problems 314

Section 31.1

Impacted Teeth and Their Removal

Excerpted from "Preparing for Third Molar Removal," by the Warren Grant Magnuson Clinical Center, National Institutes of Health (www .cc.nih.gov), 1999. This document was reviewed by David A. Cooke, M.D., May 29, 2008.

Reasons for Removing Third Molars

Third molars are usually removed when they are impacted. Teeth are impacted when there is not enough room for them in the mouth. Removal should take place before the surrounding jaw bone has hardened and before any major changes have taken place in the jaw.

Other reasons why third molars would be removed are the following:

- recurrent infections or cysts around the tooth that cause bone loss and weakening of the jaw bone;

- third molars causing damage to an adjacent tooth; or

- third molars crowding other teeth, causing them to shift out of line.

Third molars are usually removed before people reach the age of 30.

Complications from Surgery

As with any operation, complications are possible during third molar removal. These complications include delayed healing of the extraction site (dry socket), infection, perforation of the lining of the sinuses located in the upper jaw, damage to the teeth, or temporarily or permanently altered sensation of the lower lip, chin, or tongue.

A rare complication of oral surgery is a fractured jaw. There may also be side effects from the local anesthetic used during surgery. Possible, though rare, adverse reactions include temporary facial paralysis, a bruise, injection into a vein, and allergic reactions.

Some patients have experienced one or more of the following transient adverse effects from the pain medication used after surgery: drowsiness, dizziness, nausea, vomiting, and allergic reactions.

On the Day of Surgery

Before Surgery

Your primary nurse will ask you some routine questions and take your vital signs (temperature, pulse, respiration rate, blood pressure). If you have any questions or concerns about your surgery, please ask them at that time.

You will be taken to one of the operatories where the surgery will be performed. An IV (intravenous) line will be placed in your arm. This device will enable the staff to obtain blood samples and administer medications without having to give you many needle sticks. The IV will remain in place after surgery or until the necessary blood samples have been drawn.

After Surgery and throughout the Day

After surgery, you should plan to rest at home for the remainder of the day. If you have been given a sedative, lie down at home until it has completely worn off. Reading, watching television, and taking a nap are examples of quiet activities that you may enjoy until bedtime.

The sedative that you received during surgery, as well as certain medicines, may cause drowsiness and dizziness after the operation. Because of these effects, do not drive a car, operate machinery, drink alcoholic beverages, or expose yourself to safety hazards.

Proper mouth care after oral surgery will speed healing and reduce complications. The following suggestions are offered to help you recover quickly and safely from oral surgery.

Bleeding

Expect some bleeding to occur: oozing may continue for 24 hours. To help stop the bleeding, gently bit on folded gauze for an hour as needed during the first 24 hours. If bleeding has not subsided after 24 hours, contact the clinic. So that bleeding does not worsen, engage in nonstrenous quiet activities.

Protecting the Blood Clot

• Do not rinse, spit, brush your teeth, or use a mouthwash.

- Do not exercise strenuously for 7 to 10 days after surgery.
- Do not pick at the surgical site.
- Do not use a straw.
- Do not use a Waterpik.
- Do not drink alcoholic or carbonated beverages.
- If you smoke, do not do so for 24 hours or longer.
- Do not chew tobacco for 1 week.

Smoking or chewing tobacco will greatly increase your postoperative problems.

Swelling

Expect swelling, especially if your surgery was difficult. You may even see some bruising on your cheek. Use ice bags immediately and for the next 24 hours. Apply them at regular intervals: put the ice bags on for 30 minutes and take them off for 15 minutes. If you had teeth removed on both sides, alternate a single ice pack from side to side every 15 minutes. Keep your head elevated on two or three pillows while you rest or sleep. The swelling will peak in 2 to 3 days and should subside after that. If you notice any increase in swelling after the first 48 hours, a fever, a bad taste in your mouth, or pus, you may have an infection. Call the clinic or your oral surgeon and arrange to be seen that day.

Pain

After oral surgery, you may feel some discomfort. It can be eased by taking pain medications as directed. Take the first dose of medication when your lower lip begins to tingle or when you begin to feel pain. Take your next dose 4 to 6 hours later as prescribed. By taking your medication every 4 to 6 hours as prescribed, you will be able to stay ahead of your pain. Stomach discomfort can be avoided by eating before you take the pain medication.

Eating

It is very important to eat and drink enough after oral surgery. The first day, eat such cool, soft foods as instant breakfasts, milkshakes, yogurt, and applesauce. The next day, advance to semisoft foods when you can tolerate them. Avoid tough, hard, chewy, hot, and spicy foods.

The Day after and the Week Following Surgery

These guidelines will help you continue your recovery.

Ice Bags

If circumstances permit, continue using ice bags the morning after surgery. Do not use them for a longer period.

Heat

Starting 24 hours after surgery, apply warm, moist heat to the outside of your face several times daily for 2 to 3 days.

Oral Hygiene

Brush your teeth as best you can after meals and at bedtime. Rinse your mouth with warm salt water (1/2 teaspoon table salt in an 8-ounce glass of warm water) every 2 hours and after meals. Brushing and rinsing will help maintain oral hygiene and prevent infections.

Food

Return to your normal diet as soon as you can. While you may have some stiffness in your jaws for several days, chewing will help loosen your jaw muscles.

Medications

Continue taking your pain medications as prescribed. Since the pain should begin to diminish after 2 days, take pain medication only when needed.

Note: Certain medications may cause sleepiness and dizziness. **Do not** operate machinery, drive a car, drink alcohol, or expose yourself to safety hazards. If you feel an increase in pain after 3 or 4 days, call the clinic or your oral surgeon.

Blood

If you see any blood in nasal secretions or after blowing your nose, call the clinic or your oral surgeon.

Injection Site

If medication was given to you through your vein and you have redness, pain, irritation, or hardness at the injection site, wrap the area

313

with a warm, moist towel and call the clinic or your oral surgeon for further instructions.

Section 31.2

Removing Wisdom Teeth during Adolescence Prevents Problems

"Best to Have Wisdom Teeth Removed as a Teenager," © 2006
Medical College of Wisconsin. Reprinted with permission of Medical
College of Wisconsin HealthLink, www.healthlink.mcw.edu.

For many Americans, having their wisdom teeth removed is part of growing up. Wisdom teeth, also known as third molars, are the last teeth to erupt, or push through the gum. This usually occurs during the teenage years and, according to many dentists, that's the best time to have them removed.

Why remove new teeth if they aren't causing any trouble? Because they're likely to trigger problems eventually, says Mary Lou (Ma'Lou) Sabino, D.D.S., Assistant Professor of Oral and Maxillofacial Surgery, part of the Medical College of Wisconsin Department of Surgery. And after age 25, extracting wisdom teeth becomes much more complicated than if it's done when patients are between about 15 to 20 years old.

"It's easier when you're younger, because the bony structures under the teeth are still forming and relatively soft," says Dr. Sabino. "After 25, bones have hardened, and extractions can become more difficult," she says. "And the healing process is usually faster in younger patients."

Wisdom teeth are sort of an evolutionary throwback, left over from the time when early man's diet consisted of unrefined food that required considerably more chewing than the modern diet. It's thought they got their name because with age comes wisdom (and wisdom teeth).

Often, wisdom teeth cannot erupt normally because the jaw is not large enough to accommodate them plus all the other teeth that are growing in. Wisdom teeth that are not fully erupted are termed "impacted," because they either remain below the jaw line or don't grow in properly.

Potential Problems

Some of the problems wisdom teeth can trigger include:

- **Gum infection (pericoronitis):** When wisdom teeth don't fully erupt, food and bacteria can collect under the gum and cause local inflammation, which can produce bad breath, pain, swelling, and difficulty opening the mouth. Such an infection could even trigger life-threatening problems, Dr. Sabino says. "When gum tissue becomes inflamed, it can develop a secondary infection or abscess that can rapidly travel to areas where it compromises breathing. This is a medical emergency."

- **Decay:** Saliva, bacteria, and food particles can collect around an impacted wisdom tooth, causing it, or the adjacent tooth, to decay.

- **Periodontal problems:** Even a fully erupted wisdom tooth can emerge crooked and press against the next tooth, Dr. Sabino says. That can shift the alignment of other teeth. And because these teeth are more difficult to clean, it can also lead to cavities on the back of the adjacent molar.

Impacted wisdom teeth can vary depending on their level of eruption, Dr. Sabino notes. The least severe is a soft-tissue impaction, where part of the tooth remains under the gum or soft tissue. Next is a partial bony impaction, where part of the tooth lies in the bony structure of the jaw. Finally, there is a full, or complete, bony impaction, where the tooth is seated entirely in the bone. Depending on the level of impaction, some extraction procedures might be covered by medical insurance, Dr. Sabino says.

Procedure Usually Brief

Many patients dread the thought of having their wisdom teeth removed, but generally all four wisdom teeth can be removed in 20 to 30 minutes, says Dr. Sabino. The procedure is performed under local anesthesia (nitrous oxide, sometimes called "laughing gas"), so the patient shouldn't feel any pain, just a sensation of pushing. In more anxious patients, intravenous sedation can be used. Patients are then sent home with instructions about aftercare and pain medication, which they might or might not require.

For the next few days after the procedure, Dr. Sabino says, some patients could experience discomfort. All patients should avoid chewing and eat only a soft diet for the next two or three days—soups, puddings, and pureed or mashed food. By the fifth day, they should be able to resume a normal diet.

"Whether a patient experiences pain after a wisdom teeth extraction procedure may depend on the level of the impaction and on the individual," says Dr. Sabino. Sometimes, a patient may develop a "dry socket." This occurs as a result of a prematurely lost blood clot, which can be very painful. Normally, the hole fills with blood that forms a clot, which eventually forms bone and fills in the space. A dry socket can occur if the clot dissolves too quickly or is dislodged. Dry sockets can usually be prevented if patients follow the post-treatment instructions provided by the dentist or oral surgeon. If a dry socket does occur, patients should call the dentist or oral surgeon for additional medication and treatment.

Like any surgery, a wisdom teeth extraction procedure carries potential risk, Dr. Sabino notes. "In addition to a dry socket, some patients experience bleeding or infection, nerve damage, or sinus perforation if the roots of the upper teeth lie close to the wall of the nasal sinuses." These complications are relatively rare, she adds.

Wisdom teeth can be removed by family dentists, but increasingly, more and more dentists refer patients—especially if their wisdom teeth are impacted, or if they are older patients—to an oral surgeon, Dr. Sabino says.

Chapter 32

Endodontic and Root Canal Treatment

Chapter Contents

Section 32.1—Root Canal Treatment 318
Section 32.2—Understanding Endodontic Surgery 321
Section 32.3—Endodontic Retreatment 324

Section 32.1

Root Canal Treatment

What Is Endodontic Treatment?

"Endo" is the Greek word for "inside" and "odont" is Greek for
"tooth." Endodontic treatment treats the inside of the tooth.

To understand endodontic treatment, it helps to know something
about the anatomy of the tooth. Inside the tooth, under the white
enamel and a hard layer called the dentin, is a soft tissue called the
pulp. The pulp contains blood vessels, nerves, and connective tissue
and creates the surrounding hard tissues of the tooth during development.

The pulp extends from the crown of the tooth to the tip of the roots
where it connects to the tissues surrounding the root. The pulp is
important during a tooth's growth and development. However, once
a tooth is fully mature it can survive without the pulp, because the
tooth continues to be nourished by the tissues surrounding it.

Why Would I Need an Endodontic Procedure?

Endodontic treatment is necessary when the pulp, the soft tissue
inside the root canal, becomes inflamed or infected. The inflammation or infection can have a variety of causes: deep decay, repeated
dental procedures on the tooth, or a crack or chip in the tooth. In addition, an injury to a tooth may cause pulp damage even if the tooth
has no visible chips or cracks. If pulp inflammation or infection is left
untreated, it can cause pain or lead to an abscess.

What Are the Signs of Needing Endodontic Treatment?

Signs to look for include pain, prolonged sensitivity to heat or cold,
tenderness to touch and chewing, discoloration of the tooth, and swelling, drainage, and tenderness in the lymph nodes as well as nearby

bone and gingival tissues. Sometimes, however, there are no symptoms.

How Does Endodontic Treatment Save the Tooth?

The endodontist removes the inflamed or infected pulp, carefully cleans and shapes the inside of the canal, a channel inside the root, then fills and seals the space. Afterwards, you will return to your dentist, who will place a crown or other restoration on the tooth to protect and restore it to full function. After restoration, the tooth continues to function like any other tooth.

Will I Feel Pain during or after the Procedure?

Many endodontic procedures are performed to relieve the pain of toothaches caused by pulp inflammation or infection. With modern techniques and anesthetics, most patients report that they are comfortable during the procedure.

For the first few days after treatment, your tooth may feel sensitive, especially if there was pain or infection before the procedure. This discomfort can be relieved with over-the-counter or prescription medications. Follow your endodontist's instructions carefully.

Your tooth may continue to feel slightly different from your other teeth for some time after your endodontic treatment is completed. However, if you have severe pain or pressure or pain that lasts more than a few days, call your endodontist.

Endodontic Procedure

Endodontic treatment can often be performed in one or two visits and involves the following steps:

1. The endodontist examines and x-rays the tooth, then administers local anesthetic. After the tooth is numb, the endodontist places a small protective sheet called a "dental dam" over the area to isolate the tooth and keep it clean and free of saliva during the procedure.

2. The endodontist makes an opening in the crown of the tooth. Very small instruments are used to clean the pulp from the pulp chamber and root canals and to shape the space for filling.

3. After the space is cleaned and shaped, the endodontist fills the root canals with a biocompatible material, usually a rubber-like

material called "gutta-percha." The gutta-percha is placed with an adhesive cement to ensure complete sealing of the root canals. In most cases, a temporary filling is placed to close the opening. The temporary filling will be removed by your dentist before the tooth is restored.

4. After the final visit with your endodontist, you must return to your dentist to have a crown or other restoration placed on the tooth to protect and restore it to full function.

If the tooth lacks sufficient structure to hold the restoration in place, your dentist or endodontist may place a post inside the tooth. Ask your dentist or endodontist for more details about the specific restoration planned for your tooth.

How Much Will the Procedure Cost?

The cost varies depending on how complex the problem is and which tooth is affected. Molars are more difficult to treat, the fee is usually more. Most dental insurance policies provide some coverage for endodontic treatment.

Generally, endodontic treatment and restoration of the natural tooth are less expensive than the alternative of having the tooth extracted. An extracted tooth must be replaced with a bridge or implant to restore chewing function and prevent adjacent teeth from shifting. These procedures tend to cost more than endodontic treatment and appropriate restoration. With root canal treatment you save your natural teeth and money.

Will the Tooth Need Any Special Care or Additional Treatment after Endodontic Treatment?

You should not chew or bite on the treated tooth until you have had it restored by your dentist. The unrestored tooth is susceptible to fracture, so you should see your dentist for a full restoration as soon as possible. Otherwise, you need only practice good oral hygiene, including brushing, flossing, and regular checkups and cleanings.

Most endodontically treated teeth last as long as other natural teeth. In a few cases, a tooth that has undergone endodontic treatment does not heal or the pain continues. Occasionally, the tooth may become painful or diseased months or even years after successful treatment. Often when this occurs, redoing the endodontic procedure can save the tooth.

What Causes an Endodontically Treated Tooth to Need Additional Treatment?

New trauma, deep decay, or a loose, cracked, or broken filling can cause new infection in your tooth. In some cases, the endodontist may discover additional very narrow or curved canals that could not be treated during the initial procedure.

Can All Teeth Be Treated Endodontically?

Most teeth can be treated. Occasionally, a tooth can't be saved because the root canals are not accessible, the root is severely fractured, the tooth doesn't have adequate bone support, or the tooth cannot be restored. However, advances in endodontics are making it possible to save teeth that even a few years ago would have been lost. When endodontic treatment is not effective, endodontic surgery may be able to save the tooth.

Section 32.2

Understanding Endodontic Surgery

"Endodontic Surgery," © 2007 American Association of Endodontists (www.aae.org). Reprinted with permission.

Why would I need endodontic surgery?

- Surgery can help save your tooth in a variety of situations.

- Surgery may be used in diagnosis. If you have persistent symptoms but no problems appear on your x-ray, your tooth may have a tiny fracture or canal that could not be detected during nonsurgical treatment. In such a case, surgery allows your endodontist to examine the entire root of your tooth, find the problem, and provide treatment.

- Sometimes calcium deposits make a canal too narrow for the instruments used in nonsurgical root canal treatment to reach the end of the root. If your tooth has this "calcification," your

321

endodontist may perform endodontic surgery to clean and seal the remainder of the canal.

- Usually, a tooth that has undergone a root canal can last the rest of your life and never need further endodontic treatment. However, in a few cases, a tooth may not heal or become infected. A tooth may become painful or diseased months or even years after successful treatment. If this is true for you, surgery may help save your tooth.

- Surgery may also be performed to treat damaged root surfaces or surrounding bone.

Although there are many surgical procedures that can be performed to save a tooth, the most common is called apicoectomy or root-end resection. When inflammation or infection persists in the bony area around the end of your tooth after a root canal procedure, your endodontist may have to perform an apicoectomy.

What is an apicoectomy?

In this procedure, the endodontist opens the gum tissue near the tooth to see the underlying bone and to remove any inflamed or infected tissue. The very end of the root is also removed.

A small filling may be placed in the root to seal the end of the root canal, and a few stitches or sutures are placed in the gingiva to help the tissue heal properly.

Over a period of months, the bone heals around the end of the root.

Are there other types of endodontic surgery?

Other surgeries endodontists might perform include dividing a tooth in half, repairing an injured root, or even removing one or more roots. Your endodontist will be happy to discuss the specific type of surgery your tooth requires.

In certain cases, a procedure called intentional replantation may be performed. In this procedure, a tooth is extracted, treated with an endodontic procedure while it is out of the mouth, and then replaced in its socket.

These procedures are designed to help you save your tooth.

Will the procedure hurt?

Local anesthetics make the procedure comfortable. Of course, you may feel some discomfort or experience slight swelling while the incision heals.

This is normal for any surgical procedure. Your endodontist will recommend appropriate pain medication to alleviate your discomfort.

Your endodontist will give you specific postoperative instructions to follow. If you have questions after your procedure, or if you have pain that does not respond to medication, call your endodontist.

Can I drive myself home?

Often you can, but you should ask your endodontist before your appointment so that you can make transportation arrangements if necessary.

When can I return to my normal activities?

Most patients return to work or other routine activities the next day. Your endodontist will be happy to discuss your expected recovery time with you.

Does insurance cover endodontic surgery?

Each insurance plan is different. Check with your employer or insurance company prior to treatment.

How do I know the surgery will be successful?

Your dentist or endodontist is suggesting endodontic surgery because he or she believes it is the best option for saving your own natural tooth. Of course, there are no guarantees with any surgical procedure. Your endodontist will discuss your chances for success so that you can make an informed decision.

What are the alternatives to endodontic surgery?

Often, the only alternative to surgery is extraction of the tooth. The extracted tooth must then be replaced with an implant, bridge, or removable partial denture to restore chewing function and to prevent adjacent teeth from shifting. Because these alternatives require surgery or dental procedures on adjacent healthy teeth, endodontic surgery is usually the most biologic and cost-effective option for maintaining your oral health.

No matter how effective modern artificial tooth replacements are—and they can be very effective—nothing is as good as a natural tooth. You've already made an investment in saving your tooth. The payoff for choosing endodontic surgery could be a healthy, functioning natural tooth for the rest of your life.

Section 32.3

Endodontic Retreatment

Why do I need another endodontic procedure?

As occasionally happens with any dental or medical procedure, a tooth may not heal as expected after initial treatment for a variety of reasons:

- Narrow or curved canals were not treated during the initial procedure.

- Complicated canal anatomy went undetected in the first procedure.

- The placement of the crown or other restoration was delayed following the endodontic treatment.

- The restoration did not prevent salivary contamination to the inside of the tooth.

In other cases, a new problem can jeopardize a tooth that was successfully treated. For example:

- New decay can expose the root canal filling material to bacteria, causing a new infection in the tooth.

- A loose, cracked, or broken crown or filling can expose the tooth to new infection.

- A tooth sustains a fracture.

What will happen during retreatment?

First, the endodontist will discuss your treatment options. If you and your endodontist choose retreatment, the endodontist will reopen your tooth to gain access to the root canal filling material. In many cases, complex restorative materials—crown, post, and core material—must be disassembled and removed to permit access to the root canals.

After removing the canal filling, the endodontist can clean the canals and carefully examine the inside of your tooth using magnification and illumination, searching for any additional canals or unusual anatomy that requires treatment.

After cleaning the canals, the endodontist will fill and seal the canals and place a temporary filling in the tooth. If the canals are unusually narrow or blocked, your endodontist may recommend endodontic surgery. This surgery involves making an incision to allow the other end of the root to be sealed.

After your endodontist completes retreatment, you will need to return to your dentist as soon as possible to have a new crown or other restoration placed on the tooth to protect and restore it to its full function.

Is retreatment the best choice for me?

Whenever possible, it is best to save your natural tooth. Retreated teeth can function well for years, even for a lifetime.

Advances in technology are constantly changing the way root canal treatment is performed, so your endodontist may use new techniques that were not available when you had your first procedure. Your endodontist may be able to resolve your problem with retreatment.

As with any dental or medical procedure, there are no guarantees. Your endodontist will discuss your options and the chances of success before beginning retreatment.

How much will the procedure cost?

The cost varies depending on how complicated the procedure will be. The procedure will probably be more complex than your first root canal treatment, because your restoration and filling material may need to be removed to accomplish the new procedure. In addition, your endodontist may need to spend extra time searching for unusual canal anatomy. Therefore, you can generally expect retreatment to cost more than the initial endodontic treatment.

While dental insurance may cover part or all of the cost for retreatment, some policies limit coverage to a single procedure on a tooth in a given period of time. Check with your employer or insurance company prior to retreatment to be sure of your coverage.

What are the alternatives to retreatment?

If nonsurgical retreatment is not an option, then endodontic surgery should be considered. This surgery involves making an incision to allow access to the tip of the root. Endodontic surgery may also be recommended in conjunction with retreatment or as an alternative. Your endodontist will discuss your options and recommend appropriate treatment.

What are the alternatives to endodontic retreatment and/or endodontic surgery?

The only other alternative is extraction of the tooth. The extracted tooth must then be replaced with an implant, bridge, or removable partial denture to restore chewing function and to prevent adjacent teeth from shifting. Because these options require extensive surgery or dental procedures on adjacent healthy teeth, they can be far more costly and time consuming than retreatment and restoration of the natural tooth.

No matter how effective tooth replacements are—nothing is as good as your own natural tooth. You've already made an investment in saving your tooth. The payoff for choosing retreatment could be a healthy, functioning natural tooth for many years to come.

Chapter 33

Prosthodontics: Extracting, Restoring, and Replacing Teeth

Chapter Contents

Section 33.1—Overview of Prosthodontic Procedures 328

Section 33.2—Dental Implants: A Solution for Replacing
Missing Teeth 331

Section 33.3—Dentures: Frequently Asked Questions 333

Section 33.4—What Are Crowns? 337

Section 33.5—Dental Bridges 339

Section 33.1

Overview of Prosthodontic Procedures

Bridges

Traditional methods to replace a missing tooth or teeth include the
fabrication of a bridge. To replace a missing tooth with a bridge, at least
one tooth on either side of the space created by the missing tooth must
be prepared for a crown. Then a false tooth is joined to the crowns, and
the entire structure is cemented to the prepared teeth. The patient cannot remove the bridge, and special aids are available to keep it clean.

Cleft Palate/Obturator

Many cleft lip and palate patients exhibit missing teeth in the area
of the cleft and would benefit from a prosthodontist's care in the management of these areas. Although most cleft palates are now successfully closed surgically, there are patients who require an obturator to
close the palatal defect, whether it is congenital or acquired. A prosthodontist possesses the skills necessary to fabricate an obturator that
will improve the patient's speech and swallowing.

Congenital and Developmental Mouth Defects

Many patients are missing certain teeth because the teeth never
developed or may be misshapen. A prosthodontist can determine the
best way to replace and/or restore these teeth. Other patients exhibit
teeth with poorly developed tooth structure throughout the mouth and
require a prosthodontist's expertise in restoring these teeth to proper
form and function.

Crowns/Caps

Crowns cover or "cap" a tooth to restore the normal function and
appearance of the tooth. Crowns may be made as all metal, porcelain

fused to metal or all-ceramic (porcelain). Crowns are indicated for teeth with very large fillings, teeth that have had a root canal, fractured teeth, and misshapen and/or discolored teeth.

Dental Implants

Today's dental implants are typically made of titanium and may be parallel-sided or tapered and may or may not have threads. These fixtures are placed into the jawbone and allowed to heal until they are "integrated" into the bone. Dental implants may be used to replace one, many, or all of a patient's teeth.

Dentures

When a patient no longer has any natural teeth, complete dentures are the traditional method to restore function and appearance. Many patients experience difficulty wearing conventional dentures because of poor stability and decreased chewing function. The use of dental implants to improve the stability and retention of dentures is becoming quite popular.

Esthetic/Cosmetic Dentistry

Many patients are interested in improving the appearance of their smile. Prosthodontists are the dental specialists who long ago determined what constitutes a pleasing smile. Teeth whitening, reshaping natural teeth, bonding of tooth-colored material to teeth, and porcelain veneers are procedures commonly used to modify a smile.

Removable Partial Dentures

When there are multiple missing teeth, weak anchor teeth, or no posterior teeth to anchor on, a removable partial denture is used to replace teeth. These restorations typically are made of a metal framework and a plastic base with teeth. They must be removed for daily cleaning and at night.

Teeth Grinding/Night Guards

Often patients who grind their teeth at night are unaware of their habit, but the forces exerted on both the teeth and the temporomandibular joint (TMJ) can be quite destructive. A custom-made night guard can protect the teeth and relieve pressure on the TMJ.

Teeth Whitening

Many products are now available for patients to whiten their teeth. These products include commercially available strips, custom fabricated trays with a beaching gel, or bleaching in a dental office using UV light or laser as the catalyst.

TMJ

Many patients use this acronym to refer to the painful symptoms related to temporomandibular joint dysfunction. Symptoms may include pain in the joint itself, pain in the muscles of mastication, and limited movement of the lower jaw.

Sleep Apnea

Sleep apnea refers to a temporary cessation of breathing while sleeping. Many times the airway is obstructed by the patient's anatomy, and the placement of a specially designed night guard that repositions the lower jaw can improve the airflow.

Veneers

Porcelain veneers are used to modify the shape and color of teeth. Veneers are thin shells of porcelain that are etched and then bonded to the enamel of the teeth. Tooth preparation is necessary to avoid over bulking of the tooth, but it is limited to the enamel and usually involves only a few surfaces of the tooth.

Section 33.2

Dental Implants:
A Solution for Replacing Missing Teeth

"Implants," © 2008 Academy of General Dentistry
(www.agd.org).Reprinted with permission.

When people lose or break their teeth, the teeth may be replaced with implants. What's involved, and what are the benefits? Read on to learn more.

What are implants?

Dental implants are artificial tooth roots that are surgically anchored to the jaw to hold a replacement tooth or bridge in place. One of the major benefits of implants is that they do not rely on neighboring teeth for support and they are permanent and stable. Implants are a good solution to tooth loss because they look and feel like natural teeth.

What are implants made of?

Implant material is made from different types of metallic and bone-like ceramic materials that are compatible with body tissues. Most implants are made of titanium, which bonds well with bone and is biocompatible, making it an ideal material for implants.

How are implants placed?

First, a general dentist, oral surgeon, or other specialist will perform surgery to place the implant's anchor in the jaw. The surgery can last several hours, and it may take as long as 6 months for the jaw bone to grow around the anchor to hold it firmly in place. Once the implant is stable and the gums have healed, the dentist or specialist makes the artificial teeth and fits them to the post portion of the anchor. Your dentist will work with you to create an implant that fits well and is comfortable and attractive.

Who places the implants?

Depending upon their training, general dentists, oral surgeons, or other specialists can place implants.

Who should get implants?

Implants are not an option for everyone. Because implants require surgery, patients must be in good health, have healthy gums, and have adequate bone structure to support the implants. While lack of adequate bone support is a limitation, additional procedures may be available to create a good implant site. People who are unable to wear dentures also may be good candidates. The success rate for implants decreases dramatically among those who suffer from chronic problems, such as clenching or bruxism, or systemic diseases, such as diabetes. Additionally, people who smoke or drink alcohol may not be good candidates. For more information, talk to your dentist.

What is the difference between implants and dentures?

While implants are permanently fixed in the mouth, dentures are removable. A conventional removable full denture depends upon support from the bone and soft tissues rather than being solidly fixed in place; as a result, dentures may not offer as much stability as implants.

How do I care for implants?

Poor oral hygiene is a main reason why some implants fail. It is important to floss and brush around implants at least twice a day. Your dentist will give you specific instructions on how to care for your new implants. Additional dental cleanings (up to four times per year) may be necessary to ensure that you retain healthy gums.

How will I adjust to implants?

Most people adjust to implants immediately; however, some people feel slight discomfort and notice differences in chewing or speech for a short time. Patients will soon see a difference in their confidence level and enjoy their new smile.

Section 33.3

Dentures: Frequently Asked Questions

What's the difference between conventional dentures and immediate dentures?

Complete dentures are called "conventional" or "immediate" according to when they are made and when they are inserted into the mouth.

Immediate dentures are inserted immediately after the removal of the remaining teeth. To make this possible, the dentist takes measurements and makes the models of the patient's jaws during a preliminary visit.

An advantage of immediate dentures is that the wearer does not have to be without teeth during the healing period. However, bones and gums can shrink over time, especially during the period of healing in the first six months after the removal of teeth. When gums shrink, immediate dentures may require rebasing or relining to fit properly. A conventional denture can then be made once the tissues have healed. Healing may take at least 6–8 weeks.

What is an overdenture?

A removable denture that fits over a small number of remaining natural teeth or implants. The natural teeth must be prepared to provide stability and support for the denture. Your dentist can determine if an overdenture would be suitable for you.

What will dentures feel like?

New dentures may feel awkward for a few weeks until you become accustomed to them. The dentures may feel loose while the muscles of your cheek and tongue learn to keep them in place.

It is not unusual to experience minor irritation or soreness. You may find that saliva flow temporarily increases. As your mouth becomes accustomed to the dentures, these problems should diminish. One or more follow-up appointments with the dentist are generally needed after a denture is inserted. If any problem persists, particularly irritation or soreness, be sure to consult your dentist.

Will dentures make me look different?

Dentures can be made to closely resemble your natural teeth so that little change in appearance will be noticeable. Dentures may even improve the look of your smile and help fill out the appearance of your face and profile.

Will I be able to eat with my dentures?

Eating will take a little practice. Start with soft foods cut into small pieces. Chew slowly using both sides of your mouth at the same time to prevent the dentures from tipping. As you become accustomed to chewing, add other foods until you return to your normal diet.

Continue to chew food using both sides of the mouth at the same time. Be cautious with hot or hard foods and sharp-edged bones or shells.

Will dentures change how I speak?

Pronouncing certain words may require practice. Reading out loud and repeating troublesome words will help. If your dentures "click" while you're talking, speak more slowly.

You may find that your dentures occasionally slip when you laugh, cough, or smile. Reposition the dentures by gently biting down and swallowing. If a speaking problem persists, consult your dentist.

How long should I wear my dentures?

Your dentist will provide instructions about how long dentures should be kept in place. During the first few days, you may be advised to wear them most of the time, including while you sleep. After the initial adjustment period, you may be instructed to remove the dentures before going to bed. This allows gum tissues to rest and promotes oral health. Generally, it is not desirable that the tissues be constantly covered by denture material.

Should I use a denture adhesive?

Denture adhesive can provide additional retention for well-fitting dentures. Denture adhesives are not the solution for old, ill-fitting dentures. A poorly fitting denture, which causes constant irritation over a long period, may contribute to the development of sores. These dentures may need a reline or need to be replaced. If your dentures begin to feel loose, or cause pronounced discomfort, consult with your dentist immediately.

How do I take care of my dentures?

Dentures are very delicate and may break if dropped even a few inches. Stand over a folded towel or a basin of water when handling dentures. When you are not wearing them, store your dentures away from children and pets.

Like natural teeth, dentures must be brushed daily to remove food deposits and plaque. Brushing helps prevent dentures from becoming permanently stained and helps your mouth stay healthy. It's best to use a brush designed for cleaning dentures. A toothbrush with soft bristles can also be used. Avoid using hard-bristled brushes that can damage dentures.

Some denture wearers use hand soap or mild dishwashing liquid, which are both acceptable for cleaning dentures. Avoid using other powdered household cleansers, which may be too abrasive. Also, avoid using bleach, as this may whiten the pink portion of the denture.

Your dentist can recommend a denture cleanser. Look for denture cleansers with the ADA Seal of Acceptance. Products with the ADA Seal have been evaluated for safety and effectiveness.

The first step in cleaning dentures is to rinse away loose food particles thoroughly. Moisten the brush and apply denture cleanser. Brush every surface, scrubbing gently to avoid damage.

Dentures may lose their shape if they are allowed to dry out. When they are not worn, dentures should be placed in a denture cleanser soaking solution or in water. Your dentist can recommend the best method. Never place dentures in hot water, which could cause them to warp.

Ultrasonic cleaners are also used to care for dentures. However, using an ultrasonic cleaner does not replace a thorough daily brushing.

Can I make minor adjustments or repairs to my dentures?

You can seriously damage your dentures and harm your health by trying to adjust or repair your dentures. A denture that is not made to fit properly can cause irritation and sores.

See your dentist if your dentures break, crack, chip, or if one of the teeth becomes loose. A dentist can often make the necessary adjustments or repairs on the same day. A person who lacks the proper training will not be able to reconstruct the denture. This can cause greater damage to the denture and may cause problems in your mouth. Glue sold over-the-counter often contains harmful chemicals and should not be used on dentures.

Will my dentures need to be replaced?

Over time, dentures will need to be relined, rebased, or remade due to normal wear. To reline or rebase a denture, the dentist uses the existing denture teeth and refits the denture base or makes a new denture base. Dentures may need to be replaced if they become loose and the teeth show signs of significant wear. Dentures become loose because a mouth naturally changes with age. Bone and gum ridges can recede or shrink, causing jaws to align differently. Shrinking ridges can cause dentures to fit less securely. Loose dentures can cause health problems, including sores and infections. A loose denture also makes chewing more difficult and may change your facial features. It's important to replace worn or poorly-fitting dentures before they cause problems.

Must I do anything special to care for my mouth?

Even with full dentures, you still need to take good care of your mouth. Every morning, brush your gums, tongue and palate with a soft-bristled brush before you put in your dentures. This removes plaque and stimulates circulation in the mouth. Selecting a balanced diet for proper nutrition is also important for maintaining a healthy mouth.

How often should I schedule dental appointments?

Your dentist will advise you about how often to visit. Regular dental checkups are important. The dentist will examine your mouth to see if your dentures continue to fit properly. The dentist also examines your mouth for signs of oral diseases including cancer.

With regular professional care, a positive attitude and persistence, you can become one of the millions of people who wear their dentures with a smile.

Section 33.4

What Are Crowns?

A crown is a restoration that covers, or "caps," a tooth to restore it to its normal shape and size, strengthening and improving the appearance of a tooth. Crowns are necessary when a tooth is generally broken down and fillings won't solve the problem. If a tooth is cracked, a crown holds the tooth together to seal the cracks so the damage doesn't get worse. Crowns are also used to restore a tooth when there isn't enough of the tooth remaining to provide support for a large filling, attach a bridge, protect weak teeth from fracturing, restore fractured teeth, or cover badly shaped or discolored teeth.

How is a crown placed?

To prepare the tooth for a crown, it is reduced so the crown can fit over it. An impression of the teeth and gums is made and sent to the lab for the crown fabrication. A temporary crown is fitted over the tooth until the permanent crown is made. On the next visit, the dentist removes the temporary crown and cements the permanent crown onto the tooth.

Will it look natural?

Yes. The dentist's main goal is to create a crown that looks like a natural tooth. That is why your dentist takes an impression. To achieve a certain look, a number of factors are considered, such as the color, bite, shape, and length of your natural teeth. Any one of these factors alone can affect your appearance.

If you have a certain cosmetic look in mind for your crown, discuss it with your dentist at your initial visit. When the procedure is complete, your teeth will not only be stronger, but they may be more attractive.

Why crowns and not veneers?

Crowns require more tooth structure removal, hence they cover more of the tooth than veneers. Crowns are customarily indicated for teeth that have sustained significant loss of structure or to replace missing teeth. Crowns may be placed on natural teeth or dental implants.

What is the difference between a cap and a crown?

There is no difference between a cap and a crown.

How long do crowns last?

Crowns should last approximately five to eight years. However, with good oral hygiene and supervision, most crowns will last for a much longer period of time. Some damaging habits like grinding your teeth, chewing ice, or fingernail biting may cause this period of time to decrease significantly.

How should I take care of my crown?

To prevent damaging or fracturing the crown, avoid chewing hard foods, ice, or other hard objects. You also want to avoid teeth grinding. Besides visiting your dentist and brushing twice a day, cleaning between your teeth is vital with crowns. Floss or interdental cleaners (specially shaped brushes and sticks) are important tools to remove plaque from the crown area where the gum meets the tooth. Plaque in that area can cause dental decay and gum disease.

Section 33.5

Dental Bridges

One or more missing teeth can adversely affect the appearance and functionality of your smile. Missing teeth can cause a change in occlusion (bite), shifting of the teeth, temporomandibular joint disorder, speech impediments, an increased risk for periodontal disease, and a greater chance of tooth decay.

Dental bridges, like implants and partial dentures, are used to replace missing teeth. There are several types of fixed dental bridges (cannot be removed), including conventional fixed bridges, cantilever bridges, and resin-bonded bridges.

Typically, conventional and cantilever bridges require shaping of the teeth surrounding a missing tooth. Crowns are then placed on the shaped teeth and attached to an artificial tooth (called a pontic).

A resin-bonded bridge requires less preparation of adjacent teeth. It is often used to replace front teeth, provided that the gums are healthy and the surrounding teeth do not have extensive dental fillings.

The Dental Bridge Procedure

During the first visit, your dentist examines the health of your gums and other teeth to evaluate if you are a candidate for a dental bridge. If you are a candidate for a dental bridge, you are given a local anesthetic so your dentist can prepare the teeth required to support the bridge. If the support teeth are decayed or badly broken down, your dentist may have to build them back up before they can be used as support teeth for a bridge.

Next, your dentist takes an impression of the prepared teeth with a putty-like material that is used to create a model of your teeth. Your bridge is fabricated based on this model by a skilled lab technician so that it precisely fits the prepared teeth. It is important that your restoration fit perfectly to avoid additional oral health problems such as tooth decay.

While your bridge is being fabricated, your dentist fits you with a temporary bridge so the teeth and gums can be protected from damage until your permanent bridge is ready.

To complete the dental bridge procedure, you must return to the dental office for a second visit to have the bridge fitted and cemented.

The Cost of Dental Bridges

The cost of dental bridges depends on several factors, including:

- the potential need for additional procedures (such as fillings or root canals) in one or two of the adjoining teeth;

- the artistic technique of the dentist and lab technician;

- the location of the dentist;

- the coverage provided by your dental insurance;

- the type of material used in the bridge; and

- the preparation of teeth involved in the bridge procedure.

Dental bridges can range in price from $1,000 to $3,000 per tooth based on the aforementioned factors. If you exercise proper dental hygiene and visit your dentist for regular checkups, your bridges can last for many years. There are a number of variables that can affect bridge longevity, though it is not uncommon for a dental bridge to last for 10 to 20 years.

Chapter 34

Orthodontics: Treating Bite Problems

Chapter Contents

Section 34.1—All about Orthodontia 342

Section 34.2—Overview of Braces and Appliances 347

Section 34.3—Straight Talk on Braces 349

Section 34.4—The Reality of Retainers 357

Section 34.1

All about Orthodontia

Just getting braces and have no idea what to expect? Had braces for a while but wonder what's going on in there? Whatever your situation is, you're not alone—millions of teens have braces. Braces are a totally normal and practically expected part of puberty (and many adults get braces, too).

Why Do People Need Braces?

To better understand why braces and other orthodontic devices are needed, it helps to talk a bit about the teeth first. You probably don't remember your very first set of tiny teeth, but you had 20 of them when you were young. (The first ones probably came in when you were about 6 months old, and you most likely had all of them by the time you reached age 3.)

As you made your way through childhood, these teeth fell out one by one, to be replaced by permanent, adult teeth. If you're 14 or older, it's pretty likely that you have 28 of your permanent teeth in place; four more will grow in as you get a little older to create a complete set of 32 teeth. These last four teeth are commonly known as "wisdom teeth."

The basic makeup of every tooth in your mouth is the same, and they all grow out of the same place: from down within the jawbones, which are surrounded by the gums. And although some people's adult teeth grow out from the gums at the right angle and with the right spacing, many people's teeth don't.

Some teeth may grow in crooked or overlapping. In other people, some teeth may grow in rotated or twisted. Some people's mouths are too small, and this crowds the teeth and causes them to shift into crooked positions.

And in some cases, a person's upper jaw and lower jaw aren't the same size. When the lower half of the jaw is too small, it makes the upper jaw hang over when the jaw is shut, resulting in a condition called an overbite. When the opposite happens (the lower half of the jaw is larger than the upper half), it's called an underbite.

All of these different types of disorders go by one medical name: malocclusion. This word comes from Latin and means "bad bite." In most cases, a "bad bite" isn't anyone's fault; crooked teeth, overbites, and underbites are often inherited traits, just like brown eyes or big feet are inherited traits.

In some cases, things like dental disease, early loss of baby or adult teeth, some types of medical problems, an accident, or a habit like prolonged thumb sucking can cause the disorders.

Malocclusion can be a problem because it interferes with proper chewing—crooked teeth that aren't aligned properly don't work as well as straight ones. Because chewing is the first part of eating and digestion, it's important that teeth can do the job. Teeth that aren't aligned correctly can also be harder to brush and keep clean, which can lead to tooth decay and cavities. And finally, many people who have crooked teeth may feel self-conscious about how they look; braces can help them feel better about their smile and whole face.

If a dentist suspects that a kid or teen needs braces or other corrective devices, he or she will refer the patient to an orthodontist. Orthodontists are dentists who have special training in the diagnosis and treatment of misaligned teeth and jaws. Most regular dentists can tell if teeth will be misaligned once a patient's adult teeth begin to come in—sometimes as early as age 6 or 7—and the orthodontist may recommend interceptive treatment therapy. (Interceptive treatment therapy involves the wearing of appliances to influence facial growth and help teeth grow in better, and helps prevent more serious problems from developing.) In many cases, the patient won't be referred to an orthodontist until closer to the teen years.

Diagnosis

First the orthodontist will need to reach a diagnosis before deciding on treatment. Reaching the diagnosis means making use of several different tools, including X-rays, photographs, and impressions.

The X-rays give the orthodontist a good idea of where the teeth are positioned and if any more teeth have yet to come through the gums. Special X-rays that are taken from 360 degrees around the head may also be ordered; this type of X-ray shows the relationships of the teeth to the jaws and the jaws to the head.

The orthodontist may also take regular photographs of the patient's face to help him or her understand these relationships better. And finally, the orthodontist may need an impression made of the patient's teeth. This is done by having the patient bite down on a mushy material that is used later to form an exact copy of the teeth.

Treatment

Once a diagnosis is made, the orthodontist can then decide on the right kind of treatment. In some cases, a removable retainer will be all that's necessary. In other rare cases (especially when there is an extreme overbite or underbite), an operation will be necessary. But in most cases, the answer is braces.

Braces straighten teeth because they do two very important things: stay in place for an extended amount of time, and exert steady pressure. It's this combination that allows braces to successfully change the arrangement of teeth in a patient's mouth, periodically adjusted by the orthodontist.

An orthodontist can outfit patients with a few different kinds of braces. Some braces are made of a lightweight metal and go around each tooth, while other metal ones are attached to the outside surfaces of the teeth with special glue. Clear braces can be attached to the outside surfaces of the teeth, as can ceramic ones that are the same color as teeth. Some patients can get newer "mini-braces," which are much smaller, or "invisible braces," which are affixed to the inside surfaces of the teeth. In many cases, the patient can choose which kind he or she wants.

Once the orthodontist puts on the braces, they will usually remain on the patient's teeth for anywhere from 6 months to 2 years. In some cases, the braces may need to remain on for more than 2 years.

After the amount of time needed for correction has been established for the patient, the orthodontist must work on the other part of the treatment: making sure the braces exert steady pressure. To achieve this, the patient must come for regular visits, usually once a month or so. During the visits, the orthodontist attaches wires, springs, or rubber bands to the braces in order to create more tension and pressure on the teeth. Sometimes the rubber bands will connect certain teeth to one another to create a kind of opposing tension.

With some teens, the orthodontist may decide that extra tension is needed outside the mouth—when braces alone aren't enough to straighten the teeth or shift the jaw. In cases like these, a patient may need to wear head or neck gear with wires that attach inside the mouth and elastic that attaches the gear to the head. Many times, a patient will only need to wear this type of gear at night or in the evening, while at home.

It may take a while, but with the right combination and timing of wires, springs, rubber bands, and sometimes head gear, the teeth will slowly but surely move into their correct positions.

During this period of time, it can help to know that you're not alone when you go for your adjustments—but that won't necessarily make you feel any better if your teeth hurt! Some of the adjustments can make your mouth feel a bit sore or uncomfortable because the tension tends to make itself felt in more places than your teeth. Most of the time, taking ibuprofen or acetaminophen can help relieve the pain. If you always have a lot of pain after your braces are adjusted, talk to your orthodontist about it; he or she may able to make the adjustments a bit differently.

Caring for Teeth with Braces

Your orthodontist will also make sure that you know how to take special care of your teeth while your braces are on. Braces, wires, springs, rubber bands, and other appliances can act like magnets for food and plaque, which can leave permanent stains on the teeth if not brushed away. Most orthodontists recommend brushing after meals with fluoride toothpaste and taking special care to remove food stuck in braces. Some orthodontists will also prescribe or recommend a fluoride mouthwash, which can get into places in a mouth with braces that a toothbrush can't.

Some people with braces find that they are more prone to canker sores (from the braces hitting the inside surface of the mouth). If this happens, an orthodontist may recommend an over-the-counter medicine that can be placed directly on the canker sore to help heal it.

Faces after Braces

After what can seem like a long time to someone who has braces, the magic day finally comes: the orthodontist takes the braces off! After your teeth are cleaned thoroughly, the orthodontist may actually want to repeat the process of taking X-rays and impressions of the teeth. This allows the orthodontist to really check the work, and in the case of X-rays, see if wisdom teeth are now visible.

In some cases, an orthodontist may recommend that a patient have the wisdom teeth pulled if they are starting to come in after the braces have been removed. The reason? The wisdom teeth can cause the newly straightened teeth to shift and move in the mouth.

And speaking of teeth shifting and moving, a very important part of a person's post-braces treatment is retention, or keeping the teeth in their new place. The truth is that most teens, after wearing braces and going for adjustments for up to 2 years or longer, don't want anything to do with the orthodontist or having appliances in their mouths. But even though the teeth have been successfully moved with braces, they are still not completely stable—they need to settle in their corrected positions until the bones, gums, and muscles adapt to the change. This is usually accomplished with the use of retainers, which work by retaining the straight position of the teeth.

Some retainers are made of clear plastic and metal wires that cover the outside surface of the teeth, whereas others are made of rubber. Most retainers need to be worn all the time for the first 6 months, then usually only during sleeping. How long a retainer must be worn depends on the patient—one person might wear it for a few months, while another might have to wear it for several years. Whatever the timeframe, retainers are very important; without them, the teeth could shift back into their old, crooked positions, making all the orthodontist's work and your years of patience useless!

The most important things to remember when you're feeling frustrated about having a face full of braces? That during every school photo where you can't be persuaded to open your mouth because of your braces, there are millions of other people experiencing the same thing. And that no matter what, your braces will come off eventually—and you'll be left with a wonderful, straight smile.

Section 34.2

Overview of Braces and Appliances

The purpose of this text is to illustrate different types of common orthodontic and orthopedic appliances. Orthodontists use many different types of appliances, the word for braces or other devices, to move or stabilize teeth and jaws. Sometimes an orthodontic treatment involves more than just moving the teeth. The official name of the specialty is orthodontics and dentofacial orthopedics. Let's look at what that means.

- Ortho- means to straighten, -dontic, or dento- means teeth, so orthodontics means to straighten teeth.

- -facial- means the face and jaws and -pedics- means "the child," so dentofacial orthopedics means to straighten or correct the face and jaws of the child.

Orthodontists do more than align teeth; they modify and correct problems with facial growth. Different orthodontic appliances are used for different purposes in an orthodontic treatment. Some are designed to primarily move teeth (orthodontic), while others are used orthopedically to modify facial growth. Some appliances have both orthodontic and orthopedic treatment effects.

Appliances come in two types: ones that are fixed, or don't come out, and ones the patient can take out. The kind the patients can take out are called removable. The orthodontist selects either fixed or removable appliances based on an individual patient's treatment needs and how much cooperation or compliance (following the orthodontist's instructions) can be expected from the patient. Removable appliances are easier to keep clean, but can be lost or misplaced. Fixed appliances are worn all the time and are often indicated for problems that require a more aggressive or time-sensitive treatment. Patients who have trouble wearing removable appliances can often be treated with fixed appliances.

Fixed Appliances

Examples of fixed orthodontic appliances are the brackets, bands, and wires most often associated with braces. Brackets can be made of metal, ceramic, or plastic or combinations of these materials. Some metal brackets are silver-colored, but some are gold-colored. Ceramic brackets are typically clear or tooth-colored and are generally used by patients who want to minimize the visibility of their braces.

Pendex appliances, distal jet appliances, and coil springs of different materials are used primarily to move teeth. Devices such as Forsus springs or Jasper jumpers are often used in place of elastics, but all share a common purpose of making upper and lower teeth fit together better. Lip bumpers may be used for patients with lower arch crowding.

Your orthodontist may also use some fixed devices to hold teeth in place while other teeth are moved. These common appliances include lingual holding arches, Nance appliances, and transpalatal arches. A quad helix is an appliance made of heavy wire that moves teeth, but can also have an orthopedic effect. These types of appliances may have other names, but have common uses.

Examples of fixed orthopedic appliances are the various types of palate expanders and functional appliances. Palatal expanders are used to make the upper jaw wider. The Hyrax and Haas expanders are examples. Functional appliances are used to normalize growth discrepancies between the upper and lower jaw. Examples of these are the Herbst appliance, twin block, and Mara appliances. These are typically worn over extended periods of time.

Removable Appliances

Removable orthodontic appliances can have many shapes and appearances. Retainers are examples of one type. Retainers usually just hold teeth in their new positions after active orthodontic treatment (braces) is complete, but springs or elastics can be added to these types of appliances to move teeth. Rubber bands, or elastics, are used in almost every treatment to help move teeth into a correct position.

Expanders and tooth movers come in many shapes and forms. The orthodontist can prescribe and construct individual appliances suited to a patient's individual and unique needs.

There are also removable orthopedic functional appliances that help correct growth discrepancies. Bionators and Frankel appliances are examples of those. Various types of headgears are also commonly used removable orthopedic correctors. Some, such as cervical pull or high pull, help to correct conditions when the lower jaw growth does not keep up with upper jaw growth, while other types, such as reverse pull headgear, face masks, and chin cups, help when upper jaw growth does not keep up with lower jaw growth.

Orthodontists select the type of appliance that suits each patient's needs from these and other appliances. As you can see, appliances can be as different as each patient seeking orthodontic treatment. You can trust your orthodontist to choose the appropriate appliance for your treatment because orthodontists have two to three academic years of university-based specialty training in orthodontics and dentofacial orthopedics.

Section 34.3

Straight Talk on Braces

From "Straight Talk on Braces," by Linda Bren, *FDA Consumer* magazine (www.fda.gov/fdac), published by the U.S. Food and Drug Administration (FDA), January 2005.

"Heavy metal bands" may conjure up images of rock music today, but many baby boomers remember them as the clunky and conspicuous devices they wore in their mouths as children to straighten their teeth.

Today's braces are a lot different from the metal-mouth look of a generation ago. "They're more aesthetic and more efficient," says Donald Joondeph, D.D.S., an associate professor of orthodontics at the University of Washington in Seattle. And they're more comfortable to wear and better at repositioning teeth, he adds.

Braces used to be put on only after all the permanent teeth came in. Today, a multitude of dental devices, or orthodontic appliances, are being used at an early age to simplify later treatment, provide a better outcome, and, in some cases, avoid braces altogether. Adults, who make up one fifth of orthodontic patients, also are opting for straighter teeth as more choices in orthodontic appliances become available.

About 4.5 million people in the United States are wearing braces or other appliances to achieve a beautiful smile and healthy teeth, according to the American Association of Orthodontists (AAO). These appliances are regulated by the Food and Drug Administration to assure their safety and effectiveness.

Not Just for Looks

Braces are more than the means to a stunning smile—they can improve dental health and function, says Susan Runner, D.D.S., chief of the Dental Devices Branch in the FDA's Center for Devices and Radiological Health. "They can be used to move teeth that are over-crowding," Runner says. Crowded or crooked teeth are harder to brush and floss, and improper cleaning can lead to tooth decay and other dental problems.

"Braces can correct severe bite problems that would hamper eating and give a greater risk of gum disease and tooth and bone loss," says Runner. Bite problems may occur when the upper and lower jaw don't come together properly. Uncorrected bite problems can cause teeth to wear down, make for difficult chewing, and put stress on the jawbone, producing pain.

Causes of Crooked Teeth

Most people do not have naturally straight teeth; in fact, the AAO estimates that up to 75 percent of people could benefit from orthodontic care.

Heredity and environmental factors are the two causes of crooked teeth and bite problems, says Terry Pracht, D.D.S., president of the AAO and an orthodontist in Westerville, Ohio. Crowding of teeth, too much space between teeth, and upper teeth that don't match lower teeth when biting down are usually inherited. But jaw-jolting accidents, as well as habits such as tongue thrusting and thumb sucking, can cause crooked teeth.

Tongue thrusting is the abnormal tendency to push the tongue onto the back of the front teeth during swallowing, causing the teeth to protrude over time.

Thumb sucking is normal in young children and isn't an orthodontic problem unless it persists when the permanent teeth come in, says Pracht. "If a child is still thumb sucking at about age 7 when the upper front teeth start to erupt, it can not only affect the teeth, but the shape of the jawbone," he says.

Then and Now

Braces work by putting pressure against the teeth, moving them gradually over time. Most of the pressure is applied by a metal wire, called an archwire, that runs on the outside of the teeth. "Rubber" bands, actually made from surgical latex, put additional pressure on the teeth that the archwire alone cannot do.

Earlier types of braces had an archwire connected to large metal bands that were individually wrapped and cemented around each tooth. "The metal bands were uncomfortable," says Pracht, adding that it used to hurt to have braces put on and adjusted. "There was a lot of pushing and shoving."

Today, the archwire is attached to tiny brackets made of metal or ceramic. The brackets are bonded with a glue-type agent to the front of the teeth. Some of the bonding agents continuously release fluoride to help protect the enamel of the teeth underneath the brackets. Metal bands may still be used on the back teeth, but they are smaller and lighter than bands used previously.

The archwire requires periodic adjustment or replacement by the orthodontist to apply continuous pressure. Today's archwires are active over longer periods of time, meaning patients don't have to visit the orthodontist as often to get their braces adjusted. "It used to be every three to four weeks; now it's every six to eight weeks," says Pracht. And archwires are much gentler. "There is some sensitivity when eating for only a day or two after an adjustment."

Archwires now are made from a heat-activated, nickel-titanium mixture originally developed by NASA to activate solar panels of spacecraft in orbit. At room temperature, the wires are very flexible, allowing them to be attached to the teeth more easily. When they warm to mouth temperature, they apply gradual and constant pressure on the teeth.

Today's braces come with more options to make them less obvious— or, if a person chooses—more obvious, with an element of fun and fashion. Most of Pracht's adult patients opt for clear or tooth-colored brackets. "They are not apparent from a distance and not very noticeable up close," he says. Some people choose gold braces. "One company markets them as jewelry for the mouth," says Pracht.

Colors are especially popular with children and teens, who will often choose the colors of their school, a favorite sports team, or holiday colors, such as pink and red for Valentine's Day and orange and black for Halloween. The colors are mainly on the elastic ties that attach the archwire to the brackets, and they can be changed when the archwire is adjusted. Archwires and rubber bands also come in a variety of hues.

For complete invisibility, braces can be fitted onto the inside of the teeth. These "lingual braces" have limitations, says Joondeph. "They can be tougher on a patient. They affect speech more and may irritate the tongue." Treatment times may also be longer than with standard braces, he says, adding that patients should talk with their orthodontists to find out if lingual braces or other options are appropriate for them.

Innovations in materials and designs have brought braces a long way since the "tin-grin" look of the past, but one thing that hasn't changed significantly is the length of time they are worn. "It's important to move the teeth gradually," says Runner. "If you move the teeth too fast, it can result in severe loosening of the teeth or tooth loss."

Braces, on average, are left on between 20 and 24 months, says Joondeph. To keep teeth straight after braces are removed, people must wear retainers. These appliances hold the teeth in their corrected position until the bones grow around the teeth to stabilize them. Since teeth tend to shift as a person ages, wearing retainers periodically may be a lifelong requirement.

Retainers can be all plastic or plastic with some metal wire. They are either fixed permanently in the mouth or are removable. Like braces, retainers come in different colors and designs. They can be roof-of-the-mouth pink or personalized with such items as sports team logos, pictures of pets, or a person's or orthodontist's phone number in case of loss.

The FDA's Role

Braces, retainers, and other orthodontic appliances are classified as medical devices, which are regulated by the FDA. "Any innovative orthodontic devices or materials require FDA review before being allowed on the market," says Runner. In this way, the FDA can assure that any new devices or materials, including bonding agents and color dyes, are safe and effective.

Some older orthodontic appliances are exempt from review because they were already on the market in 1976, the year medical device regulations went into effect. "But medical device manufacturers are still required to register with the FDA and are subject to inspections," says Runner.

As with all medical devices, braces are not risk-free. The FDA has received reports of adverse events ranging from teeth broken during bracket removal to allergic reactions involving archwire and bracket materials.

"If you're going to have an allergic reaction, it will usually be to the nickel in the wires," says Pracht. Orthodontists can fit patients with titanium wires and brackets that don't contain nickel, he says.

And as for the risk of locking braces when kissing, Pracht says it only happens in the movies. "In my 33 years of practice, I've never seen it."

A Commitment

Having braces or any other orthodontic appliance requires more frequent brushing, flossing, and general care. "Orthodontics is a serious treatment commitment," says Janie Fuller, D.D.S., M.P.H., a regulatory review officer in the FDA's Office of Surveillance and Biometrics.

"If you have poor oral hygiene, you are trading one problem for another," adds Joondeph. "Your bite may be better and your teeth straighter, but there will be significant decay."

People with braces must avoid "hard, sticky, or gooey foods," says Joondeph, such as jawbreakers, peanuts, ice cubes, caramel, and taffy. These foods can break brackets, bend wires, or get caught in the braces, causing cavities.

Fuller advises parents to clean the teeth of young children. "Children shouldn't be expected to have the dexterity to clean their teeth properly until at least 8 or 9 years old, and parents need to help even without braces," she says.

And older children must want the braces and be willing to make the commitment to their care. "The work you have to do to take care of your mouth is too hard if you don't really want braces," says Fuller. "It's not just something that you have done to you—it takes a partnership with your orthodontist for it to work."

Joondeph uses a "combination of education and prodding" with children who are reluctant to get braces. "One option is to try to convince the child it's in their best interest in the long-term. We can also try to come up with a treatment plan that would expedite treatment." There's always the option of treatment later as an adult, but by then the jaw has stopped growing and some bite problems can be corrected only with surgery, he says.

Another Straightening Option

An alternative to braces, Invisalign, was cleared by the FDA to straighten crooked teeth in people who have all of their second molars, permanent teeth that usually come in by the late teens. Invisalign uses a series of clear removable aligners instead of wires and brackets. An orthodontist takes impressions of the teeth and sends these models to the maker of Invisalign, Align Technology Inc., of Santa Clara, California. The company uses a computer-generated simulation of the desired movement of the teeth to custom-make the aligners for each patient. Each aligner is worn for about two weeks.

The aligners are removable for eating, brushing, and flossing, so unlike people who wear braces, Invisalign-wearers aren't restricted from eating hard or chewy foods. But they still must visit their orthodontist every six weeks during treatment to ensure proper progress.

The total treatment time with Invisalign averages between nine and 15 months and the average number of aligners worn during treatment is between 18 and 30, according to Align Technology. For some people, a combination of braces and Invisalign is successful, requiring less time in traditional braces.

"Invisalign is intended to have the same function as braces in terms of gradual tooth movement," says Runner. But the device is not for everybody. "It depends on the extent of the orthodontic problem, and it is not intended for younger children," she says.

"They have a place in the spectrum of orthodontic treatments for mild to moderate cases," Joondeph adds. "But they can't give us the sophisticated tooth movement and control of braces."

Appliances for Children

Other orthodontic appliances besides braces are available to help correct a broad range of tooth and jaw problems in growing children—from closing up a gap to widening the jaw to make room for new teeth to grow in properly. Some of these "functional orthodontics" are fixed in place; others are removable for brushing, eating, and sleeping.

Some children require headgear to guide the development of an improperly growing upper jaw. To move the jaw, wires must connect the upper teeth to another fixed point. Since no other teeth are strong enough to serve as a fixed point, headgear is used to anchor the upper teeth to a point outside the mouth: the head or neck. Elastic is wrapped around the top of the head or the back of the neck and connects an archwire to the upper teeth.

"Make sure the orthodontist demonstrates how to place the device and how to remove it," cautions Fuller. In one case reported to the FDA, a child was blinded in one eye and injured in the other when removing headgear improperly, causing the metal prongs from the mouthpiece to snap back into the child's face in a slingshot-like fashion.

"Never leave the office with headgear—or any other removable appliance—until you have demonstrated to the staff that you know how to remove the device safely and put it back in safely to avoid injury and to optimize treatment," says Fuller.

In some cases, a dental implant can replace the need for headgear. The implant contains a screw or pin that is inserted into the jawbone, allowing a post to protrude. The post serves as a point of stabilization to which a tooth-moving appliance is attached.

Functional orthodontics are ineffective after about age 16 for women and after age 18 for men. At these ages, the permanent teeth are in place and the jaw is set, so only braces or jaw surgery can produce straight teeth or a normal bite.

Early Is Better, But It's Never Too Late

Although healthy teeth can be moved at almost any age, the AAO recommends that children get an orthodontic exam by age 7. Many will not need treatment then, but periodic checkups can help the orthodontist detect and evaluate problems early and determine the best time to treat them.

"This is the time you can see permanent teeth erupt and you can determine the size of the teeth, the room available, and the relationship of the teeth to the jaws," says Joondeph.

In some cases, early treatment can guide jaw growth and permanent teeth into better position, avoid the need to extract teeth, and reduce abnormal swallowing or speech problems. Waiting until all the permanent teeth have come in or until facial growth is complete may make correction of some problems more difficult, as Wendy Kelly of Issaquah, Washington, will tell you.

Kelly, who didn't get braces as a child, had crowded teeth and an overbite. At 31, she was getting headaches and having problems chewing, she says. "I was only able to chew in the front of my mouth because my back teeth didn't meet when I bit down."

Joondeph, Kelly's orthodontist, informed her that braces alone wouldn't fix the problem. She also needed oral surgery to reposition the jaws so that her teeth would fit together properly. After wearing braces for 10 months, Kelly had surgery under general anesthesia, spent a night in the hospital, and continued wearing braces for several more months.

"In the old days, it was a hopeless situation," says Pracht. But today, this type of surgery, called orthognathic surgery, can improve both function and appearance for people with severe skeletal problems such as a "Dick Tracy" jaw that juts out. "It's done from inside the mouth," he says. "Nobody cuts on the face." In the early days of this surgery, the jaw was wired together for months. "Now we use little titanium screws," says Pracht, one on either side of the jaw.

"The end result is so fantastic," says Kelly, adding that her headaches are gone, she can chew without pain, and she can eat foods, such as steak, that she avoided before. But she admits that the recovery was rough. "I had a ton of pain," she says. "I was very swollen, and my jaw movement was so limited I couldn't really eat for awhile." She lost 15 pounds while recovering.

Kelly wanted to save her two girls from a similar painful experience, she says. The girls accompanied her to orthodontic appointments and got to know the staff so "they didn't have any fear" when they got their own braces at ages 7 and 9. The staff "had a very gentle way," she says, advising other parents to choose an orthodontist who talks to the child directly and explains the treatment thoroughly.

Joondeph, who treats all ages, says he has put braces on people in their 70s and 80s, as long as their gums and bones supporting the teeth are healthy. "They're the kind of people who are very vital and active," he says. "Typically, they've always wanted to have it done and for some reason they did not."

Section 34.4

The Reality of Retainers

You've probably seen a kid in the cafeteria take out his retainer before eating lunch. Carefully, he places it in a plastic container to make sure that it's safe while he eats. You can tell that this small plastic and metal mouthpiece is important to him. You might wonder why. Let's find out.

What's a Retainer?

A retainer is a piece of plastic and metal that is custom-made for each individual kid who needs one. It fits the top of the teeth and mouth. No two retainers are alike, even though many look similar. Retainers are really common. In fact, most people (kids and adults) who have braces have to wear a retainer for at least a little while after getting their braces taken off. Other people wear them to close gaps in their teeth, to help with speech problems, or to solve certain medical problems.

Why Do I Need to Wear a Retainer?

There are different reasons why you might need a retainer. The most common reason is to help your teeth stay set in their new positions after wearing braces. It's important to wear your retainer because as your body grows, your teeth do some shifting. The retainer helps to control this shifting, which occurs naturally.

After your braces are removed, your orthodontist (a special dentist who helps straighten teeth and correct jaw problems) will fit you for a retainer. He or she will tell you how long to wear it and when.

For example, you might have to wear it all day for 3 months but then only at night after that. Some kids may wear their retainer only at night right from the start, but they may have to wear it for more than a year. The retainer keeps the teeth in line and you won't even notice it while you're sleeping!

Other kids may wear retainers to close a space between their teeth or just to move one tooth. In these cases, braces aren't needed because retainers can do the job. Often, retainers will be worn for several years to close a space, for example, and then keep the gap closed by holding the teeth in place. When you wear a retainer for any reason, certain teeth may feel pressure and might even feel sore for the first few days. If you experience this, don't worry—it's completely normal.

Retainers can help many mouth problems besides shifting teeth. Sometimes they're used to help a medical problem. For example, you may have a tongue thrust (a condition where your tongue sneaks through your teeth when you talk). Some retainers, known as a crib or tongue cage retainers, are designed with small metal bars that hang down from the roof of your mouth. These retainers keep your tongue from going forward in between your teeth when you speak. Your tongue is trained to go to the roof of your mouth instead of through your teeth. The length of time kids wear a tongue cage varies depending on the kid.

Another use for retainers is to help people with temporomandibular disorder (TMD). This disorder is usually a result of a bite problem (the teeth don't meet together properly when the jaws are closed) called malocclusion (say: mal-uh-kloo-zhun) or bruxism (say: bruk-sih-zum), which is grinding your teeth while you sleep. Grinding stretches the muscles and joints in your mouth and jaws and sometimes can cause jaw pain or headaches. Retainers can help you by preventing your mouth from closing completely at night, which keeps you from grinding your teeth.

Getting Fitted for and Wearing a Retainer

This is the easy part. Your orthodontist will fit you for the retainer using a material known as alginate (say: al-juh-nate). It's a chewy, chalky kind of thick liquid that makes a mold of your teeth when you sink them into it. The fitting process is fast, painless, and doesn't even taste bad—and you can choose from different flavors.

Your finished retainer can be designed to express your style and likes. Sometimes you can have a picture such as Batman, Christmas trees, or Halloween bats on the plastic part of the retainer. Once you've been fitted for the retainer, you usually have to wait less than a week to get the real thing.

You may think your retainer feels weird at first. That's normal. But see your orthodontist for an adjustment if the retainer causes pain or cuts or rubs against your gums. At first, you'll need to get used to talking with it in your mouth. Talking slowly at first is a good way to practice and eventually, you won't even notice it's there. Dentists advise reading aloud for several minutes each day. You may also notice an increased saliva flow (more spit in your mouth) in the first few days of wearing your new retainer, which is normal.

Caring for Your Retainer

Retainers live in your mouth along with bacteria, plaque, and left-over food particles. You should clean your retainer every day, but make sure to check with your orthodontist about how your type of retainer should be cleaned (some kinds shouldn't be cleaned with toothpaste). You can also soak it in mouthwash or a denture-cleaning agent to freshen it up and kill germs.

Because the plastic of your retainer can crack if it gets too dry, you should always soak it when it isn't in your mouth. Plastic can warp easily, so don't put it in hot water or leave it near a heat source—like on your radiator, for example. Finally, do not bend the wires. Flipping the retainer around in your mouth will cause the wires to bend.

One important way to take care of your retainer is not to lose it. They are expensive and your mom or dad might have to pay for lost or damaged retainers. Worse yet, they might ask you to help pay for a new one! So look before you dump your lunch tray and try to keep it in the same spot at home when you're not wearing it. In other words, retain your retainer!

Chapter 35

Orthodontics for All Ages

Chapter Contents

Section 35.1—Space Maintenance in Young Children:
Saving Room for Permanent Teeth 362

Section 35.2—Childhood Orthodontic Treatment 363

Section 35.3—Adolescent Orthodontic Treatment 371

Section 35.4—Can Adults Wear Braces? 376

Section 35.1

Space Maintenance in Young Children: Saving Room for Permanent Teeth

Why do children lose their baby teeth?

A baby tooth usually stays in until a permanent tooth underneath
pushes it out and takes its place. Unfortunately, some children lose a
baby tooth too soon. A tooth might be knocked out accidentally or removed because of dental disease. When a tooth is lost too early, your
pediatric dentist may recommend a space maintainer to prevent future space loss and dental problems.

Why all the fuss? Baby teeth fall out eventually on their own!

Baby teeth are important to your child's present and future dental health. They encourage normal development of the jaw bones and
muscles. They save space for the permanent teeth and guide them into
position. Remember: Some baby teeth are not replaced until a child
is 12 or 14 years old.

How does a lost baby tooth cause problems for permanent teeth?

If a baby tooth is lost too soon, the teeth beside it may tilt or drift
into the empty space. Teeth in the other jaw may move up or down to
fill the gap. When adjacent teeth shift into the empty space, they create a lack of space in the jaw for the permanent teeth. So, permanent
teeth are crowded and come in crooked. If left untreated, the condition may require extensive orthodontic treatment.

What are space maintainers?

Space maintainers are appliances made of metal or plastic that are
custom fit to your child's mouth. They are small and unobtrusive in

appearance. Most children easily adjust to them after the first few days.

How does a space maintainer help?

Space maintainers hold open the empty space left by a lost tooth. They steady the remaining teeth, preventing movement until the permanent tooth takes its natural position in the jaw. It's more affordable—and easier on your child—to keep teeth in normal positions with a space maintainer than to move them back in place with orthodontic treatment.

What special care do space maintainers need?

Pediatric dentists have four rules for space maintainer care. First, avoid sticky sweets or chewing gum. Second, don't tug or push on the space maintainer with your fingers or tongue. Third, keep it clean with conscientious brushing and flossing. Fourth, continue regular dental visits.

Section 35.2

Childhood Orthodontic Treatment

"Want information about orthodontic treatment for children? (Through age 12)," © 2006 American Association of Orthodontists (www.braces.org). Reprinted with permission.

Some children as early as 5 or 6 years of age may benefit from an orthodontic evaluation. Although treatment is unusual at this early age, some preventative treatment may be indicated.

By age 7, most children have a mix of baby (primary) and adult (permanent) teeth. Some common orthodontic problems seen in children can be traced to genetics, that is, they may be inherited from their parents. Children may experience dental crowding, too much space between teeth, protruding teeth, and extra or missing teeth and sometimes jaw growth problems.

Other malocclusions (literally, "bad bite") are acquired. In other words, they develop over time. They can be caused by thumb or finger-sucking, mouth breathing, dental disease, abnormal swallowing, poor dental hygiene, the early or late loss of baby teeth, accidents, or poor nutrition. Trauma and other medical conditions such as birth defects may contribute to orthodontic problems as well. Sometimes an inherited malocclusion is complicated by an acquired problem. Whatever the cause, the orthodontist is usually able to treat most conditions successfully.

Orthodontists are trained to spot subtle problems with jaw growth and emerging teeth while some baby teeth are still present. The advantage for patients of early detection of orthodontic problems is that some problems may be easier to correct if they are found and treated early. Waiting until all the permanent teeth have come in, or until facial growth is nearly complete, may make correction of some problems more difficult. For these reasons, the AAO [American Association of Orthodontists] recommends that all children get a checkup with an orthodontist no later than age 7. While your child's teeth may appear straight to you, there could be a problem that only an orthodontist can detect. Of course, the checkup may reveal that your child's bite is fine, and that is comforting news.

Even if a problem is detected, chances are your orthodontist will take a "wait-and-see" approach, checking your child from time to time as the permanent teeth come in and the jaws and face continue to grow. For each patient who needs treatment, there is an ideal time for it to begin in order to achieve the best results. The orthodontist has the expertise to determine when the treatment time is right. The orthodontist's goal is to provide each patient with the most appropriate treatment at the most appropriate time.

In some cases, your orthodontist might find a problem that can benefit from early treatment. Early treatment may prevent more serious problems from developing and may make treatment at a later age shorter and less complicated. For those patients who have clear indications for early orthodontic intervention, early treatment gives your orthodontist the chance to:

- Guide jaw growth
- Lower the risk of trauma to protruded front teeth
- Correct harmful oral habits
- Improve appearance and self-esteem
- Guide permanent teeth into a more favorable position

- Improve the way lips meet

It's not always easy for parents to tell if their child has an orthodontic problem. Here are some signs or habits that may indicate the need for an orthodontic examination:

- Early or late loss of baby teeth
- Difficulty in chewing or biting
- Mouth breathing
- Thumb sucking
- Finger sucking
- Crowding, misplaced, or blocked out teeth
- Jaws that shift or make sounds
- Biting the cheek or roof of the mouth
- Teeth that meet abnormally or not at all
- Jaws and teeth that are out of proportion to the rest of the face

If any of these problems are noted by parents, regardless of age, it is advisable to consult an orthodontist. It is not necessary to wait until age 7 for an orthodontic checkup.

What is preventive orthodontic treatment?

Preventive orthodontic treatment is intended to keep a malocclusion ("bad bite" or crooked teeth) from developing in an otherwise normal mouth. The goal is to provide adequate space for permanent teeth to come in. Treatment may require a space maintainer to hold space for a primary (baby) tooth lost too early, or removal of primary teeth that do not come out on their own so to create room for permanent teeth.

What is interceptive orthodontic treatment?

Interceptive orthodontic treatment is performed for problems that, if left untreated, could lead to the development of more serious dental problems over time. The goal is to reduce the severity of a developing problem and eliminate the cause. The length of later comprehensive orthodontic treatment may be reduced. Examples of this kind of orthodontic treatment may include correction of thumb- and finger-sucking habits; guiding permanent teeth into desired positions through tooth removal or tooth size adjustment; or gaining or holding space for permanent teeth. Interceptive orthodontic treatment can take place when patients have primary teeth or mixed dentition (baby and permanent teeth). A patient may require more than one phase of interceptive orthodontic treatment.

What is comprehensive orthodontic treatment?

Comprehensive orthodontic treatment is undertaken for problems that involve alignment of the teeth, how the jaws function, and how the top and bottom teeth fit together. The goal of comprehensive orthodontic treatment is to correct the identified problem and restore the occlusion (the bite) to its optimum. Treatment can begin while patients have primary teeth, when they have a mix of primary and permanent teeth, or when all permanent teeth are in. Treatment may consist of one or more phases, depending on the nature of the problem being corrected and the goals for treatment.

Orthodontic care may be coordinated with other types of dental treatment that may include oral surgery (tooth extractions or jaw surgery), periodontal (gum) care, and restorative (fillings, crowns, bridges, tooth size enhancement, implants) dental care. When finished with comprehensive treatment, the patient must wear retainers to keep teeth in their new positions.

What is a space maintainer?

Baby molar teeth, also known as primary molar teeth, hold needed space for permanent teeth that will come in later. When a baby molar tooth is lost, an orthodontic device with a fixed wire is usually put between teeth to hold the space for the permanent tooth.

Why do baby teeth sometimes need to be removed?

Removing baby teeth may be necessary to allow severely crowded permanent teeth to come in at a normal time in a reasonably normal location. If the teeth are severely crowded, it may be that some unerupted permanent teeth (usually the canine teeth) will either remain impacted (teeth that should come in, but do not), or come in to a highly undesirable position. To allow severely crowded teeth to move on their own into much more desirable positions, sequential removal of baby teeth and permanent teeth (usually first premolars) can dramatically improve a severe crowding problem. This sequential extraction of teeth, called serial extraction, is typically followed by comprehensive orthodontic treatment after eruption of permanent teeth has brought about as much improvement as it can on its own.

After all the permanent teeth have come in, the extraction of selected permanent teeth may be necessary to correct crowding or to make space for necessary tooth movement to correct a bite problem. Proper extraction of teeth during orthodontic treatment should leave the patient with both excellent function and a pleasing look.

How can a child's growth affect orthodontic treatment?

Orthodontic treatment and a child's growth can complement each other. A common orthodontic problem to treat is protrusion of the upper front teeth. Quite often this problem is due in part to the lower jaw being shorter than the upper jaw. Upper teeth may also be the primary cause of the protrusion if they stick out too far. While the upper and lower jaws are growing, orthodontic appliances can be beneficial in reducing these discrepancies. A severe jaw growth discrepancy may require orthodontics and corrective surgery after jaw growth has been completed, although this is rare.

The AAO recommends that all children have a checkup with an orthodontist no later than age 7 so that growth-related problems may be identified and so that treatment can be commenced at the appropriate time for each patient.

What kinds of orthodontic appliances are typically used to reduce the severity of jaw-growth problems?

A process of dentofacial orthopedics (guiding the growth of the face and jaws) with orthodontic appliances may be used to correct jaw-growth problems. The decision about when and which appliances to use for this type of correction is based on each individual patient's problem. Some of the more common orthopedic appliances include:

- **Headgear:** This appliance applies pressure to the upper teeth and upper jaw to guide the direction of upper jaw growth and tooth eruption. The headgear may be removed by the patient and is usually worn 10 to 12 hours per day.

- **Fixed functional appliance:** The appliance is usually fixed (glued) to the upper and lower molar teeth and may not be removed by the patient. By holding the lower jaw forward, it

reduces the protrusion of the teeth while the patient is growing and helps bring the teeth together. The appliance can help
correct severe protrusion of the upper teeth.

- **Removable functional appliance:** This removable appliance holds the lower jaw forward and guides eruption of the
  teeth into a more desirable bite while helping the upper and
  lower jaws to grow in proportion to each other. Patient compliance in wearing this appliance is essential for successful improvement; the appliance cannot work unless the patient
  wears it.

- **Palatal Expansion Appliance:** A child's upper jaw may be
  too narrow for the upper teeth to fit properly with the lower
  teeth (a crossbite). When this occurs, a palatal expansion appliance can be fixed to the upper back teeth. This appliance can
  markedly expand the width of the upper jaw. For some patients,
  a wider jaw may prevent the need for extraction of permanent
  teeth.

Can my child play sports while wearing braces?

Yes. But wearing a protective mouth guard is advised while riding
a bike, skating, or playing any contact sports, whether organized
sports or a neighborhood game. Your orthodontist can recommend a
specific mouth guard.

Will braces interfere with playing musical instruments?

Playing wind or brass instruments, such as the trumpet, will
clearly require some adaptation to braces. With practice and a period
of adjustment, braces typically do not interfere with the playing of
musical instruments.

Why does orthodontic treatment time sometimes last longer than anticipated?

Estimates of treatment time can only be that—estimates. Patients
grow at different rates and will respond in their own ways to orthodontic treatment. The orthodontist has specific treatment goals in
mind, and will usually continue treatment until these goals are
achieved. Patient cooperation, however, is the single best predictor of
staying on time with treatment. Patients who cooperate by wearing
rubber bands, headgear, or other needed appliances as directed, while

taking care not to damage appliances, will most often lead to on-time and excellent treatment results.

What is patient cooperation and how important is it during orthodontic treatment?

Good "patient cooperation" means that the patient not only follows the orthodontist's instructions on wearing appliances as prescribed and tending to oral hygiene and diet, but is also an active partner in orthodontic treatment.

Successful orthodontic treatment is a "two-way street" that requires a consistent, cooperative effort by both the orthodontist and patient. To successfully complete the treatment plan, the patient must carefully clean his or her teeth, wear rubber bands, headgear, or other appliances as prescribed by the orthodontist, avoid foods that might damage braces and keep appointments as scheduled. Damaged appliances can lengthen the treatment time and may undesirably affect the outcome of treatment. The teeth and jaws can only move toward their desired positions if the patient consistently wears the forces to the teeth, such as rubber bands, as prescribed. Patients who do their part consistently make themselves look good and their orthodontist look smart.

To keep teeth and gums healthy, regular visits to the family dentist must continue during orthodontic treatment.

I recently took my child to an orthodontist for an orthodontic checkup. The orthodontist recommended treatment. Should I seek a second opinion?

You should review the recommended treatment with your family dentist. If you would like a second opinion, feel comfortable in arranging one. You may have already had more than one orthodontist recommended to you by family, friends, or your dentist. Seeking out a member of the AAO assures that your second opinion is from an educationally qualified orthodontic specialist. You should feel confident in the orthodontist and his or her staff, and trust their ability to provide you with the best possible care.

What is two-phase treatment?

Two-phase treatment simply means that the treatment is carried out in two stages. The first is the interceptive orthodontic phase and the second is the comprehensive orthodontic phase.

Some of my children's friends have already started treatment, but our orthodontist says my child should wait a while. Why is there a difference in treatment?

Each treatment plan is specific for that child and his/her specific problem. In some cases, children mature early (e.g., get their permanent teeth early) and in some cases early treatment is indicated to prevent a more severe problem from occurring. Your orthodontist is the best person to decide the most optimum treatment plan. If you have questions, you should discuss them with your orthodontist.

What do the initials mean after an orthodontist's name?

The initials after an orthodontist's name indicate the academic education of the orthodontist. For instance, D.M.D. and D.D.S. indicate that the individual is a graduate dentist. M.S. or MSc indicates that the individual has achieved a Masters in Science degree, usually associated with orthodontic training. DipOrtho indicates the individual is an orthodontist.

Are there board-certified orthodontists?

Yes, these orthodontists have completed the American Board of Orthodontics Specialty Certification exams and have met these qualifications. Board-certified orthodontists are known as Diplomates of the American Board of Orthodontics. The American Board of Orthodontics is the only orthodontic specialty certifying board recognized by the American Dental Association.

My child has an allergy to nickel. Can my child still have orthodontic treatment?

Yes, there are appliances available which are nickel-free. Please tell your orthodontist if your child has any allergies.

How can I fit the orthodontist's fee into my family budget?

Orthodontic costs and payment options can be discussed with your treating orthodontist. Your orthodontist will be able to provide you with information about insurance and other possible funding options.

Section 35.3

Adolescent Orthodontic Treatment

Most patients begin orthodontic treatment between ages 9 and 16, but this varies depending on each individual. Because teenagers are still growing, the teen years are often the optimal time to correct orthodontic problems and achieve excellent results.

Most orthodontic problems are inherited. Examples of these genetic problems are crowding, too much space between teeth, protruding upper teeth, extra or missing teeth, and some jaw growth problems.

Other malocclusions (crooked teeth) are acquired. In other words, they develop over time. They can be caused by thumb-sucking or finger-sucking as a child, mouth breathing, dental disease, abnormal swallowing, poor dental hygiene, the early or late loss of baby (primary) teeth, accidents, poor nutrition, or some medical problems.

Sometimes an inherited malocclusion is complicated by an acquired problem. But whatever the cause, the orthodontist is usually able to treat most conditions successfully.

Treatment is important because crooked or crowded teeth are hard to clean, and that may contribute to tooth decay, gum disease, and tooth loss. A bad bite can also cause abnormal wear of tooth surfaces, difficulty in chewing and/or speaking, excess stress on supporting bone and gum tissue, and possible jaw joint problems. Without treatment, problems may become worse. Orthodontic treatment to correct a problem may prove less costly than the additional dental care required to treat the problems that can develop in later years.

Then there's the emotional side of an unattractive smile. When you are not confident in the way you look, your self-esteem suffers. Teenagers whose malocclusions are left untreated may go through life feeling self-conscious, hiding their smiles with tight lips or a protective hand.

371

How do braces feel?

Most people have some discomfort after their braces are first put on or when adjusted during treatment. After the braces are on, teeth may become sore and may be tender to biting pressures for three to five days. Patients can usually manage this discomfort well with whatever pain medication they might commonly take for a headache. The orthodontist will advise patients and/or their parents what, if any, pain relievers to take. The lips, cheeks, and tongue may also become irritated for one to two weeks as they toughen and become accustomed to the surface of the braces. Orthodontic wax applied to an offending bracket will help relieve discomfort. Overall, orthodontic discomfort is short-lived and easily managed. Once patients have become accustomed to their braces, they may even forget they have them on.

Are there less noticeable braces?

Today's braces are generally less noticeable than those of the past. The brackets are smaller and are bonded directly to the teeth, minimizing the "tin grin." Brackets can be metal or clear depending on the patient's preference. In some cases, brackets may be bonded behind the teeth (lingual braces). Some of today's wires are made of "space age" materials that exert a steady, gentle pressure on the teeth, so that the tooth-moving process may be faster and more comfortable for patients. A type of clear orthodontic wire is currently in an experimental stage. Another option may be the use of a series of plastic tray aligners instead of traditional braces to correct some problems. Your orthodontist will advise which type of orthodontic appliance will best correct your problem.

Do teeth with braces need special care?

Yes. Patients with braces must be careful to avoid hard, sticky, chewy, and crunchy foods. They must not chew on pens, pencils, or fingernails because chewing on hard things can damage the braces. Damaged braces will almost always cause treatment to take longer, and will require extra trips to the orthodontist's office.

Keeping the teeth and braces clean requires more precision and time, and must be done every day if the teeth and gums are to be healthy during and after orthodontic treatment. Patients who do not keep their teeth clean may require more frequent visits to the dentist for a professional cleaning. The orthodontist and staff will teach patients how to care for their teeth, gums, and braces during treatment.

The orthodontist will tell patients (and/or their parents) how often to brush, how often to floss, and, if necessary, suggest other cleaning aids that might help the patient maintain good dental health.

A good reason to keep teeth, gums, and braces clean during orthodontic treatment is that clean, healthy teeth move more quickly! This will help keep treatment time as short as possible.

Patients who are active in contact sports, whether in organized programs or just games in the neighborhood, should wear a mouth guard. Talk with your orthodontist about the kind of mouth guard to use while braces are on.

What is patient cooperation and how important is it during orthodontic treatment?

Good "patient cooperation" means that the patient not only follows the orthodontist's instructions on oral hygiene and diet, but is also an active partner in orthodontic treatment.

Successful orthodontic treatment is a "two-way street" that requires a consistent, cooperative effort by both the orthodontist and patient. To successfully complete the treatment plan, the patient must carefully clean his or her teeth, wear rubber bands, headgear, or other appliances as prescribed by the orthodontist, avoid foods that might damage braces, and keep appointments as scheduled. Damaged appliances can lengthen the treatment time and may undesirably affect the outcome of treatment. The teeth and jaws can only move toward their desired positions if the patient consistently wears the forces to the teeth, such as rubber bands, as prescribed. Patients who do their part consistently make themselves look good and their orthodontist look smart.

To keep teeth and gums healthy, regular visits to the family dentist must continue during orthodontic treatment.

How long does treatment take?

Although every case is different, generally speaking, patients wear braces from one to three years. Treatment times vary with factors that include the severity of the problem, patient growth, gum and bone response to tooth moving forces, and how well the patient follows the orthodontists' instructions on dental hygiene, diet, and appliance wear (patient cooperation). Patients who brush and floss thoroughly and regularly; avoid hard, sticky, crunchy, and sticky foods; wear their rubber bands and/or headgear as instructed; and keep their appointments usually finish treatment on time with good results. After the braces are removed, most patients wear a retainer for some time to keep or "retain" the teeth in their new positions. The orthodontist will determine how long the retainer needs to be worn. Most patients remain under the orthodontist's supervision during the retention phase to ensure that the teeth stay properly aligned.

Why are retainers needed after orthodontic treatment?

After braces are removed, the teeth can shift out of position if they are not stabilized. Retainers are designed to hold teeth in their corrected, ideal positions until the bones and gums adapt to the treatment changes. Wearing retainers exactly as instructed is the best insurance that the treatment improvements last longer. It is normal for teeth to change with increasing age.

Will tooth alignment change later?

Studies have shown that as people age, their teeth may shift. This variable pattern of gradual shifting, called maturational change, probably slows down after the early 20s, but still continues to a degree throughout a lifetime for most people. Even children whose teeth developed into ideal alignment and bite without treatment may develop orthodontic problems as adults. The most common maturational change is crowding of the lower incisor (front) teeth. Wearing retainers as instructed after orthodontic treatment will stabilize the correction and can prevent most of this change.

What about the wisdom teeth (third molars)—should they be removed?

Research suggests that wisdom teeth do not necessarily cause teeth to shift. In most cases, removal of wisdom teeth is done for general dental health reasons rather than for orthodontic health. Your orthodontist, in consultation with your family dentist, can provide guidance regarding removal of wisdom teeth.

What happens to teeth and gums if they are not kept clean during orthodontic treatment?

Teeth can develop white spots, called "decalcification," when an individual's teeth are susceptible or when oral hygiene has been poor. If plaque is not regularly removed, the patient can develop gum disease. This is why the orthodontist, orthodontic staff, the dentist and dental hygienist stress dental hygiene—for the good of the patient's dental health.

What can I do to get my braces off sooner?

Follow the instructions your orthodontist gives you with regards to oral hygiene (keeping your teeth and gums clean) and wearing your appliances (e.g., elastics, headgear, etc.) Your cooperation may help speed up your treatment.

What will I look like with braces on?

Much will depend on the kind of braces used for your treatment. Many patients have silver-colored brackets and wires while others may have tooth-colored brackets or clear plastic aligners. Braces are much less noticeable today than they were when each tooth had a metal band around it.

Do you have any suggestions on what foods I can eat?

Choose foods that are softer. Right after you get braces or whenever they are adjusted, you may want foods that require little or no chewing such as soup and macaroni and cheese. Cut or tear sandwiches and pizza rather than biting into them.

What happens if something breaks?

If a portion of the appliance breaks, let your orthodontist know so that arrangements can be made for repairs.

My child wants to get his/her tongue pierced. Will this interfere with orthodontic treatment?

Tongue-piercing jewelry may contribute to breakage of appliances and to tooth and gum damage from contact with the stud.

Section 35.4

Can Adults Wear Braces?

Today, orthodontic treatment is a viable option for almost any adult. It is well recognized that when left untreated, many orthodontic problems may become worse. When you have a malocclusion ("bad bite"), your teeth may be crowded, excessively spaced, or may not fit together correctly. Such conditions may lead to dental health problems. Crowded teeth are hard to clean and, given time, may contribute to tooth decay, gum disease, and even tooth loss. Bad bites can also result in abnormal wearing of tooth surfaces, difficulty chewing, and damage to supporting bone and gum tissue. Poorly aligned teeth can contribute to pain in the jaw joints.

You'll be pleased to learn that orthodontic treatment will fit in with your current lifestyle—you can sing, play a musical instrument, dine out, kiss, and even have your picture taken. One in five orthodontic patients is an adult. The AAO estimates that more than 1,000,000 adults in the United States and Canada are receiving treatment from orthodontists who are members of the AAO.

The rate of toothlessness has declined over recent decades. Our great-grandparents, for the most part, lost their teeth around age 40. Today's 25-year-old has the potential of another 75 years of keeping and using their teeth. This is a major change in dental health care (and life expectancy). Teeth that do not fit well often wear down more quickly—another reason to make sure that your teeth are in good alignment and well maintained in your adult years.

Can orthodontic treatment do for me what it does for children?

Yes. Healthy teeth can be moved at any age. Many orthodontic problems can be corrected as easily for adults as for children. Orthodontic forces move the teeth in the same way for both adults and children, but adult treatment may take longer due to the maturity of the bone. Complicating factors, such as lack of jaw growth, may create different treatment planning needs for the adult. This is why a consultation with an orthodontist, the dental specialist who aligns teeth and jaws of patients of all ages, is essential.

How does adult treatment differ from that of children and adolescents?

Adults are not growing and may have experienced some breakdown or loss of their teeth and the bone that supports the teeth. Orthodontic treatment may then be only a part of the patient's overall treatment plan. Close coordination may be required among the orthodontist, oral surgeon, periodontist, endodontist, and family dentist to assure that the treatment plan is managed well. Below are the most common characteristics that can cause adult treatment to differ from that of children.

No jaw growth: Jaw discrepancy problems, including both width and length, in the adult patient may require jaw surgery. For example, if an adult's lower jaw is too short to match properly with the upper jaw, a severe bite problem results. The amount that the teeth can be moved in some cases, with braces alone, may not correct this problem. Establishing a proper bite relationship could require jaw surgery, which would lengthen the lower jaw and bring the lower teeth forward into the proper bite.

Gum or bone loss (periodontal breakdown): Adults are more likely to have experienced damage or loss of the gum and bone supporting their teeth (periodontal disease). Periodontal disease is a chronic bacterial infection that affects the gums and bone supporting the teeth. The word periodontal literally means "around the tooth." Many people are unaware that they have gum disease because there is usually little or no pain.

Periodontal disease can affect one tooth or many teeth. It begins when the bacteria in plaque (the sticky, colorless film that constantly forms on your teeth) causes inflammation in the gums.

The mildest form of the disease is called gingivitis. The gums redden, swell, and bleed easily. Gingivitis is often linked to inadequate oral hygiene. Gingivitis is often reversible with professional treatment and good oral home care.

Untreated gingivitis can advance to periodontitis, a more severe form of gum disease. With time, plaque can spread and grow below the gum line. Toxins produced by the bacteria in plaque irritate the gums. The toxins stimulate a chronic inflammatory response in which the body, in essence, turns on itself, and the tissues and bone that support the teeth are broken down and destroyed. Gums separate from the teeth, forming pockets (spaces between the teeth and gums) that become infected. As the disease progresses, the pockets deepen and more gum tissue and bone are destroyed. Eventually, teeth can become loose and may have to be removed.

The good news is that teeth that are properly aligned are less prone to gum disease.

Special treatment by the patient's dentist or a periodontist may be necessary before, during, and/or after orthodontic treatment. Bone loss can also limit the amount and direction of tooth movement that is advisable. Adults who have a history of or concerns about periodontal disease might also see a periodontist (a dental specialist who treats diseases of the gums and bone) on a regular basis throughout orthodontic treatment.

Worn, damaged, or missing teeth: Worn, damaged, or missing teeth can make orthodontic treatment more difficult. Teeth may gradually wear and move into positions where they can be restored only after precise orthodontic movement. Damaged or broken teeth may not look good or function well even after orthodontic treatment unless they are carefully restored by the patient's dentist. Extra space resulting from missing teeth that are not replaced may cause progressive tipping and drifting of other teeth, which worsens the bite, increases the potential for periodontal problems, and makes any treatment more difficult.

I have painful jaw muscles and jaw joints—can an orthodontist help?

One of the problems commonly associated with jaw muscle and jaw joint discomfort is bruxing, that is, habitual grinding or clenching of the teeth, particularly at night. Bruxism is a muscle habit pattern that can cause severe wearing of the teeth, and overloading and trauma to the jaw joint structures. Chronically or acutely sore and painful jaw muscles may accompany the bruxing habit. An orthodontist can help diagnose this problem. Your family dentist or orthodontist may place a bite splint or nightguard appliance that can protect the teeth and help jaw muscles relax, substantially reducing the original pain symptoms. Sometimes structural damage can require joint surgery and/or restoration of damaged teeth. Referral to a TMJ [temporomandibular joint] specialist may be suggested for some of these problems.

*My family dentist said I need to have some missing teeth
replaced, but I need orthodontic treatment first—why?*

Your dentist is probably recommending orthodontics so that he or
she might treat you in the best manner possible to bring you to optimal dental health. Many complicated tooth restorations, such as
crowns, bridges, and implants, can be best accomplished when the
remaining teeth are properly aligned and the bite is correct.

When permanent teeth are lost, it is common for the remaining
teeth to drift, tip, or shift. This movement can create a poor bite and
uneven spacing that cannot be restored properly unless the missing
teeth are replaced. Tipped teeth usually need to be straightened so
they can withstand normal biting pressures in the future.

*My teeth have been crooked for many years—why should I
have orthodontic treatment now?*

It's never too late. Orthodontic treatment, when indicated, is a positive step—especially for adults who have endured a long-standing problem. Orthodontic treatment can restore good function. And teeth that
work better usually look better, too. A healthy, beautiful smile can improve self-esteem, no matter the age.

Is orthodontic treatment affordable?

Patients are finding that braces are more affordable today than
ever. The cost of orthodontic treatment will depend on many factors,
including the severity of the problem, its complexity and the length
of treatment. Your orthodontist will be glad to discuss the cost with
you before treatment begins. Most orthodontists have a variety of convenient payment plans. Often there are combined plans available for
parents and children who have treatment at the same time. In addition, many dental insurance plans now include orthodontic benefits.
Dollar for dollar, when you consider the lifetime benefits of orthodontics, it is truly a great value.

*I am pregnant and want to begin orthodontic treatment. Is
this OK?*

Pregnancy brings on bodily changes that can affect the mouth. Soft
tissues such as gums become much more susceptible to infection. The
possible need for x-rays during the pregnancy is not advised. Discuss
this question with your medical practitioner/physician and orthodontist before you start orthodontic treatment.

My orthodontist wants to do something called enamel stripping to make my teeth smaller. I have never heard of this. Is this something new? Is it safe?

This procedure goes by many names: enamel stripping; interproximal reduction; slenderizing; reproximation and selective reduction. The goal is to remove some of the outer tooth surface (enamel) to acquire more space for your teeth. The procedure has been used in orthodontic treatment since the 1940s and has been shown to be safe and effective. Some studies among patients who have had this procedure show that it neither makes teeth more susceptible to tooth decay nor does it predispose patients to gum disease.

I see ads for perfect teeth in only one or two visits to the dentist. Will that give me straight teeth?

Crooked teeth should be evaluated by an orthodontist so that the most appropriate treatment plan can be suggested.

Chapter 36

Cosmetic Dentistry: Improving Your Teeth's Appearance

Chapter Contents

Section 36.1—How Can My Dentist Improve My Smile?......... 382

Section 36.2—What Should You Ask Your Dentist about
Tooth Whitening Treatments? 384

Section 36.3—Veneers 386

Section 36.4—Enamel Microabrasion 387

Section 36.5—Decorative Dental Grills: Wearers Should
Be Careful 389

Section 36.1

How Can My Dentist Improve My Smile?

"How Can My Dentist Improve My Smile?," © 2007 Academy
of General Dentistry (www.agd.org). Reprinted with permission.

From subtle changes to major repairs, your dentist can perform a variety of procedures to improve your smile. There are many techniques and options to treat teeth that are discolored, chipped, misshapen, or missing. Your dentist can reshape your teeth, close spaces, restore worn or short teeth, or alter the length of your teeth. Common procedures include bleaching, bonding, crowns, veneers, and reshaping and contouring.

These improvements are not always just cosmetic. Many of these treatments can improve oral problems, such as your bite.

Bleaching

Bleaching is a common and popular chemical process used to whiten teeth. Some people get their teeth bleached to make stains disappear, while other just want a whiter shade.

Discoloration occurs in the enamel and can be caused by medication, coffee, tea, and cigarettes. Discoloration also can be hereditary or due simply to getting older.

Bleaching can be performed by your dentist in the office or, under dental supervision, at home. Many patients enjoy bleaching at home because it is more convenient. Treatment begins when your dentist creates a custom mouthpiece to ensure the correct amount of whitening solution is used and that your teeth are properly exposed. Typically, whitening at home takes two to four weeks, depending on the desired shade you wish to achieve. Whitening in the office may call for one or more 45-minute to one-hour visits to your dentist's office.

Bonding

Bonding is tooth-colored material used to fill in gaps or change the color of teeth. Requiring a single office visit, bonding lasts several years.

Bonding is more susceptible to staining or chipping than other forms of restoration. When teeth are chipped or slightly decayed, bonded composite resins may be the material of choice. Bonding also is used as a tooth-colored filling for small cavities. Additionally, it can be used to close spaces between teeth or cover the entire outside surface of a tooth to change its color and shape.

Crowns

Crowns, also known as caps, cover a tooth to restore it to its normal shape and appearance. Due to their cost, they are used in cases where other procedures will not be effective. Crowns have the longest life expectancy of all cosmetic restorations, but are the most time-consuming.

Veneers

Veneers are thin pieces of porcelain or plastic placed over the front teeth to change the color or shape of your teeth. Veneers are used on teeth with uneven surfaces or are chipped, discolored, oddly shaped, unevenly spaced, or crooked. Little or no anesthesia is needed. Veneers are used to treat some of the same problems as bonding.

This treatment is an alternative to crowns, which are more expensive. The procedure requires your dentist to take an impression of your tooth. Before the custom-made veneer is cemented directly onto the tooth, your dentist will lightly buff the tooth to compensate for the added thickness of the veneer. Once the cement is between the veneer and your tooth, a light beam is used to harden it. Porcelain veneers require more than one visit because they are fabricated in a laboratory. Veneers have a longer life expectancy and color stability than bonding.

Contouring and Reshaping

Tooth reshaping and contouring is a procedure to correct crooked teeth, chipped or irregularly shaped teeth, or even overlapping teeth in a single session. Tooth reshaping and contouring is commonly used to alter the length, shape, or position of your teeth. Contouring teeth may also help correct small problems with bite. It is common for bonding to be combined with tooth reshaping.

This procedure is ideal for candidates with normal, healthy teeth but who want subtle changes to their smile. Your dentist will take x-rays to evaluate the size and location of the pulp of each tooth to ensure that there's enough bone between the teeth to support them.

Which Procedure Is Right for Me?

Your dentist can answer any questions you may have about techniques used to improve your smile. The condition of your teeth and desired result you want often dictates the best procedure. If you are considering a treatment, there are a few questions you can ask your dentist before deciding if a particular procedure is right for you.

- What will the changes look like?
- What should I expect through the course of treatment?
- What type of maintenance will be required?

Section 36.2

What Should You Ask Your Dentist about Tooth Whitening Treatments?

What should you ask your dentist?

You may want to start by speaking with your dentist. He or she can tell you whether whitening procedures would be effective for you. Whiteners may not correct all types of discoloration. For example, yellowish hued teeth will probably bleach well, brownish-colored teeth may bleach less well, and grayish-hued teeth may not bleach well at all. Likewise, bleaching may not enhance your smile if you have had bonding or tooth-colored fillings placed in your front teeth. The whitener will not affect the color of these materials, and they will stand out in your newly whitened smile. In these cases, you may want to investigate other options, like porcelain veneers or dental bonding.

What is in-office bleaching?

If you are a candidate for bleaching, your dentist may suggest a procedure that can be done in his or her office. This procedure is called chairside bleaching and may require more than one office visit. Each visit may take from 30 minutes to one hour.

During chairside bleaching, the dentist will apply either a protective gel to your gums or a rubber shield to protect the oral soft tissues. A bleaching agent is then applied to the teeth, and a special light may be used to enhance the action of the agent. Lasers have been used during tooth whitening procedures to enhance the action of the whitening agent.

What are at-home procedures and products?

There are several types of products available for use at home, which can either be dispensed by your dentist or purchased over-the-counter.

Bleaching solutions: These products contain peroxide(s), which actually bleach the tooth enamel. These products typically rely on percent carbamide peroxide as the bleaching agent, carbamide peroxide comes in several different concentrations (10%, 16%, 22%).

Peroxide-containing whiteners typically come in a gel and are placed in a mouth guard. Usage regimens vary. Some products are used for about twice a day for 2 weeks, and others are intended for overnight use for 1-2 weeks. If you obtain the bleaching solution from your dentist, he or she can make a custom-fitted mouth guard for you that will fit your teeth precisely. Currently, only dentist-dispensed home-use 10% carbamide peroxide tray-applied gels carry the ADA [American Dental Association] Seal.

You also may want to speak with your dentist should any side effects become bothersome. For example, teeth can become sensitive during the period when you are using the bleaching solution. In many cases, this sensitivity is temporary and should lessen once the treatment is finished. Some people also experience soft tissue irritation—either from a tray that doesn't fit properly or from solution that may come in contact with the tissues. If you have concerns about such side effects, you should discuss them with your dentist.

Toothpastes: All toothpastes help remove surface stain through the action of mild abrasives. "Whitening" toothpastes in the ADA Seal of Acceptance program have special chemical or polishing agents that provide additional stain removal effectiveness. Unlike bleaches, these ADA Accepted products do not alter the intrinsic color of teeth.

How should I choose a whitening product?

When selecting a whitener or any dental product, be sure to look for the ADA Seal of Acceptance—your assurance that they have met ADA standards of safety and effectiveness.

Section 36.3

Veneers

"Veneers: A Facelift for Your Teeth," *Word of Mouth*, Summer-Fall 2005. © 2005 Massachusetts Dental Society (www.massdental.org). Reprinted with permission.

With the abundance of makeover reality television shows and contests for free makeovers populating the airwaves, odds are that you have heard the term "veneers" in recent months. In many of these "extreme" makeover cases, veneers are used to fix badly stained front teeth and improve less-than-perfect smiles. But how do you know if veneers are the right choice for you?

Before deciding how best to treat stained front teeth, a professional cleaning is in order to determine whether the staining is from too many cups of coffee, a lot of red wine, or just too many years on earth. Front teeth that have been stained over the years can often be made more attractive with dental treatment. Depending on the degree of discoloration and the shape of the teeth, bleaching may be the best option. However, tooth whitening can only lighten the color of the teeth; when the size and shape of the teeth require adjustments to improve their appearance, either veneers or full crowns need to be considered. And when dramatic changes to the shape or position of the teeth are necessary, full crowns are a better choice.

Veneers are very much like artificial fingernails in that they are glued to the front surface of the eight upper front teeth. They produce a smooth, attractive surface on the front of the teeth, the part that shows when you smile. Sometimes, this can be accomplished without removing any of the tooth surfaces. However, most of the time, the front surface of the teeth has to be shaved down to make room for enough plastic or porcelain to cover the stain and to achieve a natural look. It's important to remember that this procedure is permanent. Unlike artificial fingernails, you can't take veneers off if you don't like them.

For younger people, treating only the upper teeth with bleach, veneers, or crowns is often adequate because that is all that shows when they speak or smile. As we age, however, we tend to see more and more of the lower teeth and less of the upper teeth. Therefore, for older people, just treating the upper front teeth does not usually achieve the desired result.

Consult your dentist if you have any questions about veneers or any other cosmetic dentistry procedure.

Section 36.4

Enamel Microabrasion

"Enamel Microabrasion," © 2008 American Academy of
Pediatric Dentistry (www.aapd.org). Reprinted with permission.

What is microabrasion?

In microabrasion, dentists carefully rub a compound on the teeth to remove superficial stains and discoloration.

Why are my child's teeth discolored?

A number of conditions can cause discoloration of permanent teeth. For example, trauma to a baby tooth, an infection around a baby tooth, and high fevers or prolonged chronic illnesses during childhood can cause discolorations. Fluoride can also cause some white or brown discolorations of teeth when a child receives a high dose over a period of time.

Some teeth have a deeper, irreversible stain or discoloration, the result of trauma, root canal therapy, or medications such as tetracycline. These deep stains are not improved by microabrasion.

Will microabrasion work for my child?

The success of microabrasion depends on a number of factors, especially the type and extent of discoloration. So, it is difficult to predict when microabrasion will remove a discoloration completely from a tooth. Pediatric dentists have learned that brown or dark stains are removed readily in most cases. White discolorations are often improved; sometimes they are totally eliminated. Other times, white discolorations are very persistent and not removed completely with microabrasion.

Some teeth have a "speckled" appearance, showing a lot of white spots all over the tooth. These teeth may be improved with microabrasion. By removing the bright white spots, the teeth will have a slightly darker, but more even, natural color.

What if microabrasion doesn't work?

Microabrasion is a safe, minimal treatment of discolored teeth. Attempting microabrasion does not eliminate any of the alternatives for treatment. Other treatments for discolored teeth are plastic or porcelain veneers or porcelain crowns. These options are less affordable and more extensive than microabrasion because they require some tooth preparation. So, it's wise to consider microabrasion as your first choice of treatment for discolored teeth.

Section 36.5

Decorative Dental Grills: Wearers Should Be Careful

"Dental Grills (Grillz or Fronts)," http://www.ada.org/
public/topics/grills.asp. © 2008 American Dental Association.
All rights reserved. Reprinted with permission.

Some celebrities have been flashing more than clean, white teeth at their fans. Under the spotlight, the glint from their mouths comes from "grills" or "grillz"—decorative covers often made of gold, silver, or jewel-encrusted precious metals that snap over one or more of their teeth.

Grills, sometimes called "fronts," generally are removable but some wearers have had their teeth altered with gold crowns to permanently resemble a grill. And some have tried to attach their grill with permanent cement—something that is not meant for internal use and can damage the teeth and tissues!

At present there are no studies that show that grills are harmful to the mouth—but there are no studies that show that their long-term wear is safe, either. Some grills are made from non-precious (base) metals that may cause irritation or metal-allergic reactions.

Boy Meets Grill

The trend toward tooth coverings was boosted in recent years by hip-hop icons and rappers such as Nelly and Paul Wall. Although wealthy musicians and some athletes have spent thousands of dollars to decorate their teeth with grills made of gold and platinum, most teenagers and young adults who want to emulate these celebrities do so by purchasing inexpensive do-it-yourself kits online or purchasing them from local jewelers. Some jewelers and other "grill" vendors are unaware that, in some states, taking an impression of someone's mouth is considered dentistry, which requires a license.

Wearers should be especially careful about brushing and flossing to prevent potential problems. Food and other debris may become trapped between the teeth and the grill allowing bacteria to collect and produce acids. The acids can cause tooth decay and harm gum tissue. Bacteria may also contribute to bad breath. There also is the potential for grills to irritate surrounding oral tissues and to wear the enamel away on the opposing teeth.

To prevent problems, wearers should limit the amount of time spent wearing removable grills.

If you already wear a grill, you should remove it before eating. It should be cleaned daily to remove plaque bacteria and food debris. Avoid using jewelry cleaners or any products that are dangerous to ingest.

If you are considering getting a dental grill, make sure you talk to your dentist first. Find out exactly what materials the grill is made of and avoid creating a breeding ground for bacteria. Grills might be trendy for the moment, but "pearly whites" will never go out of style.

Part Six

Jaw and Mouth Disorders

Chapter 37

Trigeminal Neuralgia: A Common Cause of Orofacial Pain

What is trigeminal neuralgia?

Trigeminal neuralgia (TN), also called tic douloureux, is a chronic pain condition that affects the trigeminal or 5th cranial nerve, one of the largest nerves in the head. The disorder causes extreme, sporadic, sudden burning or shock-like face pain that lasts anywhere from a few seconds to as long as two minutes per episode. These attacks can occur in quick succession. The intensity of pain can be physically and mentally incapacitating.

The trigeminal nerve is one of 12 pairs of cranial nerves that originate at the base of the brain. The nerve has three branches that conduct sensations from the upper, middle, and lower portions of the face, as well as the oral cavity, to the brain. The ophthalmic, or upper, branch supplies sensation to most of the scalp, forehead, and front of the head. The maxillary, or middle, branch passes through the cheek, upper jaw, top lip, teeth and gums, and to the side of the nose. The nerve's mandibular, or lower, branch passes through the lower jaw, teeth, gums, and bottom lip. More than one nerve branch can be affected by the disorder.

What causes trigeminal neuralgia?

The presumed cause of TN is a blood vessel pressing on the trigeminal nerve as it exits the brainstem. This compression causes the wearing

"Trigeminal Neuralgia Fact Sheet," from the National Institute of Neurological Disorders and Stroke (NINDS, www.ninds.nih.gov), part of the National Institutes of Health, May 9, 2008.

away of the protective coating around the nerve (the myelin sheath). TN may be part of the normal aging process—as blood vessels lengthen they can come to rest and pulsate against a nerve. TN symptoms can also occur in people with multiple sclerosis, a disease caused by the deterioration of myelin throughout the body, or may be caused by damage to the myelin sheath by compression from a tumor. This deterioration causes the nerve to send abnormal signals to the brain. In some cases the cause is unknown.

What are its symptoms?

TN is characterized by a sudden, severe, electric shock-like, stabbing pain that is typically felt on one side of the jaw or cheek. Pain may occur on both sides of the face, although not at the same time. The attacks of pain, which generally last several seconds and may repeat in quick succession, come and go throughout the day. These episodes can last for days, weeks, or months at a time and then disappear for months or years. In the days before an episode begins, some patients may experience a tingling or numbing sensation or a somewhat constant and aching pain.

The intense flashes of pain can be triggered by vibration or contact with the cheek (such as when shaving, washing the face, or applying makeup), brushing teeth, eating, drinking, talking, or being exposed to the wind. The pain may affect a small area of the face or may spread. The bouts of pain rarely occur at night, when the patient is sleeping.

Patients are considered to have Type 1 TN if more than 50 percent of the pain they experience is sudden, intermittent, sharp and stabbing, or shock-like. These patients may also have some burning sensation. Type 2 TN involves pain that is constant, aching, or burning more than 50 percent of the time.

TN is typified by attacks that stop for a period of time and then come back. The attacks often worsen over time, with fewer and shorter pain-free periods before they recur. The disorder is not fatal, but can be debilitating. Due to the intensity of the pain, some patients may avoid daily activities because they fear an impending attack.

Who is affected?

TN occurs most often in people over age 50, but it can occur at any age. The disorder is more common in women than in men. There is some evidence that the disorder runs in families, perhaps because of an inherited pattern of blood vessel formation.

How is TN diagnosed?

There is no single test to diagnose TN. Diagnosis is generally based on the patient's medical history and description of symptoms, a physical exam, and a thorough neurological examination by a physician. Other disorders, such as post-herpetic neuralgia, can cause similar facial pain, as do syndromes such as cluster headaches. Injury to the trigeminal nerve (perhaps the result of sinus surgery, oral surgery, stroke, or facial trauma) may produce neuropathic pain, which is characterized by dull, burning, and boring pain. Because of overlapping symptoms, and the large number of conditions that can cause facial pain, obtaining a correct diagnosis is difficult, but finding the cause of the pain is important as the treatments for different types of pain may differ.

Most TN patients undergo a standard magnetic resonance imaging scan to rule out a tumor or multiple sclerosis as the cause of their pain. This scan may or may not clearly show a blood vessel on the nerve. Magnetic resonance angiography, which can trace a colored dye that is injected into the bloodstream prior to the scan, can more clearly show blood vessel problems and any compression of the trigeminal nerve close to the brainstem.

How is it treated?

Treatment options include medicines, surgery, and complementary approaches. Anticonvulsant medicines—used to block nerve firing—are generally effective in treating TN. These drugs include carbamazepine, oxcarbazepine, topiramate, clonazepam, phenytoin, lamotrigine, and valproic acid. Gabapentin or baclofen can be used as a second drug to treat TN and may be given in combination with other anticonvulsants.

Tricyclic antidepressants such as amitriptyline or nortriptyline are used to treat pain described as constant, burning, or aching. Typical analgesics and opioids are not usually helpful in treating the sharp, recurring pain caused by TN. If medication fails to relieve pain or produces intolerable side effects such as excess fatigue, surgical treatment may be recommended.

Several neurosurgical procedures are available to treat TN. The choice among the various types depends on the patient's preference, physical well-being, previous surgeries, presence of multiple sclerosis, and area of trigeminal nerve involvement (particularly when the upper/ophthalmic branch is involved). Some procedures are done on an outpatient basis, while others may involve a more complex operation that is performed under general anesthesia. Some degree of facial numbness is expected after most of these procedures, and TN

395

might return despite the procedure's initial success. Depending on the procedure, other surgical risks include hearing loss, balance problems, infection, and stroke.

A rhizotomy is a procedure in which select nerve fibers are destroyed to block pain. A rhizotomy for TN causes some degree of permanent sensory loss and facial numbness. Several forms of rhizotomy are available to treat TN:

- **Balloon compression** works by injuring the insulation on nerves that are involved with the sensation of light touch on the face. The procedure is performed in an operating room under general anesthesia. A tube called a cannula is inserted through the cheek and guided to where one branch of the trigeminal nerve passes through the base of the skull. A soft catheter with a balloon tip is threaded through the cannula and the balloon is inflated to squeeze part of the nerve against the hard edge of the brain covering (the dura) and the skull. After 1 minute the balloon is deflated and removed, along with the catheter and cannula. Balloon compression is generally an outpatient procedure, although sometimes the patient may be kept in the hospital overnight.

- **Glycerol injection** is generally an outpatient procedure in which the patient is sedated intravenously. A thin needle is passed through the cheek, next to the mouth, and guided through the opening in the base of the skull to where all three branches of the trigeminal nerve come together. The glycerol injection bathes the ganglion (the central part of the nerve from which the nerve impulses are transmitted) and damages the insulation of trigeminal nerve fibers.

- **Radiofrequency thermal lesioning** is usually performed on an outpatient basis. The patient is anesthetized and a hollow needle is passed through the cheek to where the trigeminal nerve exits through a hole at the base of the skull. The patient is awakened and a small electrical current is passed through the needle, causing tingling. When the needle is positioned so that the tingling occurs in the area of TN pain, the patient is then sedated and that part of the nerve is gradually heated with an electrode, injuring the nerve fibers. The electrode and needle are then removed and the patient is awakened.

- **Stereotactic radiosurgery** uses computer imaging to direct highly focused beams of radiation at the site where the trigeminal nerve exits the brainstem. This causes the slow formation of a lesion on the nerve that disrupts the transmission of pain signals to the brain. Pain relief from this procedure may take several months. Patients usually leave the hospital the same day or the next day following treatment.

Microvascular decompression is the most invasive of all surgeries for TN, but it also offers the lowest probability that pain will return. This inpatient procedure, which is performed under general anesthesia, requires that a small opening be made behind the ear. While viewing the trigeminal nerve through a microscope, the surgeon moves away the vessels that are compressing the nerve and places a soft cushion between the nerve and the vessels. Unlike rhizotomies, there is usually no numbness in the face after this surgery. Patients generally recuperate for several days in the hospital following the procedure. A neurectomy, which involves cutting part of the nerve, may be performed during microvascular decompression if no vessel is found to be pressing on the trigeminal nerve. Neurectomies may also be performed by cutting branches of the trigeminal nerve in the face. When done during microvascular decompression, a neurectomy will cause permanent numbness in the area of the face that is supplied by the nerve or nerve branch that is cut. However, when the operation is performed in the face, the nerve may grow back and in time sensation may return.

Some patients choose to manage TN using complementary techniques, usually in combination with drug treatment. These therapies offer varying degrees of success. Options include acupuncture, biofeedback, vitamin therapy, nutritional therapy, and electrical stimulation of the nerves.

Chapter 38

Bruxism (Teeth Grinding and Clenching)

When you look in on your sleeping child, you want to hear the sounds of sweet dreams: easy breathing and perhaps an occasional sigh. But some parents hear the harsher sounds of gnashing and grinding teeth, called bruxism, which is common in kids.

What Is Bruxism?

Bruxism is the medical term for the grinding of teeth or the clenching of jaws, especially during deep sleep or while under stress. It comes from the Greek word "brychein," which means to gnash the teeth. Three out of every 10 kids will grind or clench, experts say, with the highest incidence in children under 5.

Causes of Bruxism

Though studies have been done, no one knows why bruxism happens. But in some cases, kids may grind because the top and bottom teeth aren't aligned properly. Others do it as a response to pain, such

"Bruxism (Teeth Grinding or Clenching)," September 2007, reprinted with permission from www.kidshealth.org. Copyright © 2007 The Nemours Foundation. This information was provided by KidsHealth, one of the largest resources online for medically reviewed health information written for parents, kids, and teens. For more articles like this one, visit www.KidsHealth.org, or www.TeensHealth.org. This document was reviewed by: Lisa A. Goss, R.D.H., B.S., and Charlie J. Inga, D.D.S.

as an earache or teething. Kids might grind their teeth as a way to ease the pain, just as they might rub a sore muscle. Most kids outgrow these fairly common causes for grinding.

Stress—usually nervous tension or anger—is another cause. For instance, your child may be worrying about a test at school or experiencing a change in routine (a new sibling or a new teacher). Even arguing with parents and siblings can cause enough stress to prompt teeth grinding or jaw clenching. Some kids who are hyperactive also experience bruxism.

Effects of Bruxism

Generally, bruxism doesn't hurt a child's teeth. Many cases go undetected with no adverse effects, though some may result in mild morning headaches or earaches. Most often, however, the condition can be more bothersome to you and others in your home because of the grinding sound.

In some extreme circumstances, nighttime grinding and clenching can wear down tooth enamel, chip teeth, increase temperature sensitivity, and cause severe facial pain and jaw problems, such as temporomandibular joint disease (TMJ). Most kids who grind, however, do not have TMJ problems unless their grinding and clenching is chronic.

Diagnosing Bruxism

Lots of kids who grind their teeth aren't even aware of it, so it's often siblings or parents who identify the problem.

Some signs to watch for:

- grinding noises when your child is sleeping
- complaints of a sore jaw or face in the morning
- thumb sucking
- fingernail biting
- gnawing on pencils and toys
- chewing the inside of the cheek

If you think your child is grinding his or her teeth, visit the dentist, who will examine the teeth for chipped enamel and unusual wear and tear, and spray air and water on the teeth to check for unusual sensitivity.

If damage is detected, the dentist will ask your child a few questions, such as:

- How do you feel before bed?

- Are you worried about anything at home or school?

- Are you angry with someone?

- What do you do before bed?

The exam will help the dentist determine whether the grinding is caused by anatomical (misaligned teeth) or psychological (stress) factors and come up with an effective treatment plan.

Treating Bruxism

Most kids outgrow bruxism, but a combination of parental observation and dental visits can help keep the problem in check until they do.

In cases where the grinding and clenching make a child's face and jaw sore or damage the teeth, dentists may prescribe a special night guard. Molded to a child's teeth, the night guard is similar to the protective mouthpieces worn by football players. Though a mouthpiece may take some getting used to, positive results happen quickly.

Helping Kids with Bruxism

Whether the cause is physical or psychological, kids might be able to control bruxism by relaxing before bedtime—for example, by taking a warm bath or shower, listening to a few minutes of soothing music, or reading a book.

For bruxism that's caused by stress, try to find out what's upsetting your child and find a way to help. For example, a kid who is worried about being away from home for a first camping trip might need reassurance that mom or dad will be nearby if anything happens.

If the issue is more complicated, such as moving to a new town, discuss your child's concerns and try to ease any fears. If you're concerned about your child's emotional state, talk to your doctor.

In rare cases, basic stress relievers aren't enough to stop bruxism. If your child has trouble sleeping or is acting differently than usual, your child's dentist or doctor may suggest a psychological assessment. This can help determine the cause of the stress and an appropriate course of treatment.

How Long Does Bruxism Last?

Childhood bruxism is usually outgrown by adolescence. Most kids stop grinding when they lose their baby teeth because permanent teeth are much more sensitive to pain. However, a few children do continue to grind into adolescence. And if the bruxism is caused by stress, it will continue until the stress is relieved.

Preventing Bruxism

Because some bruxism is a child's natural reaction to growth and development, most cases can't be prevented. Stress-induced bruxism can be avoided, however, by talking with kids regularly about their feelings and helping them deal with stress.

Chapter 39

Temporomandibular Joint and Muscle Disorders

Temporomandibular joint and muscle disorders, commonly called "TMJ," are a group of conditions that cause pain and dysfunction in the jaw joint and the muscles that control jaw movement. We don't know for certain how many people have TMJ disorders, but some estimates suggest that over 10 million Americans are affected. The condition appears to be more common in women than men.

For most people, pain in the area of the jaw joint or muscles does not signal a serious problem. Generally, discomfort from these conditions is occasional and temporary, often occurring in cycles. The pain eventually goes away with little or no treatment. Some people, however, develop significant, long-term symptoms.

If you have questions about TMJ disorders, you are not alone. Researchers, too, are looking for answers to what causes these conditions and what are the best treatments. Until we have scientific evidence for safe and effective treatments, it's important to avoid, when possible, procedures that can cause permanent changes in your bite or jaw.

What Is the Temporomandibular Joint?

The temporomandibular joint connects the lower jaw, called the mandible, to the bone at the side of the head—the temporal bone. If you place your fingers just in front of your ears and open your mouth,

Excerpted from "TMJ Disorders," by the National Institute of Dental and Craniofacial Research (NIDCR, www.nidcr.nih.gov), part of the National Institutes of Health, June 2006. NIH Publication No. 06-3487.

403

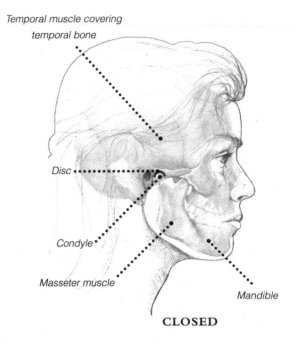

Temporal muscle covering temporal bone

Disc

Condyle

Masseter muscle

Mandible

CLOSED

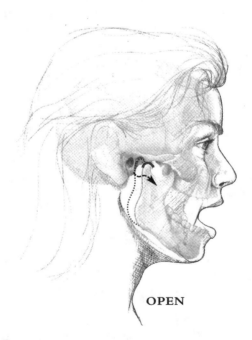

OPEN

Figure 39.1. When the mouth is closed and open.

you can feel the joints. Because these joints are flexible, the jaw can move smoothly up and down and side to side, enabling us to talk, chew, and yawn. Muscles attached to and surrounding the jaw joint control its position and movement.

When we open our mouths, the rounded ends of the lower jaw, called condyles, glide along the joint socket of the temporal bone. The condyles slide back to their original position when we close our mouths. To keep this motion smooth, a soft disk lies between the condyle and the temporal bone. This disk absorbs shocks to the jaw joint from chewing and other movements.

The temporomandibular joint is different from the body's other joints. The combination of hinge and sliding motions makes this joint among the most complicated in the body. Also, the tissues that make up the temporomandibular joint differ from other load-bearing joints, like the knee or hip. Because of its complex movement and unique makeup, the jaw joint and its controlling muscles can pose a tremendous challenge to both patients and health care providers when problems arise.

What Are TMJ Disorders?

Disorders of the jaw joint and chewing muscles—and how people respond to them—vary widely. Researchers generally agree that the conditions fall into three main categories:

1. Myofascial pain, the most common temporomandibular disorder, involves discomfort or pain in the muscles that control jaw function.

2. Internal derangement of the joint involves a displaced disk, dislocated jaw, or injury to the condyle.

3. Arthritis refers to a group of degenerative/inflammatory joint disorders that can affect the temporomandibular joint.

A person may have one or more of these conditions at the same time. Some people have other health problems that co-exist with TMJ disorders, such as chronic fatigue syndrome, sleep disturbances, or fibromyalgia, a painful condition that affects muscles and other soft tissues throughout the body. It is not known whether these disorders share a common cause.

People who have a rheumatic disease, such as rheumatoid arthritis, may develop TMJ disease as a secondary condition. Rheumatic diseases refer to a large group of disorders that cause pain, inflammation, and stiffness in the joints, muscles, and bone. Both rheumatoid arthritis and some TMJ disorders involve inflammation of the tissues that line the joints. The exact relationship between these conditions is not known.

How jaw joint and muscle disorders progress is not clear. Symptoms worsen and ease over time, but what causes these changes is not known. Most people have relatively mild forms of the disorder. Their symptoms improve significantly, or disappear spontaneously, within weeks or months. For others, the condition causes long-term, persistent, and debilitating pain.

What Causes TMJ Disorders?

Trauma to the jaw or temporomandibular joint plays a role in some TMJ disorders. But for most jaw joint and muscle problems, scientists don't know the causes. For many people, symptoms seem to start without obvious reason. Research disputes the popular belief that a bad bite or orthodontic braces can trigger TMJ disorders. Because the condition is more common in women than in men, scientists are exploring a possible link between female hormones and TMJ disorders.

There is no scientific proof that clicking sounds in the jaw joint lead to serious problems. In fact, jaw clicking is common in the general population. Jaw noises alone, without pain or limited jaw movement, do not indicate a TMJ disorder and do not warrant treatment.

The roles of stress and tooth grinding as major causes of TMJ disorders are also unclear. Many people with these disorders do not grind their teeth, and many long-time tooth grinders do not have painful joint symptoms. Scientists note that people with sore, tender chewing muscles are less likely than others to grind their teeth because it causes pain. Researchers also found that stress seen in many persons with jaw joint and muscle disorders is more likely the result of dealing with chronic jaw pain or dysfunction than the cause of the condition.

What Are the Signs and Symptoms?

A variety of symptoms may be linked to TMJ disorders. Pain, particularly in the chewing muscles and/or jaw joint, is the most common symptom. Other likely symptoms include:

- radiating pain in the face, jaw, or neck;
- jaw muscle stiffness;

- limited movement or locking of the jaw;
- painful clicking, popping, or grating in the jaw joint when opening or closing the mouth; and
- a change in the way the upper and lower teeth fit together.

How Are TMJ Disorders Diagnosed?

There is no widely accepted, standard test now available to correctly diagnose TMJ disorders. Because the exact causes and symptoms are not clear, identifying these disorders can be difficult and confusing. Currently, health care providers note the patient's description of symptoms, take a detailed medical and dental history, and examine problem areas, including the head, neck, face, and jaw. Imaging studies may also be recommended.

You may want to consult your doctor to rule out known causes of pain. Facial pain can be a symptom of many other conditions, such as sinus or ear infections, various types of headaches, and facial neuralgias (nerve-related facial pain). Ruling out these problems first helps in identifying TMJ disorders.

How Are TMJ Disorders Treated?

Because more studies are needed on the safety and effectiveness of most treatments for jaw joint and muscle disorders, experts strongly recommend using the most conservative, reversible treatments possible. Conservative treatments do not invade the tissues of the face, jaw, or joint, or involve surgery. Reversible treatments do not cause permanent changes in the structure or position of the jaw or teeth. Even when TMJ disorders have become persistent, most patients still do not need aggressive types of treatment.

Conservative Treatments

Because the most common jaw joint and muscle problems are temporary and do not get worse, simple treatment is all that is usually needed to relieve discomfort.

Self-Care Practices: There are steps you can take that may be helpful in easing symptoms, such as:

- eating soft foods;
- applying ice packs;

- avoiding extreme jaw movements (such as wide yawning, loud singing, and gum chewing);

- learning techniques for relaxing and reducing stress; and

- practicing gentle jaw stretching and relaxing exercises that may help increase jaw movement. Your health care provider or a physical therapist can recommend exercises if appropriate for your particular condition.

Pain Medications: For many people with TMJ disorders, short-term use of over-the-counter pain medicines or nonsteroidal anti-inflammatory drugs (NSAIDs), such as ibuprofen, may provide temporary relief from jaw discomfort. When necessary, your dentist or doctor can prescribe stronger pain or anti-inflammatory medications, muscle relaxants, or antidepressants to help ease symptoms.

Stabilization Splints: Your doctor or dentist may recommend an oral appliance, also called a stabilization splint or bite guard, which is a plastic guard that fits over the upper or lower teeth. Stabilization splints are the most widely used treatments for TMJ disorders. Studies of their effectiveness in providing pain relief, however, have been inconclusive. If a stabilization splint is recommended, it should be used only for a short time and should not cause permanent changes in the bite. If a splint causes or increases pain, stop using it and see your health care provider.

The conservative, reversible treatments described are useful for temporary relief of pain—they are not cures for TMJ disorders. If symptoms continue over time, come back often, or worsen, tell your doctor.

Irreversible Treatments

Irreversible treatments that have not been proven to be effective—and may make the problem worse—include orthodontics to change the bite; crown and bridge work to balance the bite; grinding down teeth to bring the bite into balance, called "occlusal adjustment"; and repositioning splints, also called orthotics, which permanently alter the bite.

Surgery: Other types of treatments, such as surgical procedures, invade the tissues. Surgical treatments are controversial, often irreversible, and should be avoided where possible. There have been no long-term clinical trials to study the safety and effectiveness of surgical treatments for TMJ disorders. Nor are there standards to identify people who would most likely benefit from surgery. Failure to respond to conservative treatments, for example, does not automatically mean that surgery is necessary. If surgery is recommended, be sure to have the doctor explain to you, in words you can understand, the reason for the treatment, the risks involved, and other types of treatment that may be available.

Implants: Surgical replacement of jaw joints with artificial implants may cause severe pain and permanent jaw damage. Some of these devices may fail to function properly or may break apart in the jaw over time. If you have already had temporomandibular joint surgery, be very cautious about considering additional operations. Persons undergoing multiple surgeries on the jaw joint generally have a poor outlook for normal, pain-free joint function. Before undergoing any surgery on the jaw joint, it is extremely important to get other independent opinions and to fully understand the risks.

The U.S. Food and Drug Administration (FDA) monitors the safety and effectiveness of medical devices implanted in the body, including artificial jaw joint implants. Patients and their health care providers can report serious problems with TMJ implants to the FDA through MedWatch at www.fda.gov/medwatch or telephone toll-free at 800-332-1088.

If You Think You Have a TMJ Disorder

Remember that for most people, discomfort from TMJ disorders will eventually go away on its own. Simple self-care practices are often effective in easing symptoms. If treatment is needed, it should be based on a reasonable diagnosis, be conservative and reversible, and be customized to your special needs. Avoid treatments that can cause permanent changes in the bite or jaw. If irreversible treatments are recommended, be sure to get a reliable, independent second opinion.

Because there is no certified specialty for TMJ disorders in either dentistry or medicine, finding the right care can be difficult. Look for a health care provider who understands musculoskeletal disorders (affecting muscle, bone, and joints) and who is trained in treating pain conditions. Pain clinics in hospitals and universities are often a good source of advice, particularly when pain continues over time and interferes with daily life. Complex cases, often marked by prolonged, persistent, and severe pain; jaw dysfunction; co-existing conditions; and diminished quality of life, likely require a team of experts from various fields, such as neurology, rheumatology, pain management, and others, to diagnose and treat this condition.

Chapter 40

Oral Cancer

Chapter Contents

Section 40.1—Oral Cancer Overview 412
Section 40.2—The Oral Cancer Exam Step-by-Step 414
Section 40.3—Novel Device Shows Potential in Better
           Detecting Oral Cancer 415

Section 40.1

Oral Cancer Overview

"Oral Cancer," from the National Institute of Dental and
Craniofacial Research (NIDCR, www.nidcr.nih.gov), part of the
National Institutes of Health, November 14, 2007.

About Oral Cancer

The term oral cancer includes cancers of the mouth and the pharynx, part of the throat. About two thirds of oral cancers occur in the mouth and about one third are found in the pharynx.

Oral cancer will be diagnosed in an estimated 28,000 Americans this year and will cause approximately 7,000 deaths. It is the 6th most common cancer in men and the 14th most common cancer in women.

Oral cancer can spread quickly. On average, 59 percent of those with the disease will survive more than five years.

Oral cancer most often occurs in people over the age of 40 and affects twice as many men as women.

Lower Your Risk

Most oral cancer is preventable. Seventy-five percent of oral cancers are related to tobacco use, alcohol use, or use of both substances together. Using both tobacco and alcohol puts you at much greater risk than using either substance alone.

- Do not use tobacco products—cigarettes, chew or snuff, pipes, or cigars. Tobacco in all forms plays a role in oral cancers.

- If you drink alcohol, do so only in moderation. Excessive alcohol use can increase your risk of oral cancer.

- Use lip balm that contains sunscreen. Exposure to sunlight is a risk factor for lip cancer.

- Eat plenty of fruits and vegetables. Eating lots of fruits and vegetables as part of a low-fat, high fiber diet may help reduce cancer risk. The National Cancer Institute suggests eating at least five servings of fruits and vegetables a day.

Possible Signs and Symptoms

See a dentist or physician if any of the following symptoms last for more than two weeks.

- a sore, irritation, lump, or thick patch in your mouth, lip, or throat;

- a white or red patch in your mouth;

- a feeling that something is caught in your throat;

- difficulty chewing or swallowing;

- difficulty moving your jaw or tongue;

- numbness in your tongue or other areas of your mouth;

- swelling of your jaw that causes dentures to fit poorly or become uncomfortable; or

- pain in one ear without hearing loss.

Early Detection

It is important to find oral cancer as early as possible when it can be treated more successfully.

- An oral cancer examination can detect early signs of cancer. Oral cancer exams are painless and quick—and take only a few minutes.

- Your regular dental checkup is an excellent opportunity to have the exam.

- During the exam, your dentist or dental hygienist will check your face, neck, lips, and entire mouth for possible signs of cancer.

- Some parts of the pharynx are not visible during an oral cancer exam. Talk to your dentist about whether a specialist should check your pharynx.

Section 40.2

The Oral Cancer Exam Step-by-Step

"The Oral Cancer Exam," from the National Institute of Dental and Craniofacial Research (NIDCR, www.nidcr.nih.gov), part of the National Institutes of Health, November 9, 2007.

An oral cancer exam is painless and quick—it takes only a few minutes. Your regular dental checkup is an excellent opportunity to have the exam.

Here's what to expect:

1. Preparing for the exam: If you have dentures (plates) or partials, you will be asked to remove them.

2. Your health care provider will inspect your face, neck, lips, and mouth to look for any signs of cancer.

3. With both hands, he or she will feel the area under your jaw and the side of your neck, checking for lumps that may suggest cancer.

4. He or she will then look at and feel the insides of your lips and cheeks to check for possible signs of cancer, such as red and/or white patches.

5. Next, your provider will have you stick out your tongue so it can be checked for swelling or abnormal color or texture.

6. Using gauze, he or she will then gently pull your tongue to one side, then the other, to check the base of your tongue. The underside of your tongue will also be checked.

7. In addition, he or she will look at the roof and floor of your mouth, as well as the back of your throat.

8. Finally, your provider will put one finger on the floor of your mouth and, with the other hand under your chin, gently press down to check for lumps or sensitivity.

Section 40.3

Novel Device Shows Potential in Better Detecting Oral Cancer

"Novel Device Shows Potential in Better Detecting Oral Cancer,"
from the National Institute of Dental and Craniofacial Research
(NIDCR, www.nidcr.nih.gov), part of the National Institutes of
Health, April 10, 2006.

Researchers supported by the National Institute of Dental and Craniofacial Research, part of the National Institutes of Health, report today their initial success using a customized optical device that allows dentists to visualize in a completely new way whether a patient might have a developing oral cancer.

Called a Visually Enhanced Lesion Scope (VELscope), this simple, handheld device emits a cone of blue light into the mouth that excites various molecules within our cells, causing them to absorb the light energy and re-emit it as visible fluorescence. Remove the light, and the fluorescence of the tissue is no longer visible.

Because changes in the natural fluorescence of healthy tissue generally reflect light-scattering biochemical or structural changes indicative of developing tumor cells, the VELscope allows dentists to shine a light onto a suspicious sore in the mouth, look through an attached eyepiece, and watch directly for changes in color. Normal oral tissue emits a pale green fluorescence, while potentially early tumor, or dysplastic, cells appear dark green to black.

Testing the device in 44 people, the results of which are published online in the *Journal of Biomedical Optics,* the scientists found they could distinguish correctly in all but one instance between normal and abnormal tissue. Their diagnoses were confirmed to be correct by biopsy and standard pathology.

"The natural fluorescence of the mouth is invisible to the naked eye," said Dr. Miriam Rosin, a senior author on the paper and a cancer biologist at the British Columbia Cancer Research Center in Vancouver, Canada. "The VELscope literally brings this natural fluorescence to light, helping dentists to answer in a more informed way a common question in daily practices: To biopsy or not to biopsy."

Because developing tumors in the mouth are often easily visible, public health officials have long advocated early detection of oral cancer. But determining whether a suspicious sore is benign or potentially cancerous has remained scientifically problematic. "A major reason is looks alone can be deceiving," said Rosin, referring to the common practice of diagnosing cancer based on the general appearance and staining patterns of tissue biopsy. "What's been badly needed in screening for oral cancer is a way to visualize the biological information within and let it tell you whether or not a lesion is likely to become cancerous."

Rosin said the VELscope goes a long way toward answering this unmet need. "Historically, the problem in developing a fluorescence-reading instrument has been largely organizational," said Rosin, a leader of the British Columbia Oral Cancer Prevention Program. "No one scientific discipline possesses sufficient expertise to build such a sophisticated imaging device, and the needed interdisciplinary groups weren't forming to tackle the problem."

This lack of communication changed a few years ago when Rosin broached the subject to Dr. Calum MacAulay, the head of the British Columbia Cancer Research Center's cancer imaging program and who has extensive training in physics, pathology, and engineering imaging devices. Based on these discussions, MacAulay and post-doctoral fellow Pierre Lane agreed to begin the technologically challenging process of designing a hand-held device that also would be user friendly in the dentist's office.

Starting with a crude, light-emitting box and a pair of goggles that their group had previously cobbled together to visualize skin cancer, Lane and MacAulay gradually progressed to the one-step device reported today. "We essentially refined and integrated the box-and-goggles concept into one device," said MacAulay, who also works closely with a corporate partner that would like to commercialize the VELscope. "The box was molded into the lightweight, hand-held structure, a flexible cord attaches the examination light, and the goggles became the view finder that allows dentists to directly evaluate lesions in real time."

In their study, the scientists evaluated 50 tissue sites from 44 people. All sites were biopsied, and pathologists classified seven as normal, 11 had severe dysplasia, and 33 biopsies were oral squamous cell carcinoma. Reading the fluorescence patterns of the 50 sites, the group correctly identified all of the normal biopsies, 10 of the severe dysplasias, and all of the cancers. These numbers translated to 100 percent specificity and 98 percent sensitivity. Sensitivity refers to how well a test correctly identifies people who have a disease, while specificity characterizes the ability of a test to correctly identify those who are well.

Rosin said her group is now engaged in a larger follow-up study in Vancouver that will further evaluate the VELscope. "Laboratories are developing similar devices to detect lung and cervical cancer," said Rosin. "That means that the same basic technology is now being used to evaluate three tumor sites, and we can begin hopefully to pool our data and fine tune the characteristics and meaning of the changes in fluorescence."

The American Cancer Society (ACS) estimated last year that about 20,000 Americans were diagnosed with various oral cancers. The ACS also estimated that just over 5,000 Americans died from these cancers in 2005.

Chapter 41

Lip and Oral Cavity Cancer

Lip and oral cavity cancer is a disease in which malignant (cancer) cells form in the lips or mouth.

The oral cavity includes the following:

- the front two thirds of the tongue;

- the gingiva (gums);

- the buccal mucosa (the lining of the inside of the cheeks);

- the floor (bottom) of the mouth under the tongue;

- the hard palate (the roof of the mouth); and

- the retromolar trigone (the small area behind the wisdom teeth).

Most lip and oral cavity cancers start in squamous cells, the thin, flat cells that line the lips and oral cavity. These are called squamous cell carcinomas. Cancer cells may spread into deeper tissue as the cancer grows. Squamous cell carcinoma usually develops in areas of leukoplakia (white patches of cells that do not rub off).

Tobacco and alcohol use can affect the risk of developing lip and oral cavity cancer.

Excerpted from PDQ® Cancer Information Summary. National Cancer Institute; Bethesda, MD. Lip and Oral Cavity Cancer Treatment (PDQ®): Patient Version. Updated 06/2008. Available at: http://cancer.gov. Accessed June 19, 2008.

Risk factors for lip and oral cavity cancer include the following:

- using tobacco products;

- heavy alcohol use;

- being exposed to sunlight;

- being male; and

- being infected with human papillomavirus (HPV).

Possible signs of lip and oral cavity cancer include a sore or lump on the lips or in the mouth.

These and other symptoms may be caused by lip and oral cavity cancer. Other conditions may cause the same symptoms. A doctor should be consulted if any of the following problems occur:

- a sore on the lip or in the mouth that does not heal;

- a lump or thickening on the lips or gums or in the mouth;

- a white or red patch on the gums, tongue, tonsils, or lining of the mouth;

- bleeding, pain, or numbness in the lip or mouth;

- change in voice;

- loose teeth or dentures that no longer fit well;

- trouble chewing or swallowing or moving the tongue or jaw;

- swelling of jaw; and

- sore throat or feeling that something is caught in the throat.

Lip and oral cavity cancer may not have any symptoms and is sometimes found during a regular dental exam.

Tests that examine the mouth and throat are used to detect (find), diagnose, and stage lip and oral cavity cancer.

The following tests and procedures may be used:

- **Physical exam of the lips and oral cavity:** An exam to check the lips and oral cavity for abnormal areas. The doctor or dentist will feel the entire inside of the mouth with a gloved finger and examine the oral cavity with a small long-handled mirror and lights. This will include checking the insides of the cheeks and lips; the gums; the roof and floor of the mouth; and the top, bottom, and sides of the tongue. The neck will be felt for swollen lymph nodes. A history of the patient's health habits and past illnesses and medical and dental treatments will also be taken.

- **Endoscopy:** A procedure to look at organs and tissues inside the body to check for abnormal areas. An endoscope (a thin, lighted tube) is inserted through an incision (cut) in the skin or opening in the body, such as the mouth. Tissue samples and lymph nodes may be taken for biopsy.

- **X-rays of the head, neck, and chest:** An x-ray is a type of energy beam that can go through the body and onto film, making a picture of areas inside the body.

- **Biopsy:** The removal of cells or tissues so they can be viewed under a microscope by a pathologist. If leukoplakia is found, cells taken from the patches are also checked under the microscope for signs of cancer.

- **MRI (magnetic resonance imaging):** A procedure that uses a magnet, radio waves, and a computer to make a series of detailed pictures of areas inside the body. This procedure is also called nuclear magnetic resonance imaging (NMRI).

- **CT scan (CAT scan):** A procedure that makes a series of detailed pictures of areas inside the body, taken from different angles. The pictures are made by a computer linked to an x-ray machine. A dye may be injected into a vein or swallowed to help the organs or tissues show up more clearly. This procedure is also called computed tomography, computerized tomography, or computerized axial tomography.

- **Exfoliative cytology:** A procedure to collect cells from the lip or oral cavity. A piece of cotton, a brush, or a small wooden stick is used to gently scrape cells from the lips, tongue, mouth, or throat. The cells are viewed under a microscope to find out if they are abnormal.

- **Barium swallow:** A series of x-rays of the esophagus and stomach. The patient drinks a liquid that contains barium (a silver-white metallic compound). The liquid coats the esophagus and x-rays are taken. This procedure is also called an upper GI [gastrointestinal] series.

- **PET scan (positron emission tomography scan):** A procedure to find malignant tumor cells in the body. A small amount

421

of radionuclide glucose (sugar) is injected into a vein. The PET scanner rotates around the body and makes a picture of where glucose is being used in the body. Malignant tumor cells show up brighter in the picture because they are more active and take up more glucose than normal cells do.

Certain factors affect prognosis (chance of recovery) and treatment options.

Prognosis (chance of recovery) depends on the following:

- the stage of the cancer;

- where the tumor is in the lip or oral cavity; and

- whether the cancer has spread to blood vessels.

For patients who smoke, the chance of recovery is better if they stop smoking before beginning radiation therapy.

Treatment options depend on the following:

- the stage of the cancer;

- the size of the tumor and where it is in the lip or oral cavity;

- whether the patient's appearance and ability to talk and eat can stay the same; and

- the patient's age and general health.

Patients who have had lip and oral cavity cancer have an increased risk of developing a second cancer in the head or neck. Frequent and careful follow-up is important. Clinical trials are studying the use of retinoid drugs to reduce the risk of a second head and neck cancer.

After lip and oral cavity cancer has been diagnosed, tests are done to find out if cancer cells have spread within the lip and oral cavity or to other parts of the body.

The process used to find out if cancer has spread within the lip and oral cavity or to other parts of the body is called staging. The information gathered from the staging process determines the stage of the disease. It is important to know the stage in order to plan treatment. The results of the tests used to diagnose lip and oral cavity cancer are also used to stage the disease.

There are three ways that cancer spreads in the body.

The three ways that cancer spreads in the body are:

- Through tissue. Cancer invades the surrounding normal tissue.

- Through the lymph system. Cancer invades the lymph system and travels through the lymph vessels to other places in the body.

- Through the blood. Cancer invades the veins and capillaries and travels through the blood to other places in the body.

When cancer cells break away from the primary (original) tumor and travel through the lymph or blood to other places in the body, another (secondary) tumor may form. This process is called metastasis. The secondary (metastatic) tumor is the same type of cancer as the primary tumor. For example, if breast cancer spreads to the bones, the cancer cells in the bones are actually breast cancer cells. The disease is metastatic breast cancer, not bone cancer.

Treatment Option Overview

There are different types of treatment for patients with lip and oral cavity cancer.

Different types of treatment are available for patients with lip and oral cavity cancer. Some treatments are standard (the currently used treatment), and some are being tested in clinical trials. A treatment clinical trial is a research study meant to help improve current treatments or obtain information on new treatments for patients with cancer. When clinical trials show that a new treatment is better than the standard treatment, the new treatment may become the standard treatment. Patients may want to think about taking part in a clinical trial. Some clinical trials are open only to patients who have not started treatment.

Patients with lip and oral cavity cancer should have their treatment planned by a team of doctors who are expert in treating head and neck cancer.

Treatment will be overseen by a medical oncologist, a doctor who specializes in treating people with cancer. Because the lips and oral cavity are important for breathing, eating, and talking, patients may need special help adjusting to the side effects of the cancer and its treatment. The medical oncologist may refer the patient to other health professionals with special training in the treatment of patients with head and neck cancer. These include the following:

- head and neck surgeon;

- radiation oncologist;

- dentist;

- speech therapist;
- dietitian;
- psychologist;
- rehabilitation specialist; and
- plastic surgeon.

Two types of standard treatment are used.

Surgery

Surgery (removing the cancer in an operation) is a common treatment for all stages of lip and oral cavity cancer. Surgery may include the following:

Wide local excision: Removal of the cancer and some of the healthy tissue around it. If cancer has spread into bone, surgery may include removal of the involved bone tissue.

Neck dissection: Removal of lymph nodes and other tissues in the neck. This is done when cancer may have spread from the lip and oral cavity.

Plastic surgery: An operation that restores or improves the appearance of parts of the body. Dental implants, a skin graft, or other plastic surgery may be needed to repair parts of the mouth, throat, or neck after removal of large tumors.

Even if the doctor removes all the cancer that can be seen at the time of the surgery, some patients may be given chemotherapy or radiation therapy after surgery to kill any cancer cells that are left. Treatment given after the surgery, to increase the chances of a cure, is called adjuvant therapy.

Radiation Therapy

Radiation therapy is a cancer treatment that uses high-energy x-rays or other types of radiation to kill cancer cells. There are two types of radiation therapy. External radiation therapy uses a machine outside the body to send radiation toward the cancer. Internal radiation therapy uses a radioactive substance sealed in needles, seeds, wires, or catheters that are placed directly into or near the cancer. The way the radiation therapy is given depends on the type and stage of the cancer being treated.

For patients who smoke, radiation therapy works better when smoking is stopped before beginning treatment. It is also important for patients to have a dental exam before radiation therapy begins, so that existing problems can be treated.

New types of treatment are being tested in clinical trials.

Chemotherapy

Chemotherapy is a cancer treatment that uses drugs to stop the growth of cancer cells, either by killing the cells or by stopping the cells from dividing. When chemotherapy is taken by mouth or injected into a vein or muscle, the drugs enter the bloodstream and can reach cancer cells throughout the body (systemic chemotherapy). When chemotherapy is placed directly into the spinal column, an organ, or a body cavity such as the abdomen, the drugs mainly affect cancer cells in those areas (regional chemotherapy). The way the chemotherapy is given depends on the type and stage of the cancer being treated.

Hyperfractionated Radiation Therapy

Hyperfractionated radiation therapy is radiation treatment in which each day's total dose of radiation is divided into two or more smaller doses, usually given hours apart, instead of giving it all at once. This is also called superfractionated radiation therapy.

Hyperthermia Therapy

Hyperthermia therapy is a treatment in which body tissue is heated above normal temperature to damage and kill cancer cells or to make cancer cells more sensitive to the effects of radiation and certain anticancer drugs.

Patients may want to think about taking part in a clinical trial. For some patients, taking part in a clinical trial may be the best treatment choice. Clinical trials are part of the cancer research process. Clinical trials are done to find out if new cancer treatments are safe and effective or better than the standard treatment.

Many of today's standard treatments for cancer are based on earlier clinical trials. Patients who take part in a clinical trial may receive the standard treatment or be among the first to receive a new treatment.

Patients who take part in clinical trials also help improve the way cancer will be treated in the future. Even when clinical trials do not lead to effective new treatments, they often answer important questions and help move research forward.

Patients can enter clinical trials before, during, or after starting their cancer treatment.

Some clinical trials only include patients who have not yet received treatment. Other trials test treatments for patients whose cancer has not gotten better. There are also clinical trials that test new ways to stop cancer from recurring (coming back) or reduce the side effects of cancer treatment.

Follow-Up Tests May Be Needed

Some of the tests that were done to diagnose the cancer or to find out the stage of the cancer may be repeated. Some tests will be repeated in order to see how well the treatment is working. Decisions about whether to continue, change, or stop treatment may be based on the results of these tests. This is sometimes called re-staging.

Some of the tests will continue to be done from time to time after treatment has ended. The results of these tests can show if your condition has changed or if the cancer has recurred (come back). These tests are sometimes called follow-up tests or check-ups.

Chapter 42

Salivary Gland Cancer

General Information about Salivary Gland Cancer

Salivary gland cancer is a rare disease in which malignant (cancer) cells form in the tissues of the salivary glands.

The salivary glands make saliva and release it into the mouth. Saliva has enzymes that help digest food and antibodies that help protect against infections of the mouth and throat. There are three pairs of major salivary glands:

- **Parotid glands:** These are the largest salivary glands and are found in front of and just below each ear. Most major salivary gland tumors begin in this gland.

- **Sublingual glands:** These glands are found under the tongue in the floor of the mouth.

- **Submandibular glands:** These glands are found below the jawbone.

There are also hundreds of small (minor) salivary glands lining parts of the mouth, nose, and larynx that can be seen only with a microscope. Most small salivary gland tumors begin in the palate (roof of the mouth).

Excerpted from PDQ® Cancer Information Summary. National Cancer Institute; Bethesda, MD. Salivary Gland Cancer Treatment (PDQ®): Patient Version. Updated 02/2008. Available at: http://cancer.gov. Accessed June 23, 2008.

More than half of all salivary gland tumors are benign (not cancerous) and do not spread to other tissues.

Being exposed to certain types of radiation may increase the risk of salivary cancer.

Anything that increases the chance of getting a disease is called a risk factor. Having a risk factor does not mean that you will get cancer; not having risk factors doesn't mean that you will not get cancer. People who think they may be at risk should discuss this with their doctor. Although the cause of most salivary gland cancers is not known, risk factors include the following:

- older age;

- treatment with radiation therapy to the head and neck; and

- being exposed to certain substances at work.

Possible signs of salivary gland cancer include a lump or trouble swallowing.

Salivary gland cancer may not cause any symptoms. It is sometimes found during a regular dental checkup or physical exam. Symptoms caused by salivary gland cancer also may be caused by other conditions. A doctor should be consulted if any of the following problems occur:

- a lump (usually painless) in the area of the ear, cheek, jaw, lip, or inside the mouth;

- fluid draining from the ear;

- trouble swallowing or opening the mouth widely;

- numbness or weakness in the face; and

- pain in the face that does not go away.

Tests that examine the head, neck, and the inside of the mouth are used to detect (find) and diagnose salivary gland cancer.

The following procedures may be used:

- **Physical exam and history:** An exam of the body to check general signs of health. The head, neck, mouth, and throat will be checked for signs of disease, such as lumps or anything else that seems unusual. A history of the patient's health habits and past illnesses and treatments will also be taken.

- **MRI (magnetic resonance imaging):** A procedure that uses a magnet, radio waves, and a computer to make a series of detailed pictures of areas inside the body. This procedure is also called nuclear magnetic resonance imaging (NMRI).

- **CT scan (CAT scan):** A procedure that makes a series of detailed pictures of areas inside the body, taken from different angles. The pictures are made by a computer linked to an x-ray machine. A dye may be injected into a vein or swallowed to help the organs or tissues show up more clearly. This procedure is also called computed tomography, computerized tomography, or computerized axial tomography.

- **PET scan (positron emission tomography scan):** A procedure to find malignant tumor cells in the body. A small amount of radioactive glucose (sugar) is injected into a vein. The PET scanner rotates around the body and makes a picture of where glucose is being used in the body. Malignant tumor cells show up brighter in the picture because they are more active and take up more glucose than normal cells do.

- **Ultrasound exam:** A procedure in which high-energy sound waves (ultrasound) are bounced off internal tissues or organs and make echoes. The echoes form a picture of body tissues called a sonogram. The picture can be printed to be looked at later.

- **Endoscopy:** A procedure to look at organs and tissues inside the body to check for abnormal areas. For salivary gland cancer, an endoscope is inserted into the mouth to look at the mouth, throat, and larynx. An endoscope is a thin, tube-like instrument with a light and a lens for viewing.

- **Fine needle aspiration (FNA) biopsy:** The removal of tissue or fluid using a thin needle. A pathologist views the tissue or fluid under a microscope to look for cancer cells.

Because salivary gland cancer can be hard to diagnose, patients should ask to have biopsy samples checked by a pathologist who has experience in diagnosing salivary gland cancer.

Certain factors affect treatment options and prognosis (chance of recovery).

The treatment options and prognosis (chance of recovery) depend on the following:

- the stage of the cancer (especially the size of the tumor);
- the type of salivary gland the cancer is in;

- the type of cancer cells (how they look under a microscope); and
- the patient's age and general health.

After salivary gland cancer has been diagnosed, tests are done to find out if cancer cells have spread within the salivary gland or to other parts of the body.

The process used to find out if cancer has spread within the salivary glands or to other parts of the body is called staging. The information gathered from the staging process determines the stage of the disease. It is important to know the stage in order to plan treatment. The following procedures may be used in the staging process:

- **MRI (magnetic resonance imaging):** A procedure that uses a magnet, radio waves, and a computer to make a series of detailed pictures of areas inside the body. This procedure is also called nuclear magnetic resonance imaging (NMRI).

- **CT scan (CAT scan):** A procedure that makes a series of detailed pictures of areas inside the body, taken from different angles. The pictures are made by a computer linked to an x-ray machine. A dye may be injected into a vein or swallowed to help the organs or tissues show up more clearly. This procedure is also called computed tomography, computerized tomography, or computerized axial tomography.

There are three ways that cancer spreads in the body. The three ways that cancer spreads in the body are:

- **Through tissue:** Cancer invades the surrounding normal tissue.

- **Through the lymph system:** Cancer invades the lymph system and travels through the lymph vessels to other places in the body.

- **Through the blood:** Cancer invades the veins and capillaries and travels through the blood to other places in the body.

When cancer cells break away from the primary (original) tumor and travel through the lymph or blood to other places in the body, another (secondary) tumor may form. This process is called metastasis. The secondary (metastatic) tumor is the same type of cancer as the primary tumor. For example, if breast cancer spreads to the bones, the cancer cells in the bones are actually breast cancer cells. The disease is metastatic breast cancer, not bone cancer.

Treatment Option Overview

There are different types of treatment for patients with salivary gland cancer.

Different types of treatment are available for patients with salivary gland cancer. Some treatments are standard (the currently used treatment), and some are being tested in clinical trials. A treatment clinical trial is a research study meant to help improve current treatments or obtain information on new treatments for patients with cancer. When clinical trials show that a new treatment is better than the standard treatment, the new treatment may become the standard treatment. Patients may want to think about taking part in a clinical trial. Some clinical trials are open only to patients who have not started treatment.

Patients with salivary gland cancer should have their treatment planned by a team of doctors who are experts in treating head and neck cancer.

Your treatment will be overseen by a medical oncologist, a doctor who specializes in treating people with cancer. Because the salivary glands help in eating and digesting food, patients may need special help adjusting to the side effects of the cancer and its treatment. The medical oncologist may refer you to other doctors who have experience and expertise in treating patients with head and neck cancer and who specialize in certain areas of medicine. These include the following:

- head and neck surgeon;
- radiation oncologist;
- dentist;
- speech therapist;
- dietitian;
- psychologist;
- rehabilitation specialist; and
- plastic surgeon.

Three types of standard treatment are used:

Surgery

Surgery (removing the cancer in an operation) is a common treatment for salivary gland cancer. A doctor may remove the cancer and some of the healthy tissue around the cancer. In some cases, a lymphadenectomy (surgery in which lymph nodes are removed) will also be done.

Even if the doctor removes all the cancer that can be seen at the time of the surgery, some patients may be given radiation therapy after surgery to kill any cancer cells that are left. Treatment given after surgery to increase the chance of a cure is called adjuvant therapy.

Radiation Therapy

Radiation therapy is a cancer treatment that uses high-energy x-rays or other types of radiation to kill cancer cells or keep them from growing. There are two types of radiation therapy. External radiation therapy uses a machine outside the body to send radiation toward the cancer. Internal radiation therapy uses a radioactive substance sealed in needles, seeds, wires, or catheters that are placed directly into or near the cancer. The way the radiation therapy is given depends on the type and stage of the cancer being treated.

Special types of radiation may be used to treat some salivary gland tumors. These include:

- **Fast neutron radiation therapy:** Fast neutron radiation therapy is a type of high-energy external radiation therapy. A radiation therapy machine aims tiny, invisible particles, called neutrons, at the cancer cells to kill them. Fast neutron radiation therapy uses a higher-energy radiation than the x-ray type of radiation therapy. This allows the radiation therapy to be given in fewer treatments.

- **Photon-beam radiation therapy:** A type of radiation therapy that reaches deep tumors with high-energy x-rays made by a machine called a linear accelerator. This can be delivered as hyperfractionated radiation therapy, in which each day's total dose of radiation is divided into two or more smaller doses that are usually given hours apart.

Chemotherapy

Chemotherapy is a cancer treatment that uses drugs to stop the growth of cancer cells, either by killing the cells or by stopping them from dividing. When chemotherapy is taken by mouth or injected into a vein or muscle, the drugs enter the bloodstream and can reach cancer cells throughout the body (systemic chemotherapy). When chemotherapy is placed directly into the spinal column, an organ, or a body cavity such as the abdomen, the drugs mainly affect cancer cells in those areas (regional chemotherapy). The way the chemotherapy is given depends on the type and stage of the cancer being treated.

Radiosensitizers

Radiosensitizers are drugs that make tumor cells more sensitive to radiation therapy. Combining radiation therapy with radiosensitizers may kill more tumor cells.

Patients may want to think about taking part in a clinical trial. For some patients, taking part in a clinical trial may be the best treatment choice. Clinical trials are part of the cancer research process. Clinical trials are done to find out if new cancer treatments are safe and effective or better than the standard treatment.

Many of today's standard treatments for cancer are based on earlier clinical trials. Patients who take part in a clinical trial may receive the standard treatment or be among the first to receive a new treatment.

Patients who take part in clinical trials also help improve the way cancer will be treated in the future. Even when clinical trials do not lead to effective new treatments, they often answer important questions and help move research forward.

Patients can enter clinical trials before, during, or after starting their cancer treatment.

Some clinical trials only include patients who have not yet received treatment. Other trials test treatments for patients whose cancer has not gotten better. There are also clinical trials that test new ways to stop cancer from recurring (coming back) or reduce the side effects of cancer treatment.

Follow-Up Tests May Be Needed

Some of the tests that were done to diagnose the cancer or to find out the stage of the cancer may be repeated. Some tests will be repeated in order to see how well the treatment is working.

Decisions about whether to continue, change, or stop treatment may be based on the results of these tests. This is sometimes called re-staging.

Some of the tests will continue to be done from time to time after treatment has ended. The results of these tests can show if your condition has changed or if the cancer has recurred (come back). These tests are sometimes called follow-up tests or checkups.

Chapter 43

Dry Mouth and
Burning Mouth Syndrome

Chapter Contents

Section 43.1—Dry Mouth 436
Section 43.2—Burning Mouth Syndrome 439

Section 43.1

Dry Mouth

Excerpted from "Dry Mouth," by the National Institute on Aging
(NIA, www.nia.nih.gov), part of the National Institutes of Health,
December 17, 2007.

What Is Dry Mouth?

Dry mouth is the feeling that there is not enough saliva in the mouth. Everyone has dry mouth once in a while—if they are nervous, upset, under stress, or taking certain medications. But if you have dry mouth all or most of the time, see a dentist or physician. Many older adults have dry mouth, but it is not a normal part of aging.

Saliva does more than keep your mouth wet. It protects teeth from decay, helps heal sores in your mouth, and prevents infection by controlling bacteria, viruses, and fungi in the mouth.

Saliva helps digest food and helps us chew and swallow. Saliva is involved in taste perception as well. Each of these functions of saliva is hampered when a person has dry mouth.

Dry mouth can be uncomfortable. Some people notice a sticky, dry feeling in the mouth. Others notice a burning feeling or difficulty while eating. The throat may feel dry, too, making swallowing difficult and choking common. Also, people with dry mouth may get mouth sores, cracked lips, and a dry, rough tongue.

What Causes Dry Mouth?

People get dry mouth when the glands in the mouth that make saliva are not working properly. Because of this, there might not be enough saliva to keep your mouth healthy. There are several reasons why these glands, called salivary glands, might not work right.

More than 400 medicines, including some over-the-counter medications, can cause the salivary glands to make less saliva, or to change the composition of the saliva so that it can't perform the functions it should. As an example, medicines for urinary incontinence, allergies, high blood pressure, and depression often cause dry mouth.

436

Some diseases can affect the salivary glands. Dry mouth can occur in patients with diabetes and Parkinson disease. Dry mouth is the hallmark symptom of the fairly common autoimmune disease Sjögren syndrome.

Sjögren syndrome can occur either by itself or with another autoimmune disease like rheumatoid arthritis or lupus. Salivary and tear glands are the major targets of the syndrome and the result is a decrease in production of saliva and tears. The disorder can occur at any age, but the average person with the disorder is in his or her late 50s. Women with the disorder outnumber men 9 to 1.

Certain cancer treatments can affect the salivary glands. Head and neck radiation therapy can cause the glands to produce little or no saliva. Chemotherapy may cause the salivary glands to produce thicker saliva, which makes the mouth feel dry and sticky. Injury to the head or neck can damage the nerves that tell salivary glands to make saliva.

Treatment for Dry Mouth

Dry mouth treatment will depend on what is causing the problem. If you think you have dry mouth, see your dentist or physician. He or she can help to determine what is causing your dry mouth. If your dry mouth is caused by medicine, your physician might change your medicine or adjust the dosage.

If your salivary glands are not working right but can still produce some saliva, your dentist or physician might give you a medicine that helps the glands work better. Your dentist or physician might also suggest that you use artificial saliva to keep your mouth wet.

Drinking water or sugarless drinks often will make chewing and swallowing easier when eating. Avoid drinks with caffeine such as coffee, tea, and some sodas. Caffeine can dry out the mouth.

Don't use tobacco or alcohol. They dry out the mouth. Chew sugarless gum or suck on sugarless hard candy to stimulate saliva flow. Be aware that spicy or salty foods may cause pain in a dry mouth. Finally, use a humidifier at night to promote moisture in the air while you sleep.

Scientists are exploring the potential use of gene therapy—replacing, manipulating, or supplementing nonfunctional genes with healthy genes—to treat salivary gland dysfunction. The idea is to transfer additional or replacement genes into the salivary glands of people with Sjögren syndrome and cancer patients whose salivary glands were damaged during radiation treatment. The hope is that these genes will increase the production of saliva and eliminate the chronic parched sensation that bothers people with dry mouth conditions.

Research efforts are also under way to develop an artificial salivary gland for patients who have lost all salivary gland function. The first-generation artificial gland will be a tiny tube lined with cells that have been engineered to produce saliva-like fluid. Made of biodegradable material, the tube would be inserted into the inside of the cheek. All the components for the artificial gland have been developed and are now being tested with the goal of producing a prototype within a few years.

Keep Your Mouth Healthy

If you have dry mouth, you need to be extra careful to keep your teeth healthy. Saliva helps protect teeth from decay. But without enough saliva, you may be more likely to develop tooth decay or other infections in the mouth. Here are some tips for keeping your mouth healthy.

- Brush your teeth with an extra-soft toothbrush after every meal and at bedtime. If brushing hurts, soften the bristles in warm water.

- Floss your teeth gently every day. If your gums bleed and hurt, avoid the areas that are bleeding or sore, but keep flossing your other teeth, and see your dentist as soon as possible.

- Always use toothpaste with fluoride in it. Most toothpastes sold at grocery and drug stores have fluoride in them.

- Avoid sticky, sugary foods. If you do eat them, brush immediately afterward.

- Do not use mouthwashes with alcohol in them. Alcohol can dry out the mouth.

- Visit your dentist for a checkup at least twice a year—and more frequently if you have dry mouth. Your dentist might give you a special fluoride solution that you can rinse with to help keep your teeth healthy.

Section 43.2

Burning Mouth Syndrome

"Burning Mouth Syndrome" is from the National Institute on
Dental and Craniofacial Research (NIDCR, www.nidcr.nih.gov),
part of the National Institutes of Health, October 2007.

Burning mouth syndrome (BMS) is a painful, frustrating condition
often described as a scalding sensation in the tongue, lips, palate, or
throughout the mouth.

Although BMS can affect anyone, it occurs most commonly in
middle-aged or older women.

BMS often occurs with a range of medical and dental conditions,
from nutritional deficiencies and menopause to dry mouth and allergies. But their connection is unclear, and the exact cause of burning
mouth syndrome cannot always be identified with certainty.

Signs and Symptoms

Moderate to severe burning in the mouth is the main symptom of
BMS and can persist for months or years. For many people, the burning sensation begins in late morning, builds to a peak by evening, and
often subsides at night. Some feel constant pain; for others, pain comes
and goes. Anxiety and depression are common in people with burning mouth syndrome and may result from their chronic pain.

Other symptoms of BMS include:

• tingling or numbness on the tip of the tongue or in the mouth;

• bitter or metallic changes in taste; and

• dry or sore mouth.

Causes

There are a number of possible causes of burning mouth syndrome,
including:

• damage to nerves that control pain and taste;

- hormonal changes;
- dry mouth, which can be caused by many medicines and disorders such as:
  - Sjögren syndrome or diabetes;
  - nutritional deficiencies;
  - oral candidiasis, a fungal infection in the mouth;
  - acid reflux;
  - poorly fitting dentures or allergies to denture materials; and
  - anxiety and depression.

In some people, burning mouth syndrome may have more than one cause. But for many, the exact cause of their symptoms cannot be found.

Diagnosis

A review of your medical history, a thorough oral examination, and a general medical examination may help identify the source of your burning mouth. Tests may include:

- blood work to look for infection, nutritional deficiencies, and disorders associated with BMS such as diabetes or thyroid problems;
- oral swab to check for oral candidiasis; and
- allergy testing for denture materials, certain foods, or other substances that may be causing your symptoms.

Treatment

Treatment should be tailored to your individual needs. Depending on the cause of your BMS symptoms, possible treatments may include:

- adjusting or replacing irritating dentures;
- treating existing disorders such as diabetes, Sjögren syndrome, or a thyroid problem to improve burning mouth symptoms;
- recommending supplements for nutritional deficiencies;
- switching medicine, where possible, if a drug you are taking is causing your burning mouth;

- prescribing medications to:
  - relieve dry mouth;
  - treat oral candidiasis;
  - help control pain from nerve damage; and
  - relieve anxiety and depression.

When no underlying cause can be found, treatment is aimed at the symptoms to try to reduce the pain associated with burning mouth syndrome.

Helpful Tips

You can also try these self-care tips to help ease the pain of burning mouth syndrome.

- Sip water frequently.
- Suck on ice chips.
- Avoid irritating substances like hot, spicy foods; mouthwashes that contain alcohol; and products high in acid, like citrus fruits and juices.
- Chew sugarless gum.
- Brush your teeth/dentures with baking soda and water.
- Avoid alcohol and tobacco products.

Talk with your dentist and doctor about other possible steps you can take to minimize the problems associated with burning mouth syndrome.

Chapter 44

Bad Breath (Halitosis)

Twenty-five percent of the population suffers from chronic halitosis. Halitosis can be a very embarrassing problem and can seriously affect one's business and social life.

If you don't brush and floss daily, particles of food remain in the mouth collecting bacteria, which can cause bad breath. The surface of the tongue is one of the major breeding grounds for bacteria that attack the teeth and gums, causing bad breath. Therefore, brushing your tongue daily can greatly reduce mouth odor.

Many of us are so busy we can barely catch our breath. But for the millions of Americans who suffer from chronic halitosis, or bad breath, the joys of everyday life can be anything but breathtaking.

It is estimated that nearly $10 billion is spent each year to treat bad breath; much of it is wasted. According to the Massachusetts Dental Society, some products on the market only solve bad breath problems temporarily.

Chronic halitosis sufferers should consult their dentist first before buying products that claim to solve bad breath problems.

Chronic bad breath can be caused by a number of things. Before someone starts spending money on products that may not work on a long-term basis, it's really important that a dentist diagnose the source of the problem first. A dentist will then be able to recommend or prescribe specific products or medications that can help.

"Take Your Bad Breath Away," © Massachusetts Dental Society (www .massdental org). Reprinted with permission. The date of this document is unknown.

Medical Disorder

The origin of halitosis varies. Bad breath may be the sign of a medical disorder, such as a local infection in the respiratory tract (nose, throat, windpipe, lungs), chronic sinusitis, postnasal drip, chronic bronchitis, diabetes, gastrointestinal disturbance, liver, or kidney ailment. Therefore, if your dentist determines that your mouth is healthy, you may be referred to your family doctor or a specialist to determine the cause of bad breath.

Medications and Foods

Taking certain medications may play a role in mouth odor. In addition, certain foods, such as onions and garlic, can be absorbed into the bloodstream and then move into the lungs, where it is expelled, causing bad breath. Keeping a log of foods eaten and medications taken will help your dentist make a determination on what to recommend for the problem.

Another bad breath culprit is the use of tobacco products. Not only does tobacco cause bad breath, stain teeth, reduce one's ability to taste foods, and irritate gum tissues, but tobacco users are more likely to suffer from periodontal disease and are at greater risk for developing oral cancer. If you use tobacco, ask your dentist for tips on kicking the habit.

Dry Mouth

Bad breath may also be caused by dry mouth, which takes place when the flow of saliva decreases. Saliva is essential for cleaning the mouth and removing particles that may cause odor. Dry mouth can be caused by some medications or by constantly breathing through the mouth. To help, a dentist may suggest using sugarless candy to increase fluid intake.

Periodontal or Gum Disease

It's also important to remember that bad breath may be a sign of something more serious, such as periodontal or gum disease. If gum disease is diagnosed, a general dentist may refer you to a periodontist, a specialist in gum disease. One of the warning signs of gum disease is persistent bad breath. Periodontal disease is caused by plaque—a sticky, colorless film of bacteria that forms on the teeth. Gum disease can cause gum tissues to pull away from the teeth and form pockets. At times, only a professional periodontal cleaning can remove extensive bacteria and plaque.

Although many people may be anxious to solve their mouth odor with a quick fix, the MDS cautions consumers about some breath products on the market. Mouthwashes are generally cosmetic and do not have a long-lasting effect on bad breath. Over-the-counter mouthwashes and breath mints help get rid of a temporary mouth odor. However, if a person frequently has to use a mouthwash or mint to cover up breath problems, his or her dentist may suggest a special antimicrobial mouthwash.

However, there are some antiseptic mouth rinse products, approved by the American Dental Association, that have been shown to reduce plaque and gingivitis and that have breath-freshening properties. Instead of just temporarily solving breath odor, these products actually kill germs that cause halitosis. You can learn more about these products by visiting the consumer section of the ADA website (www.ada.org).

Whatever the source of the mouth odor, the Massachusetts Dental Society suggests that maintaining good oral health is necessary to avoid many dental problems, including bad breath, before they occur.

Chapter 45

Canker Sores

If you've ever had those open, shallow sores in your mouth and taken a gulp of orange juice—ouch!—you know what a pain canker sores can be. You're not alone, either. About one in five people get recurrent canker sores. So what can you do about them? Read on to find out.

What is a canker sore?

Canker sores, also known as aphthous ulcers, are small sores that occur inside the mouth. You can get them on the tongue and on the inside of the cheeks and lips—the parts of the mouth that can move. They usually pop up alone, but sometimes they show up in small clusters.

Your mouth might tingle or burn before the actual sore appears. Soon, a small red bump rises. Then after a day or so it bursts, leaving an open, shallow white or yellowish wound with a red border. The sores are often painful and can be up to an inch across, although most of them are much smaller. Occasionally, someone who gets canker sores may also develop a fever and feel sluggish and uncomfortable.

"Canker Sores," April 2006, reprinted with permission from www.kidshealth .org. Copyright © 2006 The Nemours Foundation. This information was provided by KidsHealth, one of the largest resources online for medically reviewed health information written for parents, kids, and teens. For more articles like this one, visit www.KidsHealth.org, or www.TeensHealth.org. This text was reviewed by Garrett B. Lyons, Sr., D.D.S., and Lisa A. Goss, R.D.H., B.S.

The good news is that canker sores are not contagious like some other mouth sores, such as cold sores. So you can't spread canker sores by sharing food or kissing someone. Cold sores, however, are caused by the herpes simplex virus, which can pass from person to person. If you have a sore and you're wondering if it's of the cold or canker variety, just look at where it's located. Cold sores usually appear outside the mouth, around the lips, chin, or nostrils. Canker sores, on the other hand, are always found inside the mouth.

You can also have spots in your mouth when you have an infection such as chickenpox or measles. In some cases of these diseases the rash actually spreads into the mouth. But someone with chickenpox or measles would find spots on other parts of the body as well, easily distinguishing those rashes from canker sores.

What causes canker sores?

No one is certain what causes canker sores. They often first appear between the ages of 10 and 20, although they can occur at any time in a person's life. One thing that doctors have noticed is that although the sores are not contagious, they can run in families. That means if your parents or siblings get canker sores, the genes you share with them make it more likely that you'll develop the sores, too.

There may be a connection between canker sores and stress. If the sores show up around exam time or some other big event in your life, it may be a sign of how much stress you're under. In addition, about twice as many women as men get them. Doctors think that may be due to the difference in male and female hormones, especially because women often get them during certain times in their menstrual cycle. Some research suggests that using products containing sodium lauryl sulfate (SLS), a foaming agent found in most toothpastes and mouthwashes, can be associated with canker sores. Dietary deficiencies, such as not getting enough iron or vitamin B12, may also contribute to some cases of canker sores.

How are they treated?

Most canker sores will heal on their own in a few days to a couple of weeks. While you're waiting for them to disappear, there are some things you can do:

- Various over-the-counter medicines can help to take the sting out of canker sores. Carbamide peroxide is a combination of peroxide and glycerin that cleans and coats the sore to protect it.

Other over-the-counter remedies have benzocaine, menthol, and eucalyptol in them. These need to be applied repeatedly and may sting at first, but they can numb the sore and cut down on how long it lasts.

• Try brushing and rinsing with toothpastes and mouthwashes that do not contain SLS.

• Some homemade mouthwashes can ease pain as well. Try rinsing your mouth four times a day with a mixture of 2 ounces of hydrogen peroxide and 2 ounces of water or a combination of 4 ounces of water mixed with 1 teaspoon (5 milliliters) of salt and 1 teaspoon of baking soda. Swish the mixture in your mouth for about a minute and then spit it out—do not swallow it!

• Dabbing a mixture of equal parts water and hydrogen peroxide directly on the sore, followed by a bit of milk of magnesia, may reduce discomfort and speed healing.

• Some doctors suggest putting wet black tea bags on sores. Black tea contains tannin, a substance that can relieve pain. You can also find tannin in some over-the-counter medicines.

You'll want to watch what you eat when you have a canker sore. Spicy foods and acidic foods such as lemons or tomatoes can be extremely painful on these open wounds. So can anything sharp, such as nuts or potato chips, which can poke or rub the sore. Be careful when you brush your teeth, too. It's important to keep your mouth clean, but brushing the sore itself with a toothbrush will make it worse.

If you have canker sores that do not get better after a few weeks, if the sores keep coming back, or if they make you feel so sick that you don't want to eat, see your doctor or dentist. Your doctor may want to do blood tests to find out if another condition—such as a vitamin deficiency, a problem with your immune system, or even a food allergy—could be contributing to the sores.

Your doctor or dentist may prescribe a topical medicine or special mouthwash to help heal the sores. If the medicine needs to be applied directly to the sore, first blot the area dry with a tissue. Use a cotton swab to apply a small amount of the medication, and do not eat or drink for at least 30 minutes to make sure that the medicine is not immediately washed away. For severe mouth sores, your doctor or dentist may suggest other medications.

Although they can certainly be a pain, in most cases canker sores aren't that big of a deal.

Chapter 46

Infections That
Affect the Lip and Mouth

Chapter Contents

Section 46.1—Cold Sores (Herpes Simplex Virus-1) 452
Section 46.2—Oral Thrush (Oropharyngeal Candidiasis) 455

Section 46.1

Cold Sores (Herpes Simplex Virus-1)

"Cold Sores (HSV-1)," August 2005, reprinted with permission from www.kidshealth.org. Copyright © 2005 The Nemours Foundation. This information was provided by KidsHealth, one of the largest resources online for medically reviewed health information written for parents, kids, and teens. For more articles like this one, visit www.KidsHealth.org, or www TeensHealth.org. This text was reviewed by Larissa Hirsch, M.D.

Neal knew something weird was going on. A few days before, his lip started tingling and felt a little numb. He didn't pay much attention to it then, but now there was a certain throbbing something on his lip and it wasn't pretty. At first Neal thought it was a zit because it was red and tender, but then it blistered and opened up. Neal had a cold sore.

Maybe you've heard of a fever blister—a cold sore is the same thing. They're pretty common and lots of people get them. So what exactly are cold sores and what causes them?

What's a cold sore?

Cold sores, which are small and somewhat painful blisters that usually show up on or around a person's lips, are caused by the herpes simplex virus-1 (HSV-1). But they don't just show up on the lips. They can sometimes be inside the mouth, on the face, or even inside or on the nose. These places are the most common, but sores can appear anywhere on the body, including the genital area.

Genital herpes isn't typically caused by HSV-1; it's caused by another type of the herpes simplex virus called herpes simplex virus-2 (HSV-2) and is spread by sexual contact. But even though HSV-1 typically causes sores around the mouth and HSV-2 causes genital sores, these viruses can cause sores in either place.

What causes a cold sore?

HSV-1 is very common—if you have it, chances are you picked it up when you were a kid. Most people who are infected with the herpes simplex virus got it during their preschool years, most likely from close contact with someone who has it or getting kissed by an adult with the virus.

Although a person who has HSV-1 doesn't always have sores, the virus stays in the body and there's no permanent cure.

When someone gets infected with HSV-1, the virus makes its way through the skin and into a group of nerve cells called a ganglion (pronounced: gang-glee-in). The virus moves in here, takes a long snooze, and every now and then decides to wake up and cause a cold sore. But not everyone who gets the herpes simplex virus develops cold sores. In some people, the virus stays dormant (asleep) permanently.

What causes the virus to "wake up" or reactivate? The truth is, no one knows for sure. A person doesn't necessarily have to have a cold to get a cold sore—they can be brought on by other infections, fever, stress, sunlight, cold weather, hormone changes in menstruation or pregnancy, tooth extractions, and certain foods and drugs. In a lot of people, the cause is unpredictable.

Here's how a cold sore develops:

- The herpes simplex virus-1, which has been lying dormant in the body, reactivates or "wakes up."

- The virus travels toward the area where the cold sore decides to show up (like a person's lip) via the nerve endings.

- The area below the skin's surface, where the cold sore is going to appear, starts to tingle, itch, or burn.

- A red bump appears in the area about a day or so after the tingling.

- The bump blisters and turns into a cold sore.

- After a few days, the cold sore dries up and a yellow crust appears in its place.

- The scab-like yellow crust falls off and leaves behind a pinkish area where it once was.

- The redness fades away as the body heals and sends the herpes simplex virus back to "sleep."

How do cold sores spread?

Cold sores are really contagious. If you have a cold sore, it's very easy to infect another person with HSV-1. The virus spreads through direct contact—through skin contact or contact with oral or genital secretions (like through kissing). Although the virus is most contagious when a sore is present, it can still be passed on even if you can't see a sore. HSV-1 can also be spread by sharing a cup or eating utensils with someone who has it.

453

In addition, if you or your partner gets cold sores on the mouth, the herpes simplex virus-1 can be transmitted during oral sex and cause herpes in the genital area.

Herpes simplex virus-1 also can spread if a person touches the cold sore and then touches a mucous membrane or an area of the skin with a cut on it. Mucous membranes are the moist, protective linings made of tissue that are found in certain areas of your body like your nose, eyes, mouth, and vagina. So it's best to not mess with a cold sore—don't pick, pinch, or squeeze it.

Actually, it's a good idea to not even touch active cold sores. If you do touch an active cold sore, don't touch other parts of your body. Be especially careful about touching your eyes—if it gets into the eyes, HSV-1 can cause a lot of damage. Wash your hands as soon as possible. In fact, if you have a cold sore or you're around someone with a cold sore, try to wash your hands frequently.

If they aren't taken care of properly, cold sores can develop into bacterial skin infections. And they can actually be dangerous for people whose immune systems are weakened (such as infants and people who have cancer or HIV/AIDS [human immunodeficiency virus/acquired immunodeficiency syndrome]) as well as those with eczema. For people with any of these conditions, an infection triggered by a cold sore can actually be life threatening.

How are cold sores diagnosed and treated?

Cold sores normally go away on their own within 7 to 10 days. And although no medications can make the infection go away, prescription drugs and creams are available that can shorten the length of the outbreak and make the cold sore less painful.

If you have a cold sore, it's important to see your doctor if:

- you have another health condition that has weakened your immune system

- the sores don't heal by themselves within 7 to 10 days

- you get cold sores frequently

- you have signs of a bacterial infection, such as fever, pus, or spreading redness

To make yourself more comfortable when you have cold sores, you can apply ice or anything cool to the area. You also can take an over-the-counter pain reliever, such as acetaminophen or ibuprofen.

Section 46.2

Oral Thrush (Oropharyngeal Candidiasis)

Excerpted from "Oropharyngeal Candidiasis," by the Centers for Disease Control and Prevention, Division of Foodborne, Bacterial and Mycotic Diseases (DFBMD, www.cdc.gov/ncidod/dbmd), October 6, 2005.

What is oropharyngeal candidiasis (OPC)?

Candidiasis of the mouth and throat, also known as a "thrush" or oropharyngeal candidiasis (OPC), is a fungal infection that occurs when there is overgrowth of fungus called *Candida. Candida* is normally found on skin or mucous membranes. However, if the environment inside the mouth or throat becomes imbalanced, *Candida* can multiply. When this happens, symptoms of thrush appear. *Candida* overgrowth can also develop in the esophagus, and is called *Candida* esophagitis, or esophageal candidiasis.

How common is OPC and who can get it?

OPC can affect normal newborns, persons with dentures, and people who use inhaled corticosteroids. It occurs more frequently and more severely in people with weakened immune systems, particularly in persons with AIDS [acquired immunodeficiency syndrome] and people undergoing treatment for cancer. *Candida* esophagitis usually occurs in people with weakened immune systems. It is very unusual in otherwise healthy people.

How do I get OPC?

Most cases of OPC are caused by the person's own *Candida* organisms which normally live in the mouth or digestive tract. A person has symptoms when overgrowth of *Candida* organisms occurs.

What are the symptoms of OPC?

People with OPC infection usually have painless, white patches in the mouth. Others may have redness and soreness of the inside of the mouth. Cracking at the corners of the mouth, known as angular cheilitis, may occur. Symptoms of *Candida* esophagitis may include pain and difficulty swallowing. Other conditions can cause similar symptoms, so it is important to see your doctor.

How is OPC diagnosed?

OPC is often diagnosed based on the clinical appearance of the mouth and by taking a scraping of the white patches and looking at it under a microscope. A culture may also be performed. Because *Candida* organisms are normal inhabitants of the human mouth, a positive culture by itself does not make the diagnosis.

How is OPC treated?

Prescription treatments include clotrimazole troches or lozenges and nystatin suspension (nystatin "swish and swallow"). Another commonly prescribed treatment is oral fluconazole. For infection which does not respond to these treatments, there are a number of other antifungal drugs that are available.

What will happen if a person does not seek treatment for OPC?

Symptoms, which may be uncomfortable, may persist. In rare cases, invasive candidiasis may occur.

Can OPC become resistant to treatment?

Yes, OPC and *Candida* esophagitis can become resistant to antifungal treatment over time. Therefore, it is important to see your doctor for evaluation if you think you have OPC or *Candida* esophagitis.

Chapter 47

Taste and Smell Disorders

Taste Disorders

If you experience a taste problem, it is important to remember that you are not alone. More than 200,000 people visit a physician for such a chemosensory problem each year. Many more taste disorders go unreported.

Many people who have taste disorders also notice problems with their sense of smell.

How does our sense of taste work?

Taste belongs to our chemical sensing system, or the chemosenses. The complex process of tasting begins when tiny molecules released by the substances around us stimulate special cells in the nose, mouth, or throat. These special sensory cells transmit messages through nerves to the brain, where specific tastes are identified.

Gustatory or taste cells react to food and beverages. These surface cells in the mouth send taste information to their nerve fibers. The taste cells are clustered in the taste buds of the mouth, tongue, and throat. Many of the small bumps that can be seen on the tongue contain taste buds.

This chapter contains text excerpted from "Taste Disorders," by the National Institute on Deafness and Other Communication Disorders (NIDCD, www.nidcd .nih.gov), part of the National Institutes of Health, March 2002, and "Smell Disorders," by the NIDCD, March 2002. Both documents were reviewed by David A. Cooke, M.D., May 11, 2008.

Another chemosensory mechanism, called the common chemical sense, contributes to appreciation of food flavor. In this system, thousands of nerve endings—especially on the moist surfaces of the eyes, nose, mouth, and throat—give rise to sensations like the sting of ammonia, the coolness of menthol, and the irritation of chili peppers.

We can commonly identify at least five different taste sensations: sweet, sour, bitter, salty, and umami (the taste elicited by glutamate, which is found in chicken broth, meat extracts, and some cheeses). In the mouth, these tastes, along with texture, temperature, and the sensations from the common chemical sense, combine with odors to produce a perception of flavor. It is flavor that lets us know whether we are eating a pear or an apple. Some people are surprised to learn that flavors are recognized mainly through the sense of smell. If you hold your nose while eating chocolate, for example, you will have trouble identifying the chocolate flavor—even though you can distinguish the food's sweetness or bitterness. That is because the distinguishing characteristic of chocolate, for example, what differentiates it from caramel, is sensed largely by its odor.

What are the taste disorders?

The most common true taste complaint is phantom taste perceptions. Additionally, testing may demonstrate a reduced ability to taste sweet, sour, bitter, salty, and umami, which is called hypogeusia. Some people can detect no tastes, called ageusia. True taste loss is rare; perceived loss usually reflects a smell loss, which is often confused with a taste loss.

In other disorders of the chemical senses, the system may misread and or distort an odor, a taste, or a flavor. Or a person may detect a foul taste from a substance that is normally pleasant tasting.

What causes taste disorders?

Some people are born with chemosensory disorders, but most develop them after an injury or illness. Upper respiratory infections are blamed for some chemosensory losses, and injury to the head can also cause taste problems.

Loss of taste can also be caused by exposure to certain chemicals such as insecticides and by some medicines. Taste disorders may result from oral health problems and some surgeries (e.g., third molar extraction and middle ear surgery). Many patients who receive radiation therapy for cancers of the head and neck develop chemosensory disorders.

How are taste disorders diagnosed?

The extent of a chemosensory disorder can be determined by measuring the lowest concentration of a chemical that a person can detect or recognize. A patient may also be asked to compare the tastes of different chemicals or to note how the intensity of a taste grows when a chemical's concentration is increased.

Scientists have developed taste testing in which the patient responds to different chemical concentrations. This may involve a simple "sip, spit, and rinse" test, or chemicals may be applied directly to specific areas of the tongue.

Are taste disorders serious?

Yes. A person with a taste disorder is challenged not only by quality-of-life issues, but also deprived of an early warning system that most of us take for granted. Taste helps us detect spoiled food or beverages and, for some, the presence of food to which we're allergic. Perhaps more serious, loss of the sense of taste can also lead to depression and a reduced desire to eat.

Abnormalities in chemosensory function may accompany and even signal the existence of several diseases or unhealthy conditions, including obesity, diabetes, hypertension, malnutrition, and some degenerative diseases of the nervous system such as Parkinson disease, Alzheimer disease, and Korsakoff psychosis.

Can taste disorders be treated?

Yes. If a certain medication is the cause of a taste disorder, stopping or changing the medicine may help eliminate the problem. Some patients, notably those with respiratory infections or allergies, regain their sense of taste when the illness resolves. Often the correction of a general medical problem can also correct the loss of taste. Occasionally, recovery of the chemosenses occurs spontaneously.

What research is being done?

The NIDCD supports basic and clinical investigations of chemosensory disorders at institutions across the nation. Some of these studies are conducted at several chemosensory research centers, where scientists work together to unravel the secrets of taste disorders.

Some of the most recent research on our sense of taste focuses on identifying the key receptors in our taste cells and how they work in order to form a more complete understanding of the gustatory system, particularly how the protein mechanisms in G-protein-coupled receptors work. Advances in this area may have great practical uses, such as the creation of medicines and artificial food products that allow older adults with taste disorders to enjoy food again. Future research may examine how tastes change in both humans and animals. Some of this research will focus on adaptive taste changes over long periods in different animal species, while other research will examine why we accept or have an aversion to different tastes. Beyond this, scientists feel future gustatory research may also investigate how taste affects various processing activities in the brain. Specifically, how taste interacts with memory, influences hormonal feedback systems, and its role in the eating decisions and behavior.

Already, remarkable progress has been made in establishing the nature of changes that occur in taste senses with age. It is now known that age takes a much greater toll on smell than on taste. Also, taste cells (along with smell cells) are the only sensory cells that are regularly replaced throughout a person's life span—taste cells usually last about 10 days. Scientists are examining these phenomena which may provide ways to replace damaged sensory and nerve cells.

What can I do to help myself?

Proper diagnosis by a trained professional, such as an otolaryngologist, is important. These physicians specialize in disorders of the head and neck, especially those related to the ear, nose, and throat. Diagnosis may lead to treatment of the underlying cause of the disorder. Many types of taste disorders are curable, and for those that are not, counseling is available to help patients cope.

Smell Disorders

Every year, thousands of people develop problems with their sense of smell. In fact, more than 200,000 people visit a physician each year for help with smell disorders or related problems. If you experience a problem with your sense of smell, call your doctor. This information explains smell and smell disorders.

Many people who have smell disorders also notice problems with their sense of taste.

How does our sense of smell work?

The sense of smell is part of our chemical sensing system, or the chemosenses. Sensory cells in our nose, mouth, and throat have a role in helping us interpret smells, as well as taste flavors. Microscopic molecules released by the substances around us (foods, flowers, etc.) stimulate these sensory cells. Once the cells detect the molecules they send messages to our brains, where we identify the smell.

Olfactory, or smell nerve cells, are stimulated by the odors around us—the fragrance of a gardenia or the smell of bread baking. These nerve cells are found in a small patch of tissue high inside the nose, and they connect directly to the brain. Our sense of smell is also influenced by something called the common chemical sense. This sense involves nerve endings in our eyes, nose, mouth, and throat, especially those on moist surfaces. Beyond smell and taste, these nerve endings help us sense the feelings stimulated by different substances, such as the eye-watering potency of an onion or the refreshing cool of peppermint.

It's a surprise to many people to learn that flavors are recognized mainly through the sense of smell. Along with texture, temperature, and the sensations from the common chemical sense, the perception of flavor comes from a combination of odors and taste. Without the olfactory cells, familiar flavors like coffee or oranges would be harder to distinguish.

What are the smell disorders?

People who experience smell disorders experience either a loss in their ability to smell or changes in the way they perceive odors. As for loss of the sense of smell, some people have hyposmia, which is when their ability to detect odor is reduced. Other people can't detect odor at all, which is called anosmia. As for changes in the perception of odors, some people notice that familiar odors become distorted. Or, an odor that usually smells pleasant instead smells foul. Still other people may perceive a smell that isn't present at all.

What causes smell disorders?

Smell disorders have many causes, some clearer than others. Most people who develop a smell disorder have recently experienced an illness or an injury. Common triggers are upper respiratory infections and head injuries.

Among other causes of smell disorders are polyps in the nasal cavities, sinus infections, hormonal disturbances, or dental problems. Exposure to certain chemicals, such as insecticides and solvents, and some medicines have also been associated with smell disorders. People with head and neck cancers who receive radiation treatment are also among those who experience problems with their sense of smell.

How are smell disorders diagnosed?

Doctors and scientists have developed tests to determine the extent and nature of a person's smell disorder. Tests are designed to measure the smallest amount of odor patients can detect as well as their accuracy in identifying different smells. In fact, an easily administered "scratch and sniff" test allows a person to scratch pieces of paper treated to release different odors, sniff them, and try to identify each odor from a list of possibilities. In this way, doctors can easily determine whether patients have hyposmia, anosmia, or another kind of smell disorder.

Are smell disorders serious?

Yes. Like all of our senses, our sense of smell plays an important part in our lives. The sense of smell often serves as a first warning signal, alerting us to the smoke of a fire or the odor of a natural gas leak and dangerous fumes. Perhaps more important is that our chemosenses are sometimes a signal of serious health problems. Obesity, diabetes, hypertension, malnutrition, Parkinson disease, Alzheimer disease, multiple sclerosis, and Korsakoff psychosis are all accompanied or signaled by chemosensory problems like smell disorders.

Can smell disorders be treated?

Yes. Some people experience relief from smell disorders. Since certain medications can cause a problem, adjusting or changing that medicine may ease its effect on the sense of smell. Others recover their ability to smell when the illness causing their olfactory problem resolves. For patients with nasal obstructions such as polyps, surgery can remove the obstructions and restore airflow. Not infrequently, people enjoy a spontaneous recovery because olfactory neurons may regenerate following damage.

What research is being done?

The NIDCD supports basic and clinical investigations of chemosensory disorders at institutions across the nation. Some of these studies are conducted at several chemosensory research centers, where scientists are making advances that help them understand our olfactory system and may lead to new treatments for smell disorders.

Some of the most recent research into our sense of smell is also the most exciting. Though a complete understanding of the uniquely sophisticated olfactory system is still in progress, recent studies on how receptors recognize odors, together with new technology, have revealed some long-hidden secrets to how the olfactory system manages to detect and discriminate between the many chemical compounds that form odors. Besides uncovering the physical mechanisms our bodies use to accomplish the act of identifying smell, these findings are helping scientists view the system as a model for other molecular sensory systems in the body. Further, scientists are confident that they are now laying the foundation to understanding the finest details about our sense of smell—research that may help them understand how smell affects and interacts with other physiological processes.

Since scientists began studying the olfactory system, much has been discovered about how our chemosenses work, especially in how they're affected by aging. Like other senses in our bodies, our sense of smell can be greatly affected simply by our growing older. In fact, scientists have found that the sense of smell begins to decline after age 60. Women at all ages are generally more accurate than men in identifying odors, although smoking can adversely affect that ability in both men and women.

Another area of discovery has been the olfactory system's reaction to different medications. Like our sense of taste, our sense of smell can be damaged by certain medicine. Surprisingly, other medications, especially those prescribed for allergies, have been associated with an improvement of the sense of smell. Scientists are working to find out why this is so and develop drugs that can be used specifically to help restore the sense of smell to patients who've lost it. Also, smell cells (along with taste cells) are the only sensory cells that are regularly replaced throughout the life span. Scientists are examining these phenomena, which may provide ways to replace these and other damaged sensory and nerve cells. NIDCD's research program goals for chemosensory sciences include:

- promoting the regeneration of sensory and nerve cells;

- appreciating the effects of the environment (such as gasoline fumes, chemicals, and extremes of relative humidity and temperature) on smell and taste;

- preventing the effects of aging;

- preventing infectious agents and toxins from reaching the brain through the olfactory nerve;

- developing new diagnostic tests;

- understanding associations between chemosensory disorders and altered food intake in aging as well as in various chronic illnesses; and

- improving treatment methods and rehabilitation strategies.

What can I do to help myself?

The best thing you can do is see a doctor. Proper diagnosis by a trained professional, such as an otolaryngologist, is important. These physicians specialize in disorders of the head and neck, especially those related to the ear, nose, and throat. Diagnosis may lead to an effective treatment of the underlying cause of your smell disorder. Many types of smell disorders are curable, and for those that are not, counseling is available to help patients cope.

Part Seven

Health Conditions
That Impact Oral Care

Chapter 48

Autoimmune Diseases That Cause Oral Complications

Chapter Contents

Section 48.1—Sjögren Syndrome 468
Section 48.2—Pemphigus 476

Section 48.1

Sjögren Syndrome

Excerpted from "Sjögren's Syndrome," from the National Institute of Arthritis and Musculoskeletal and Skin Diseases (NIAMS, www.niams.nih.gov), part of the National Institutes of Health, December 2006.

What Is Sjögren Syndrome?

Sjögren syndrome is an autoimmune disease—that is, a disease in which the immune system turns against the body's own cells. Normally, the immune system works to protect us from disease by destroying harmful invading organisms like viruses and bacteria. In the case of Sjögren syndrome, disease-fighting cells attack various organs, most notably the glands that produce tears and saliva (the lacrimal and salivary glands). Damage to these glands causes a reduction in both the quantity and quality of their secretions. This results in symptoms that include dry eyes and dry mouth. In technical terms, the form of eye dryness associated with Sjögren syndrome is called keratoconjunctivitis sicca, or KCS, and the symptoms of dry mouth are called xerostomia. Your doctor may use these terms when talking to you about Sjögren syndrome.

When organs other than the lacrimal and salivary glands are affected, this is known as extraglandular involvement. Usually, this occurs in patients with primary Sjögren syndrome. Manifestations include joint inflammation; particular forms of autoimmune thyroid, kidney, liver, lung, and skin disease; and changes in nerve function of the upper or lower limbs. A small proportion of patients may progress to a form of malignant lymphoma.

You might hear Sjögren syndrome called a rheumatic disease. This means it causes inflammation in joints, muscles, skin, and other organs. Like rheumatoid arthritis and systemic lupus erythematosus, it is also considered one of the autoimmune connective tissue diseases. These conditions affect the framework of the body (joints, muscles, and skin).

What Are the Symptoms of Sjögren Syndrome?

Sjögren syndrome can cause many symptoms. The main ones are:

- **Dry eyes:** Eyes affected by Sjögren syndrome may burn or itch. Some people say it feels like they have sand in their eyes. Others have trouble with blurry vision, or are bothered by bright light, especially fluorescent lighting.

- **Dry mouth:** Dry mouth may feel chalky or like your mouth is full of cotton. It may be difficult to swallow, speak, or taste. Because you lack the protective effects of saliva, you may develop more dental decay (cavities) and mouth infections.

As noted above, both primary and secondary Sjögren syndrome can also affect other parts of the body, causing symptoms such as:

- multiple sites of joint and muscle pain;

- prolonged dry skin;

- skin rashes on the extremities;

- chronic dry cough;

- vaginal dryness;

- numbness or tingling in the extremities; and

- prolonged fatigue that interferes with daily life.

What Causes Dryness in Sjögren Syndrome?

Often in the autoimmune attack causing Sjögren syndrome, white blood cells called lymphocytes initially will target and damage the glands that produce tears and saliva. Although no one knows exactly how this occurs, the damaged glands produce tears and saliva that are diminished in both quantity and quality, leading to the symptoms of dryness of the eyes and mouth.

Who Gets Sjögren Syndrome?

Sjögren syndrome can affect people of either sex and of any age, but most cases occur in women. The average age for onset is late 40s, but in rare cases, Sjögren syndrome is diagnosed in children.

What Causes Sjögren Syndrome?

Researchers think Sjögren syndrome is caused by a combination of genetic and environmental factors. Several different genes appear to be involved, but scientists are not certain exactly which ones are linked to the disease, since different genes seem to play a role in different people. For example, there is one gene that predisposes Caucasians to the disease. Other genes are linked to Sjögren syndrome in people of Japanese, Chinese, and African American descent. Simply having one of these genes will not cause a person to develop the disease. Some sort of trigger must activate the immune system.

Scientists think that the trigger may be a viral or bacterial infection. It might work like this: A person who has a Sjögren-associated gene gets a viral infection. The virus stimulates the immune system to act, but the gene alters the attack, sending fighter cells (lymphocytes) to the glands of the eyes and mouth. Once there, the lymphocytes attack healthy cells, causing the inflammation that damages the glands and keeps them from working properly. This is an example of autoimmunity. These fighter cells are supposed to die after their attack in a natural process called apoptosis, but in people with Sjögren syndrome, they continue to attack, causing further damage. Scientists think that resistance to apoptosis may be genetic.

The possibility that the endocrine and nervous systems play a role in the disease is also under investigation.

How Is Sjögren Syndrome Diagnosed?

Your doctor will diagnose Sjögren syndrome based on your medical history, a physical exam, and results from clinical or laboratory tests. While reviewing your medical history, your doctor will ask questions about your general health, specific symptoms you are experiencing, and medical problems you and your family members have or have had. Your doctor will also ask about any medications you are taking and about lifestyle habits such as smoking or alcohol consumption. During the exam, your doctor will check for clinical signs of Sjögren syndrome, such as indications of mouth dryness, or signs of other connective tissue diseases.

Depending on what your doctor finds during the history and exam, he or she may want to perform some tests or refer you to a specialist to establish the diagnosis of Sjögren syndrome and/or to see how severe the problem is and whether the disease is affecting other parts of the body as well.

Some common eye and mouth tests are:

- **Schirmer test:** This test measures tears to see how the lacrimal (tear) glands are working. The doctor puts thin paper strips under the lower eyelids and measures the amount of wetness on

470

the paper after 5 minutes. People with Sjögren syndrome usually produce less than 8 millimeters of tears.

- **Slit lamp examination:** This test, in which an ophthalmologist uses equipment to magnify and carefully examine the eye, shows how severe the dryness is and whether the outside of the eye is inflamed.

- **Staining with vital dyes (rose bengal or lissamine green):** These tests show the extent to which dryness has damaged the surface of the eye. To perform one of these tests, the doctor puts a drop of a liquid containing a dye into the lower eyelid. The dye stains the surface of the eye, highlighting any areas of injury, thereby allowing the doctor to see with the slit lamp how much damage has occurred on the surface of the eye.

- **Mouth exam:** The doctor will look outside the mouth for signs of major salivary gland swelling and inside the mouth for signs of dryness. Signs of dry mouth include a dry, sticky lining (called oral mucosa); dental caries (cavities) in characteristic locations; thick saliva, or none at all coming out of the major salivary ducts; redness of the mouth lining, often associated with a smooth, burning tongue; and sores at the corners of the lips. The doctor might also try to get a sample of saliva, to check its quality and see how much of it the glands are producing.

- **Lip biopsy:** This test is the best way to find out whether dry mouth is caused by Sjögren syndrome. To perform this test the doctor removes tiny minor salivary glands from the inside of the lower lip and examines them under the microscope. If the glands contain white blood cells in a particular pattern, the test is positive for the salivary component of Sjögren syndrome.

Because there are many causes of dry eyes and dry mouth (including many common medications, other diseases, or previous treatment such as radiation of the head or neck), the doctor needs a thorough history from the patient, and additional tests to see whether other parts of the body are affected. These tests may include:

- **Routine blood tests:** The doctor will take a blood sample to look for levels of different types of blood cells, check blood sugar level, and see how the liver and kidneys are working.

- **Other blood tests:** Various blood tests may be performed to check for antibodies and other immunological substances often found in the blood of people with Sjögren syndrome. Antibodies are gamma globulin molecules, called immunoglobulins, which are important for fighting infection. Everyone has these in their blood, but people with Sjögren syndrome usually have too many of them. Antibodies that are directed against the individual making them are called auto antibodies. Antibodies that may be present in people with Sjögren syndrome include the following.

- **Immunoglobulins:** The three main classes of immunoglobulins can be measured to see if there is a general increase in antibodies.

- **Anti-thyroid antibodies:** Auto antibodies against the thyroid gland are created when white blood cells (lymphocytes) migrate into the thyroid gland, causing thyroiditis (inflammation of the thyroid), a common problem in people with Sjögren syndrome.

- **Rheumatoid factors (RF):** These are auto antibodies commonly found in the blood of people with rheumatoid arthritis as well as in people with Sjögren syndrome and other autoimmune connective tissue diseases.

- **Antinuclear antibodies (ANAs):** These are auto antibodies directed at the cells' nuclei. The presence of ANAs in the blood can indicate an autoimmune disorder, including Sjögren syndrome.

- **Sjögren antibodies, anti-SS-A (or -Ro) and anti-SS-B (or -La):** These are specific antinuclear antibodies that occur commonly, but not always, in people with Sjögren syndrome.

- **Chest x-ray:** Sjögren syndrome can cause inflammation in the lungs, so the doctor may want to take an x-ray to check them.

- **Urinalysis:** The doctor will probably test a sample of your urine to see how well the kidneys are working.

What Type of Doctor Diagnoses and Treats Sjögren Syndrome?

Because the symptoms of Sjögren syndrome develop gradually and are similar to those of many other diseases, getting a diagnosis can take time; in fact, it may take years to diagnose Sjögren syndrome. During those years, depending on the symptoms, a person could see a number of doctors, any of whom could diagnose the disease and be involved in its treatment. Usually, a rheumatologist (a doctor who specializes in diseases of the joints, muscles, and bones) will coordinate treatment among a number of specialists. In a recent survey of a large number of Sjögren syndrome patients, the doctors making their first diagnoses were identified as follows, in order of decreasing frequency:

- rheumatologist;

- primary care physician/internist;

- ophthalmologist (eye specialist);

- otolaryngologist (ear, nose, and throat specialist);

- dentist (oral care specialist);

- neurologist (nerve and brain specialist);

- allergist (allergic disease specialist);

- endocrinologist (endocrine disease specialist); and

- oncologist (cancer specialist).

How Is Sjögren Syndrome Treated?

Treatment can vary from person to person, depending on what parts of the body are affected. But in all cases, the doctor will help relieve your symptoms, especially dryness. For example, you can use artificial tears to help with dry eyes and saliva stimulants and mouth lubricants for dry mouth.

If you have extraglandular involvement (that is, a problem that extends beyond the moisture-producing glands of your eyes and mouth), your doctor—or the appropriate specialist—will also treat those problems. Treatment may include the following:

- nonsteroidal anti-inflammatory drugs, such as ibuprofen (Motrin, Advil) for joint or muscle pain;

- corticosteroid medications, such as prednisone, to suppress inflammation that threatens the lungs, kidneys, blood vessels, or nervous system; and

- immune-modifying drugs such as hydroxychloroquine (Plaquenil), methotrexate (Rheumatrex), and cyclophosphamide (Cytoxan) to control the overactivity of the immune system that, in severe cases, can lead to organ damage.

What Can I Do about Dry Mouth?

There are many remedies for dry mouth. You can try some of them on your own. Your doctor may prescribe others. Here are some many people find useful:

- **Chewing gum and hard candy:** If your salivary glands still produce some saliva, you can stimulate them to make more by chewing gum or sucking on hard candy. However, gum and candy must be sugar-free, because dry mouth makes you extremely prone to progressive dental decay (cavities).

- **Water:** Take sips of water or another sugar-free, noncarbonated drink throughout the day to wet your mouth, especially when you are eating or talking. Note that drinking large amounts of liquid throughout the day will not make your mouth any less dry and will make you urinate more often. You should only take small sips of liquid, but not too often. If you sip liquids every few minutes, it may reduce or remove the mucous coating inside your mouth, increasing the feeling of dryness.

- **Lip balm:** You can soothe dry, cracked lips by using oil- or petroleum-based lip balm or lipstick. If your mouth hurts, your doctor may give you medicine in a mouth rinse, ointment, or gel to apply to the sore areas to control pain and inflammation.

- **Saliva substitutes:** If you produce very little saliva or none at all, your doctor might recommend a saliva substitute. These products mimic some of the properties of saliva, which means they make the mouth feel wet. Gel-based saliva substitutes tend to give the longest relief, but as with all saliva products, their effectiveness is limited by the fact that you eventually swallow them. It is best to use these products rather than water when awakening from sleep: They reduce oral symptoms more effectively, and they do not cause excessive urine formation.

- **Prescription medications:** At least two prescription drugs stimulate the salivary glands to produce saliva. These are pilocarpine (Salagen) and cevimeline (Evoxac). The effects last for a few hours, and you can take them three or four times a day. However, they are not suitable for everyone, so talk to your doctor about whether they might help you. In trials of these drugs, patients have also experienced some reduction in their dry eye symptoms.

474

In addition to treatments for dry mouth itself, some people need treatment for its complications. For example, people with dry mouth can easily get a mouth infection from a common yeast called *Candida*. About one third of people with Sjögren syndrome experience this infection, which is called candidiasis. Most often, it causes red patches to appear, along with a burning sensation. This occurs particularly on the tongue and corners of the lips. Candidiasis is treated with prescription antifungal drugs.

The Importance of Oral Hygiene

Natural saliva contains substances that rid the mouth of the bacteria that cause dental decay (cavities) and mouth infections, so good oral hygiene is extremely important when you have dry mouth. Here's what you can do to prevent cavities and infections:

- Visit a dentist regularly, at least twice a year, to have your teeth examined and cleaned.

- Rinse your mouth with water several times a day. Don't use mouthwash that contains alcohol, because alcohol is drying.

- Use toothpaste that contains fluoride to gently brush your teeth, gums, and tongue after each meal and before bedtime. Nonfoaming toothpaste is less drying.

- Floss your teeth every day.

- Avoid sugar between meals. That means choosing sugar-free gum, candy, and soda. If you do eat or drink sugary foods, brush your teeth immediately afterward.

- See a dentist right away if you notice anything unusual or have continuous burning or other oral symptoms.

- Ask your dentist whether you need to take fluoride supplements, use a fluoride gel at night, or have a varnish put on your teeth to protect the enamel.

Medicines and Dryness

Certain drugs can contribute to eye and mouth dryness. If you take any of the drugs listed below, ask your doctor whether they could be causing symptoms. However, don't stop taking them without asking your doctor—he or she may already have adjusted the dose to help protect you against drying side effects or chosen a drug that's least likely to cause dryness. Drugs that can cause dryness include:

- antihistamines;
- decongestants;
- diuretics;
- some antidiarrhea drugs;
- some antipsychotic drugs;
- tranquilizers;
- some blood pressure medicines; and
- antidepressants.

Section 48.2

Pemphigus

Excerpted from "Pemphigus," by the National Institute of Arthritis and Musculoskeletal and Skin Diseases (NIAMS, www.niams.nih.gov), part of the National Institutes of Health, April 2007.

What Is Pemphigus?

Pemphigus is a group of rare autoimmune diseases that cause blistering of the skin and mucous membranes (mouth, nose, throat, eyes, and genitals). Some forms of the disease, including the most common form, may be fatal if left untreated.

What Causes Pemphigus?

Normally, our immune system produces antibodies that attack viruses and harmful bacteria to keep us healthy. In people with pemphigus, however, the immune system mistakenly attacks the cells in the epidermis, or top layer of the skin, and the mucous membranes. The immune system produces antibodies against proteins in the skin known as desmogleins. These proteins form the glue that keeps skin cells attached to keep the skin intact. When desmogleins are attacked, skin cells separate from each other and fluid can collect between the layers of skin, forming blisters that do not heal. In some cases, these blisters can cover a large area of skin.

It is unclear what triggers the disease, although it appears that some people have a genetic susceptibility. Environmental agents may trigger the development of pemphigus in people who are likely to be affected by the disease because of their genes. In rare cases, it may be triggered by certain medications. In those cases, the disease usually goes away when the medication is stopped.

Is Pemphigus Contagious?

Pemphigus is not contagious. It does not spread from person to person.

Is Pemphigus Hereditary?

Though there can be a genetic predisposition to develop pemphigus, there is no indication the disease is hereditary.

Who Gets Pemphigus?

Pemphigus affects people across racial and cultural lines. Research has shown that certain ethnic groups (such as the eastern European Jewish community and people of Mediterranean descent) are more susceptible to pemphigus. A particular type of pemphigus occurs more frequently in people who live in the rain forests of Brazil.

Men and women are equally affected. Research studies suggest a genetic predisposition to the disease. Although the onset usually occurs in middle-aged and older adults, all forms of the disease may occur in young adults and children.

What Are the Different Types of Pemphigus?

There are several types of pemphigus and other similar blistering disorders. The type of disease depends on what level in the skin the blisters form and where they are located on the body. Blisters always occur on or near the surface of the skin, which is called the epidermis. People with pemphigus vulgaris, for example, have blisters that occur within the lower layer of the epidermis, while people with pemphigus foliaceus have blisters that form in the topmost layer. The type of antibody that is attacking the skin cells may also define the type of disease present.

- **Pemphigus vulgaris** is the most common type of pemphigus in the United States. Soft and limp blisters appear on healthy-looking skin and mucous membranes. The sores almost always start in the mouth. The blisters of pemphigus vulgaris form within the deep layer of the epidermis, and are often painful. Blistered skin becomes so fragile that it may peel off by rubbing a finger on it. The blisters normally heal without scarring, but pigmented spots may remain for a number of months.

- **Pemphigus vegetans** is a form of pemphigus with thick sores in the groin and under the arms.

- **Pemphigus foliaceus** involves crusted sores or fragile blisters that often appear first on the face and scalp and later on the chest and other parts of the body. Unlike pemphigus vulgaris, blisters do not form in the mouth. The sores are superficial and often itchy, and are rarely as painful as pemphigus vulgaris blisters. There may also be loose, moist scales on the skin. IgA pemphigus is a blistering disorder in which a different type of antibody binds to the cell surface of epidermal cells. This disease is different from other forms of pemphigus because it involves a different type of antibody (called IgA) than other types. The disease may result in blisters similar to those seen in pemphigus foliaceus, or it may involve many small bumps containing pus. This is the most benign, or least harmful, form of pemphigus.

- **Paraneoplastic pemphigus** is a rare disease that is distinct from pemphigus, but shares some features of it. It occurs in people with certain types of cancer, including some lymphomas and leukemias. It often involves severe ulcers of the mouth and lips, cuts and scarring of the lining of the eye and eyelids, and skin blisters. Because the antibodies also bind the airways, patients may develop life-threatening problems in the lungs. This disease is different from pemphigus, and the antibodies in the blood are different. Special tests may be needed to identify paraneoplastic pemphigus.

What Is Pemphigoid, and How Is It Different from Pemphigus?

Pemphigoid is also a blistering disorder caused by autoimmune problems that result in an attack on the skin cells by a person's own antibodies. Pemphigoid produces a split in the cells where the epidermis and dermis, the layer below the epidermis, meet, causing deep, tense blisters that do not break easily.

Pemphigus, on the other hand, causes a separation within the epidermis, and the blisters are soft, limp, and easily broken. Pemphigoid is seen most often in the elderly and may be fatal. Usually, both pemphigus and pemphigoid are treated with similar medications. Severe cases may require different treatment.

How Is Pemphigus Diagnosed?

A diagnosis of pemphigus has several parts:

- A visual examination by a dermatologist. The doctor will take a complete history and physical exam, noting the appearance and location of the blisters.

- A blister biopsy. A sample of a blister is removed and examined under the microscope. The doctor will look for cell separation that is characteristic of pemphigus, and will also determine the layer of skin in which the cells are separated.

- Direct immunofluorescence. A biopsy of a skin sample is treated in the laboratory with a chemical compound to find the abnormal desmoglein antibodies that attack the skin. The specific type of antibodies that form may indicate what type of pemphigus exists.

- Indirect immunofluorescence. Sometimes called an antibody titre test, a sample of blood is tested to measure pemphigus antibody levels in the blood and help determine the severity of the disease. Once treatment begins, this blood test may also be used to find out if treatment is working.

Pemphigus is a serious disease, and it is important to do all of these tests to confirm a diagnosis. No single test is right all of the time.

Because it is rare, pemphigus is often the last disease considered during diagnosis. Early diagnosis may permit successful treatment with only low levels of medication, so consult a doctor if you have persistent blisters on the skin or in the mouth. In the most common form of pemphigus (pemphigus vulgaris), the mouth is often the first place that blisters or sores appear.

What Type of Doctor Treats Pemphigus?

Pemphigus is a rare disease of the skin; therefore, dermatologists are the doctors best equipped to diagnose and treat people with pemphigus.

If you have blisters in the mouth, a dentist can provide guidance for maintaining good oral health. This is important for preventing gum disease and tooth loss.

How Is Pemphigus Treated?

Treatment for pemphigus vulgaris involves using one or more drugs. High-dose oral corticosteroids, such as prednisone or prednisolone, are the main treatment for pemphigus. These are anti-inflammatory medicines that suppress the immune system. High doses are often required to bring pemphigus under control. To minimize the side effects patients may experience, once the disease begins to subside the corticosteroid levels are reduced slowly to the lowest level required to prevent new blisters or sores from appearing. Many patients will go into complete remission with treatment, although this may take a number of years. Other patients will need to continue to take small doses of medication to keep the disease under control. Prednisone is usually taken by mouth, but can also be injected into a vein, muscle, or directly into a blister. The route depends on the type and severity of disease. Usually, a corticosteroid cream will be used directly on the blisters.

To keep the levels of corticosteroid use to a minimum, immunosuppressive drugs are often added to a patient's treatment. These are drugs that stop or slow down the immune system's response to what it sees as an attack on the body. They include:

- mycophenolate mofetil (CellCept);
- azathioprine (Imuran);
- cyclophosphamide (Cytoxan); and
- methotrexate.

Other drugs that may be used include:

- dapsone (DDS); and
- antibiotics such as tetracycline.

All of these medications can cause serious side effects. You should see your doctor regularly for blood and urine tests. Be sure to report any problems or side effects you experience to the doctor. With prolonged high-dose corticosteroid therapy, common side effects include susceptibility to life-threatening infections, delayed wound healing, osteoporosis, cataracts, glaucoma, type 2 diabetes, loss of muscle mass, peptic ulcers, swelling of the face and upper back, and salt and water retention. To reduce the risk of osteoporosis, bone density measurements are taken, and patients with low bone density are prescribed medications such as alendronate (Fosamax) or risedronate (Actonel). Extra calcium and vitamin D intake, exercise, and stopping smoking are also recommended. For diabetes caused by steroid use, patients must be on a low sugar diet and may need to take antidiabetic medications.

The immunosuppressive drugs that are used to treat pemphigus can also increase the chances of developing an infection and may cause anemia, a decrease in the white blood cells in the blood, inflammation of the liver, nausea, vomiting, or allergic reactions.

People with severe pemphigus that cannot be controlled with corticosteroids may undergo plasmapheresis, a treatment in which the blood containing the damaging antibodies is removed and replaced with blood that is free of antibodies. Such patients can also be treated with IVIg, or intravenous immunoglobulin, which is given daily for 3 to 5 days, every 2 to 4 weeks for 1 to several months. Plasmapheresis and IVIg are both very expensive treatments, since they require large amounts of donated and specially processed blood. Scientists have reported success in treating difficult cases of pemphigus vulgaris with a combination of IVIg and rituximab, a cancer medication.

The treatment prescribed will depend on the type of pemphigus and the severity of the disease. Work closely with your doctor to devise the treatment regimen that works best for you. Because the medications used to treat pemphigus are strong medications with potentially serious side effects, every doctor that you see should be made aware of the type and amount of medications you are taking.

It may take several months to years for the ulcers and blisters of pemphigus vulgaris to disappear after treatment has begun because circulating antibodies remain in the blood for a long time. Lesions in the mouth are particularly slow to heal. Blisters in the mouth can make brushing the teeth painful, leaving you prone to gum disease and tooth loss. A dentist can offer approaches that enable you to maintain healthy teeth and gums. Avoiding spicy, hard, and acidic foods will help, since those foods can irritate or trigger the blisters. If you are taking corticosteroids, you should receive advice for maintaining a diet low in calories, fat, and sodium, and high in potassium and calcium.

What Is the Prognosis for People Who Have Pemphigus?

The outlook for people with pemphigus has changed dramatically in the past 40 years. A person diagnosed with pemphigus vulgaris in the 1960s faced the reality that they had a disease that was rare, usually fatal, poorly understood, with no good treatment options. Today, through medical research supported by the National Institutes of Health (NIH), the picture is dramatically better. The disease is now rarely fatal, and the majority of deaths occur from infections.

For most people with pemphigus, the disease can be controlled with corticosteroids and other medications, and these medications can eventually be completely discontinued. However, as described earlier, these medications can cause side effects that can sometimes be serious. Pemphigus and its treatments can be debilitating and cause lost time at work, weight loss, loss of sleep, and emotional distress. The International Pemphigus Foundation provides patient support services to help people with the disease cope with its effects.

Chapter 49

Oral Health and Bone Disease

Chapter Contents

Section 49.1—Osteoporosis 484
Section 49.2—Bisphosphonate-Associated Osteonecrosis
of the Jaw 486

Section 49.1

Osteoporosis

Excerpted from "Oral Health and Bone Health," by the National Institute of Arthritis and Musculoskeletal Diseases (NIAMS, www.niams.nih.gov), part of the National Institutes of Health, November 2005.

Osteoporosis and tooth loss are health concerns that affect many older men and women. Osteoporosis is a disease in which the bones become less dense and more prone to fracture. This disease can affect any bone in the body, although the bones in the hip, spine, and wrist are most often affected. In the United States today, 10 million individuals already have osteoporosis and 34 million more have low bone mass, placing them at increased risk for this disease.

Research suggests that there is a link between osteoporosis and bone loss in the jaw. The bone in the jaw supports and anchors our teeth. When the jaw bone becomes less dense, tooth loss can occur. Tooth loss affects approximately one-third of adults 65 years and older.

Skeletal Bone Density and Dental Concerns

The portion of the jaw bone that supports our teeth is known as the alveolar process. Several studies have found that the loss of alveolar bone is linked to an increase in loose teeth (tooth mobility) and tooth loss. Women with osteoporosis are three times more likely to experience tooth loss than those who do not have the disease.

Low bone density in the jaw can result in other dental problems as well. For example, older women with osteoporosis may be more likely to have difficulty with loose or ill-fitting dentures and may have less optimal outcomes from oral surgical procedures.

Periodontal Disease and Bone Health

It is estimated that periodontal disease affects up to 80 percent of men and women in the United States. Periodontitis is a chronic infection that affects the gums and the bones that support the teeth. Bacteria and the body's own immune system break down the bone and connective tissue that hold teeth in place. The teeth may eventually become loose, fall out, or have to be removed.

While tooth loss is a well-documented consequence of periodontitis, the relationship between periodontitis and skeletal bone density is less clear. However, some studies have found a strong and direct relationship between bone loss, periodontitis, and tooth loss. It is possible that the loss of alveolar bone mineral density leaves bone more susceptible to periodontal bacteria, increasing the risk for periodontitis and tooth loss.

The Role of the Dentist and Dental X-Rays

Research supported by the National Institute of Arthritis and Musculoskeletal and Skin Diseases (NIAMS) suggests that dental x-rays may be used as a screening tool for osteoporosis. Researchers found that dental x-rays were highly effective in distinguishing people with osteoporosis from those with normal bone density.

Since many people see their dentist more regularly then their doctor, dentists are in a unique position to help identify people with low bone density and to encourage them to talk to their doctors about their bone health. Dental concerns that may indicate low bone density include loose teeth, gums detaching from the teeth or receding gums, and ill-fitting or loose dentures.

The Effects of Osteoporosis Treatments on Oral Health

It is not known whether osteoporosis treatments have the same beneficial effect on oral health as they do on other bones in the skeleton. While additional research is needed to fully clarify the relationship between osteoporosis and oral bone loss, scientists are hopeful that efforts to optimize skeletal bone density will have a favorable impact on dental health.

Of concern is the fact that bisphosphonates, a group of medications available for the treatment of osteoporosis, have been linked to the development of osteonecrosis of the jaw (ONJ). The risk of ONJ has been greatest in those receiving large doses of intravenous bisphosphonates, a therapy used to treat cancer. The occurrence of ONJ is rare in individuals taking oral forms of the medication for osteoporosis treatment.

Taking Steps for Healthy Bones

There are many important steps you can to take to optimize your bone health:

- Eat a well-balanced diet rich in calcium and vitamin D.

- Live a healthy lifestyle. Don't smoke, and if you choose to drink alcohol, do so in moderation.

- Engage in regular physical activity or exercise. Weight-bearing activities, such as walking, jogging, dancing, and lifting weights, are the best for strong bones.

- Report any problems with loose teeth, detached or receding gums, and loose or ill-fitting dentures to your dentist and doctor.

Section 49.2

Bisphosphonate-Associated Osteonecrosis of the Jaw

Excerpted from "Bisphosphonate-Associated Osteonecrosis of the Jaw: Pathophysiology and Epidemiology," from the National Institute of Dental and Craniofacial Research (NIDCR, www.nidcr.nih.gov), part of the National Institutes of Health, May 2006.

The bisphosphonates are a class of drugs that inhibit the activities and functions of osteoclasts (bone resorbing cells) and perturb the differentiation of osteoblasts (bone forming cells). Intravenous bisphosphonates are primarily used to treat bone erosion and hypercalcemia associated with bone metastasis, Paget's disease, and multiple myeloma. Oral bisphosphonates are used to prevent bone loss and are prescribed for patients with osteoporosis or osteopenia. In 2003, the first report surfaced in the literature that suggests an association of ONJ with bisphosphonate use. Since then, several other reports have come to light strengthening this association. Whether bisphosphonates are causal to the development of ONJ remains to be determined. Most incidences are related to intravenous bisphosphonate use in cancer patients, but several cases are associated with oral bisphosphonates as well. Patients with ONJ present with painful, exposed, and necrotic bone, which may occur following dental procedures or spontaneously, and involving predominantly the mandible. These lesions are non-healing or slow to heal, and often complicated by secondary infection. Therefore, this is a significant clinical problem of potentially broad health impact, yet with complete lack of etiological and sufficiently powered epidemiological studies.

Bisphosphonates have been in use for almost 30 years.

The pathophysiological mechanisms underlying ONJ are unknown although several cellular processes when altered have been implicated in contributing to the condition. For example, the resorptive power of osteoclasts is essential in bone remodeling. Although bisphosphonates inhibit bone loss, they can also inhibit normal physiological bone remodeling and turnover to the extent that local microdamage of bone architecture due to mechanical loading during chewing, or local bone defects due to tooth extraction, cannot be effectively repaired. Another possibility is that bisphosphonates, some of which demonstrate antiangiogenic properties, may cause avascular necrosis of the bone. Finally, the data trends indicate that not all bisphosphonate users will eventually develop ONJ, suggesting that individual genetic variations in drug metabolism or skeletal homeostasis may confer susceptibility or resistance to developing ONJ. Several risk factors for the development of ONJ have been implicated. These include concomitant corticosteroid therapy and chemotherapy, dental procedures such as tooth extraction, poor oral health, and dose, duration and type of bisphosphonate use.

The exact incidence of bisphosphonate-associated ONJ is unknown but ranges from 0.03% to 10.5% in published reports. This is in part due to the lack of recognition of the condition and under-reporting, and lack of well characterized sufficiently powered cohorts for epidemiological studies. However, collectively, there is an extremely low incidence of ONJ for patients receiving bisphosphonate treatment for less than 12 months, suggesting that the cumulative effects of dose and time contribute to the manifestation of this adverse event.

Currently, there are no effective treatments for ONJ. Patients may be treated non-invasively with antibiotics and chlorhexidine mouth rinses to limit the extent of the damage. Surgical intervention such as local debridement or radical resection of necrotic bone often exacerbates the condition. Discontinuation of bisphosphonate use is not an effective remedy as these compounds have long resident time in the bone.

Although a causal relationship between bisphosphonates and ONJ has not been established, and other risk and comorbid factors for ONJ exist, this is clearly a new and emerging medical and dental concern. There is an urgent need to fill a significant knowledge gap in characterizing the condition, identifying the root cause, and determining individual susceptibility for the prevention and intervention of bisphosphonate-associated ONJ. This initiative will accelerate discoveries so that we can better predict who may benefit from bisphosphonate treatment without accompanying risk of ONJ, who may be prone to adverse events, and how to overcome bisphosphonate-associated ONJ. Knowledge gained from these studies may pave the way for personalized recommendations for bisphosphonate therapy, and strategies for the prevention and intervention of bisphosphonate-associated ONJ, while also managing bone cancer pain or osteoporotic bone loss.

Chapter 50

Oral Health and Cancer Treatment

Chapter Contents

Section 50.1—Oral Complications of Cancer Treatment 490

Section 50.2—Three Good Reasons to See a Dentist before
Cancer Treatment 497

Section 50.3—Head and Neck Radiation Treatment and
Your Mouth 499

Section 50.4—Chemotherapy and Your Mouth 504

Section 50.1

Oral Complications of Cancer Treatment

Excerpted from "Oral Complications of Cancer Treatment: What the Oral Health Team Can Do," from the National Institute of Dental and Craniofacial Research (NIDCR, www.nidcr.nih.gov), part of the National Institutes of Health, November 15, 2007.

With more than 1 million new cases of cancer diagnosed each year and a shift to outpatient management, it is likely that you will see some of these patients in your practice. Because cancer treatment can affect the oral tissues, you need to know about potential oral complications. Moreover, preexisting or untreated oral disease can complicate cancer treatment. Your role in patient management can extend benefits beyond the oral cavity.

Oral complications from radiation to the head and neck or chemotherapy for any malignancy can seriously compromise patients' health and quality of life, as well as affect their ability to complete planned cancer treatment. The complications can be so debilitating that patients may tolerate only lower and less effective doses of therapy, may postpone scheduled treatments, or may have to discontinue treatment entirely. Oral complications can also lead to potentially life-threatening systemic infections. Medically necessary oral care before, during, and after cancer treatment can prevent or reduce the incidence and severity of oral complications, enhancing both patient survival and quality of life.

Oral Complications Related to Cancer Treatment

Oral complications of cancer treatment arise in various forms and degrees of severity, depending on the individual and the cancer treatment. Chemotherapy often impairs the function of bone marrow, suppressing the formation of white blood cells, red blood cells, and platelets (myelosuppression). Some cancer treatments are described as stomatotoxic because they have toxic effects on the oral tissues. Following are lists of complications common to both chemotherapy and radiation therapy, and complications specific to each type of treatment.

490

You will need to consider the possibility of these complications each time you evaluate a patient with cancer.

Oral complications common to both chemotherapy and radiation:

- **Oral mucositis:** inflammation and ulceration of the mucous membranes; can increase the risk for pain, oral and systemic infection, and nutritional compromise.

- **Infection:** viral, bacterial, and fungal; results from myelosuppression, xerostomia, and/or damage to the mucosa from chemotherapy or radiotherapy.

- **Xerostomia/salivary gland dysfunction:** dryness of the mouth because of thickened, reduced, or absent salivary flow; increases the risk of infection and compromises speaking, chewing, and swallowing. Medications other than chemotherapy can also cause salivary gland dysfunction. Persistent dry mouth increases the risk for dental caries.

- **Functional disabilities:** impaired ability to eat, taste, swallow, and speak because of mucositis, dry mouth, trismus, and infection.

- **Taste alterations:** changes in taste perception of foods, ranging from unpleasant to tasteless.

- **Nutritional compromise:** poor nutrition from eating difficulties caused by mucositis, dry mouth, dysphagia, and loss of taste.

- **Abnormal dental development:** altered tooth development, craniofacial growth, or skeletal development in children secondary to radiotherapy and/or high doses of chemotherapy before age 9.

Additional Complications of Chemotherapy

- **Neurotoxicity:** persistent, deep aching and burning pain that mimics a toothache, but for which no dental or mucosal source can be found. This complication is a side effect of certain classes of drugs, such as the vinca alkaloids.

- **Bleeding:** oral bleeding from the decreased platelets and clotting factors associated with the effects of therapy on bone marrow.

Additional Complications of Radiation Therapy

- **Radiation caries:** lifelong risk of rampant dental decay that may begin within 3 months of completing radiation treatment if changes in either the quality or quantity of saliva persist.

- **Trismus/tissue fibrosis:** loss of elasticity of masticatory muscles that restricts normal ability to open the mouth.

- **Osteonecrosis:** blood vessel compromise and necrosis of bone exposed to high-dose radiation therapy; results in decreased ability to heal if traumatized.

Who Has Oral Complications?

Oral complications occur in almost all patients receiving radiation for head and neck malignancies, in up to 75 percent of blood and marrow transplant recipients, and in nearly 40 percent of patients receiving chemotherapy. Risk for oral complications can be classified as low or high:

- **Lower risk:** Patients receiving minimally myelosuppressive or nonmyelosuppressive chemotherapy.

- **Higher risk:** Patients receiving stomatotoxic chemotherapy resulting in prolonged myelosuppression, including patients undergoing blood and marrow transplantation; and patients undergoing head and neck radiation for oral, pharyngeal, and laryngeal cancer.

Some complications occur only during treatment; others, such as xerostomia, may persist for years. Unfortunately, many patients with cancer do not receive oral care until serious complications develop.

The Role of Pretreatment Oral Care

A thorough oral evaluation by a knowledgeable dental professional before cancer treatment begins is important to the success of the regimen. Pretreatment oral care achieves the following:

- reduces the risk and severity of oral complications;

- allows for prompt identification and treatment of existing infections or other problems;

- improves the likelihood that the patient will successfully complete planned cancer treatment;

- prevents, eliminates, or reduces oral pain;

- minimizes oral infections that could lead to potentially fatal systemic infections;

- prevents or minimizes complications that compromise nutrition;

- prevents or reduces later incidence of bone necrosis;
- preserves or improves oral health;
- provides an opportunity for patient education about oral hygiene during cancer therapy;
- improves the quality of life; and
- decreases the cost of care.

With a pretreatment oral evaluation, the dental team can identify and treat problems such as infection, fractured teeth or restorations, or periodontal disease that could contribute to oral complications when cancer therapy begins. The evaluation also establishes baseline data for comparing the patient's status in subsequent examinations.

Before the exam, you will need to obtain the patient's cancer diagnosis and treatment plan, medical history, and dental history. Open communication with the patient's oncologist is essential to ensure that each provider has the information necessary to deliver the best possible care.

Evaluation

The pretreatment evaluation includes a thorough examination of hard and soft tissues, as well as appropriate radiographs to detect possible sources of infection and pathology. Also take the following steps before cancer treatment begins:

- identify and treat existing infections, carious and other compromised teeth, and tissue injury or trauma;
- stabilize or eliminate potential sites of infection;
- in adults, extract teeth that may pose a future problem or are nonrestorable to prevent later extraction-induced osteonecrosis;
- conduct a prosthodontic evaluation, if indicated. If a removable prosthesis is worn, make sure that it is well adapted to the tissue and that the patient is able to wear and clean it daily;
- instruct the patient to leave the prosthesis out of the mouth at night;
- perform oral surgery at least 2 weeks before radiation therapy begins. For patients receiving radiation treatment, this is the best time to consider surgical procedures. Oral surgery should be performed at least 7 to 10 days before the patient receives myelosuppressive chemotherapy;

- medical consultation is indicated before invasive procedures;

- remove orthodontic bands and brackets if highly stomatotoxic chemotherapy is planned or if the appliances will be in the radiation field;

- in children, consider extracting highly mobile primary teeth and teeth that are expected to exfoliate during treatment; and

- prescribe an individualized oral hygiene regimen to minimize oral complications. Patients undergoing head and neck radiation therapy should be instructed on the use of supplemental fluoride.

Education

Patient education is an integral part of the pretreatment evaluation and should include a discussion of potential oral complications. It is very important that the dental team impress on the patient that optimal oral hygiene during treatment, adequate nutrition, and avoiding tobacco and alcohol can prevent or minimize oral complications. To ensure that the patient fully understands what is required, provide detailed instructions on specific oral care practices, such as how and when to brush and floss, how to recognize signs of complications, and other instructions appropriate for the individual. Patients should understand that good oral care during cancer treatment contributes to its success.

Advice for Patients

- Gently brush teeth, gums, and tongue with an extra-soft toothbrush and fluoride toothpaste after every meal and before bed. If brushing hurts, soften the bristles in warm water.

- Follow instructions for using fluoride gel.

- Floss teeth gently every day. If gums are sore or bleeding, avoid those areas but keep flossing other teeth.

- Avoid mouthwashes containing alcohol.

- Several times a day, rinse the mouth with a baking soda and salt solution, followed by a plain water rinse. (Use 1/4 teaspoon of baking soda and 1/8 teaspoon of salt in 1 cup of warm water.)

- Exercise the jaw muscles three times a day to prevent and treat jaw stiffness.

- Open and close the mouth as far as possible without causing pain; repeat 20 times.

- Avoid candy, gum, and soda unless they are sugar-free.
- Avoid spicy or acidic foods, toothpicks, tobacco products, and alcohol.
- Keep the appointment schedule recommended by the dentist.

Supplemental Fluoride

Fluoride rinses are not adequate to prevent tooth demineralization. Instead, a high-potency fluoride gel, delivered via custom gel-applicator trays, is recommended. Several days before radiation therapy begins, patients should start a daily 5-minute application of a 1.1% neutral pH sodium fluoride gel or a 0.4% stannous fluoride (unflavored) gel. Patients with porcelain crowns or resin or glass ionomer restorations should use a neutral pH fluoride. Be sure that the trays cover all tooth structures without irritating the gingival or mucosal tissues.

For patients reluctant to use a tray, a high-potency fluoride gel should be brushed on the teeth following daily brushing and flossing. Either a 1.1% neutral pH sodium or a 0.4% stannous fluoride gel is recommended, based on the patient's type of dental restorations.

Patients with radiation-induced salivary gland dysfunction must continue lifelong daily fluoride applications.

Oral Care during Cancer Treatment

Careful monitoring of oral health is especially important during cancer therapy to prevent, detect, and treat complications as soon as possible. When treatment is necessary, consult the oncologist before any dental procedure, including dental prophylaxis.

- Examine the soft tissues for inflammation or infection and evaluate for plaque levels and dental caries.
- Review oral hygiene and oral care protocols; prescribe anti-microbial therapy as indicated.
- Provide recommendations for treating dry mouth and other complications.
  - Sip water frequently.
  - Suck ice chips or sugar-free candy.
  - Chew sugar-free gum.
  - If appropriate, use a saliva substitute spray or gel or a prescribed saliva stimulant.
  - Avoid glycerin swabs.

495

• Take precautions to protect against trauma.

• Provide topical anesthetics or analgesics as appropriate for oral pain.

Other Factors to Remember

• **Schedule dental work carefully:** If oral surgery is required, allow at least 7 to 10 days of healing before the patient receives myelosuppressive chemotherapy. Elective oral surgery should not be performed for the duration of radiation treatment.

• **Determine hematologic status:** If the patient is receiving chemotherapy, have the oncology team conduct blood work 24 hours before dental treatment to determine whether the patient's platelet count, clotting factors, and absolute neutrophil count are sufficient to recommend oral treatment.

• **Consider oral causes of fever:** Fever of unknown origin may be related to an oral infection. Remember that oral signs of infection or other complications may be altered by immunosuppression related to chemotherapy.

• **Consider prophylactic antibiotic treatment:** If the patient has a central venous catheter, consult the oncologist about implementing the American Heart Association prophylactic antibiotic regimen before any dental treatment.

Follow-Up Oral Care

Chemotherapy

Once all complications of chemotherapy have resolved, patients may be able to resume their normal dental care schedule. However, if immune function continues to be compromised, determine the patient's hematologic status before initiating any dental treatment or surgery. This is particularly important to remember for patients who have undergone blood and marrow transplantation.

Radiation Therapy

Once the patient has completed head and neck radiation therapy and acute oral complications have abated, evaluate the patient regularly (every 4 to 8 weeks, for example) for the first 6 months. Thereafter, you can determine a schedule based on the patient's needs. However, keep in mind that oral complications can continue or emerge long after radiation therapy has ended.

Section 50.2

Three Good Reasons to See a Dentist before Cancer Treatment

From the National Institute of Dental and Craniofacial Research (NIDCR, www.nidcr.nih.gov), part of the National Institutes of Health, November 9, 2007.

1. **Feel better:** Your cancer treatment may be easier if you work with your dentist and hygienist. Make sure you have a pretreatment dental checkup.

2. **Save teeth and bones:** A dentist will help protect your mouth, teeth, and jaw bones from damage caused by radiation and chemotherapy. Children also need special protection for their growing teeth and facial bones.

3. **Fight cancer:** Doctors may have to delay or stop your cancer treatment because of problems in your mouth. To fight cancer best, your cancer care team should include a dentist.

Protect Your Mouth during Cancer Treatment

Brush gently, brush often:

- Brush your teeth—and your tongue—gently with an extra-soft toothbrush.

- If your mouth is very sore, soften the bristles in warm water.

- Brush after every meal and at bedtime.

Floss gently—do it daily:

- Floss once a day to remove plaque.

- If your gums bleed and hurt, avoid the areas that are bleeding or sore, but keep flossing your other teeth.

Keep your mouth moist:

497

• Rinse often with water.

• Don't use mouthwashes with alcohol in them.

• Use a saliva substitute to help moisten your mouth.

Eat and drink with care:

• Choose soft, easy-to-chew foods.

• Protect your mouth from spicy, sour, or crunchy foods.

• Choose lukewarm foods and drinks instead of hot or icy-cold.

• Avoid alcoholic drinks.

Keep trying (quit using tobacco):

• Ask your cancer care team to help you stop smoking or chewing tobacco.

• People who quit smoking or chewing tobacco have fewer mouth problems.

When Should You Call Your Cancer Care Team about Mouth Problems?

Take a moment each day to check how your mouth looks and feels. Call your cancer care team when you first notice a mouth problem, an old problem gets worse, or you notice any changes you're not sure about.

Tips for Mouth Problems

• **Sore mouth, sore throat:** To help keep your mouth clean, rinse often with 1/4 teaspoon of baking soda and 1/8 teaspoon of salt in 1 cup of warm water. Follow with a plain water rinse. Ask your cancer care team about medicines that can help with the pain.

• **Dry mouth:** Rinse your mouth often with water, use sugar-free gum or candy, and talk to your dentist about saliva substitutes.

• **Infections:** Call your cancer care team right away if you see a sore, swelling, bleeding, or a sticky, white film in your mouth.

• **Eating problems:** Your cancer care team can help by giving you medicines to numb the pain from mouth sores and showing you how to choose foods that are easy to swallow.

- **Bleeding:** If your gums bleed or hurt, avoid flossing the areas that are bleeding or sore, but keep flossing other teeth. Soften the bristles of your toothbrush in warm water.

- **Stiffness in chewing muscles:** Three times a day, open and close your mouth as far as you can without pain. Repeat 20 times.

- **Vomiting:** Rinse your mouth after vomiting with 1/4 teaspoon of baking soda in 1 cup of warm water.

- **Cavities:** Brush your teeth after meals and before bedtime. Your dentist might have you put fluoride on your teeth to help prevent cavities.

Section 50.3

Head and Neck Radiation Treatment and Your Mouth

From the booklet "Head and Neck Radiation Treatment and Your Mouth," by the National Institute of Dental and Craniofacial Research (NIDCR, www.nidcr.nih.gov), part of the National Institutes of Health, November 9, 2007. NIH Publication No. 02-4362.

Are you being treated with radiation for cancer in your head or neck?

If so, this information can help you. While head and neck radiation helps treat cancer, it can also cause other things to happen in your mouth called side effects. Some of these problems could cause you to delay or stop treatment. This information will tell you ways to help prevent mouth problems so you'll get the most from your cancer treatment. To help prevent serious problems, see a dentist at least 2 weeks before starting radiation.

How does head and neck radiation affect the mouth?

Doctors use head and neck radiation to treat cancer because it kills cancer cells. But radiation to the head and neck can harm normal cells, including cells in the mouth. Side effects include problems with your teeth and gums; the soft, moist lining of your mouth; glands that make saliva (spit); and jaw bones.

It's important to know that side effects in the mouth can be serious.

- The side effects can hurt and make it hard to eat, talk, and swallow.

- You are more likely to get an infection, which can be dangerous when you are receiving cancer treatment.

- If the side effects are bad, you may not be able to keep up with your cancer treatment. Your doctor may need to cut back on your cancer treatment or may even stop it.

What mouth problems does head and neck radiation cause?

You may have certain side effects in your mouth from head and neck radiation. Another person may have different problems. Some problems go away after treatment. Others last a long time, while some may never go away. Problems may include:

- dry mouth;

- a lot of cavities;

- loss of taste;

- sore mouth and gums;

- infections;

- jaw stiffness; or

- jaw bone changes.

Why should I see a dentist?

You may be surprised that your dentist is important in your cancer treatment. If you go to the dentist before head and neck radiation begins, you can help prevent serious mouth problems. Side effects often happen because a person's mouth is not healthy before radiation starts. Not all mouth problems can be avoided but the fewer side effects you have, the more likely you will stay on your cancer treatment schedule.

It's important for your dentist and cancer doctor to talk to each other before your radiation treatment begins. Be sure to give your dentist your cancer doctor's phone number.

When should I see a dentist?

You need to see the dentist at least 2 weeks before your first radiation treatment. If you have already started radiation and didn't go to a dentist, see one as soon as possible.

What will the dentist and dental hygienist do?

• Check your teeth.

• Take x-rays.

• Take care of mouth problems.

• Show you how to take care of your mouth to prevent side effects.

• Show you how to prevent and treat jaw stiffness by exercising the jaw muscles three times a day. Open and close the mouth as far as possible (without causing pain) 20 times.

What can I do to keep my mouth healthy?

You can do a lot to keep your mouth healthy during head and neck radiation. The first step is to see a dentist before you start cancer treatment. Once your treatment starts, it's important to look in your mouth every day for sores or other changes. These tips can help prevent and treat a sore mouth.

Keep your mouth moist.

• Drink a lot of water.

• Suck ice chips.

• Use sugarless gum or sugar-free hard candy.

• Use a saliva substitute to help moisten your mouth.

Clean your mouth, tongue, and gums.

• Brush your teeth, gums, and tongue with an extra-soft toothbrush after every meal and at bedtime. If brushing hurts, soften the bristles in warm water.

• Use a fluoride toothpaste.

• Use the special fluoride gel that your dentist prescribes.

• Don't use mouthwashes with alcohol in them.

501

- Floss your teeth gently every day. If your gums bleed and hurt, avoid the areas that are bleeding or sore, but keep flossing your other teeth.

- Rinse your mouth several times a day with a solution of 1/4 teaspoon baking soda and 1/8 teaspoon salt in one cup of warm water. Follow with a plain water rinse.

- Dentures that don't fit well can cause problems. Talk to your cancer doctor or dentist about your dentures.

If your mouth is sore, watch what you eat and drink.

- Choose foods that are good for you and easy to chew and swallow.

- Take small bites of food, chew slowly, and sip liquids with your meals.

- Eat soft, moist foods such as cooked cereals, mashed potatoes, and scrambled eggs.

- If you have trouble swallowing, soften your food with gravy, sauces, broth, yogurt, or other liquids.

Call your doctor or nurse when your mouth hurts.

Work with them to find medicines to help control the pain.
If the pain continues, talk to your cancer doctor about stronger medicines.

Remember to stay away from:

- sharp, crunchy foods, like taco chips, that could scrape or cut your mouth;

- foods that are hot, spicy, or high in acid, like citrus fruits and juices, which can irritate your mouth;

- sugary foods, like candy or soda, that could cause cavities;

- toothpicks, because they can cut your mouth;

- all tobacco products; and

- alcoholic drinks.

Do children get mouth problems, too?

Head and neck radiation causes other side effects in children, depending on the child's age.

Problems with teeth are the most common. Permanent teeth may be slow to come in and may look different from normal teeth. Teeth may fall out. The dentist will check your child's jaws for any growth problems.

Before radiation begins, take your child to a dentist. The dentist will check your child's mouth carefully and pull loose teeth or those that may become loose during treatment. Ask the dentist or hygienist what you can do to help your child with mouth care.

Remember

- Visit your dentist before your head and neck radiation treatment starts.

- Take good care of your mouth during treatment.

- Talk to your dentist about using fluoride gel to help prevent all the cavities that head and neck radiation causes.

- Talk regularly with your cancer doctor and dentist about any mouth problems you have during and after head and neck radiation treatment.

Section 50.4

Chemotherapy and Your Mouth

From the booklet "Chemotherapy and Your Mouth," by the National Institute of Dental and Craniofacial Research (NIDCR, www.nidcr.nih.gov), part of the National Institutes of Health, November 9, 2007. NIH Publication No. 02-4361.

Are you being treated with chemotherapy for cancer?

If so, this information can help you. While chemotherapy helps treat cancer, it can also cause other things to happen in your body called side effects. Some of these problems affect the mouth and could cause you to delay or stop treatment. This information will tell you ways to help prevent mouth problems so you'll get the most from your cancer treatment. To help prevent serious problems, see a dentist at least 2 weeks before starting chemotherapy.

How does chemotherapy affect the mouth?

Chemotherapy is the use of drugs to treat cancer. These drugs kill cancer cells, but they may also harm normal cells, including cells in the mouth. Side effects include problems with your teeth and gums; the soft, moist lining of your mouth; and the glands that make saliva (spit).

It's important to know that side effects in the mouth can be serious.

- The side effects can hurt and make it hard to eat, talk, and swallow.

- You are more likely to get an infection, which can be dangerous when you are receiving cancer treatment.

- If the side effects are bad, you may not be able to keep up with your cancer treatment. Your doctor may need to cut back on your cancer treatment or may even stop it.

What mouth problems does chemotherapy cause?

You may have certain side effects in your mouth from chemotherapy. Another person may have different problems. The problems depend on the chemotherapy drugs and how your body reacts to them. You may have these problems only during treatment or for a short time after treatment ends:

- painful mouth and gums;

- dry mouth;

- burning, peeling, or swelling tongue;

- infection; and

- change in taste.

Why should I see a dentist?

You may be surprised that your dentist is important in your cancer treatment. If you go to the dentist before chemotherapy begins, you can help prevent serious mouth problems. Side effects often happen because a person's mouth is not healthy before chemotherapy starts. Not all mouth problems can be avoided but the fewer side effects you have, the more likely you will stay on your cancer treatment schedule.

It's important for your dentist and cancer doctor to talk to each other about your cancer treatment. Be sure to give your dentist your cancer doctor's phone number.

When should I see a dentist?

You need to see the dentist at least 2 weeks before chemotherapy begins. If you have already started chemotherapy and didn't go to a dentist, see one as soon as possible.

What will the dentist and dental hygienist do?

- Check your teeth.

- Take x-rays.

- Take care of mouth problems.

- Show you how to take care of your mouth to prevent side effects.

What can I do to keep my mouth healthy?

You can do a lot to keep your mouth healthy during chemotherapy. The first step is to see a dentist before you start cancer treatment. Once your treatment starts, it's important to look in your mouth every day for sores or other changes. These tips can help prevent and treat a sore mouth:

Keep your mouth moist.

- Drink a lot of water.

- Suck ice chips.

- Use sugarless gum or sugar-free hard candy.

- Use a saliva substitute to help moisten your mouth.

Clean your mouth, tongue, and gums.

- Brush your teeth, gums, and tongue with an extra-soft tooth-brush after every meal and at bedtime. If brushing hurts, soften the bristles in warm water.

- Use a fluoride toothpaste.

- Don't use mouthwashes with alcohol in them.

- Floss your teeth gently every day. If your gums bleed and hurt, avoid the areas that are bleeding or sore, but keep flossing your other teeth.

- Rinse your mouth several times a day with a solution of 1/4 tea-spoon baking soda and 1/8 teaspoon salt in one cup of warm water. Follow with a plain water rinse.

- Dentures that don't fit well can cause problems. Talk to your cancer doctor or dentist about your dentures.

If your mouth is sore, watch what you eat and drink.

- Choose foods that are good for you and easy to chew and swallow.

- Take small bites of food, chew slowly, and sip liquids with your meals.

- Eat soft, moist foods such as cooked cereals, mashed potatoes, and scrambled eggs.

- If you have trouble swallowing, soften your food with gravy, sauces, broth, yogurt, or other liquids.

Call your doctor or nurse when your mouth hurts.

- Work with them to find medicines to help control the pain.

- If the pain continues, talk to your cancer doctor about stronger medicines.

Remember to stay away from:

- sharp, crunchy foods, like taco chips, that could scrape or cut your mouth;

- foods that are hot, spicy, or high in acid, like citrus fruits and juices, which can irritate your mouth;

- sugary foods, like candy or soda, that could cause cavities;

- toothpicks, because they can cut your mouth;

- all tobacco products; and

- alcoholic drinks.

Do children get mouth problems, too?

Chemotherapy causes other side effects in children, depending on the child's age.

Problems with teeth are the most common. Permanent teeth may be slow to come in and may look different from normal teeth. Teeth may fall out. The dentist will check your child's jaws for any growth problems.

Before chemotherapy begins, take your child to a dentist. The dentist will check your child's mouth carefully and pull loose teeth or those that may become loose during treatment. Ask the dentist or hygienist what you can do to help your child with mouth care.

Remember

- Visit your dentist before your cancer treatment starts.

- Take good care of your mouth during treatment.

- Talk regularly with your cancer doctor and dentist about any mouth problems you have.

Chapter 51

Oral Health and Diabetes

What are diabetes problems?

Too much glucose in the blood for a long time can cause diabetes problems. This high blood glucose, also called blood sugar, can damage many parts of the body, such as the heart, blood vessels, eyes, and kidneys. Heart and blood vessel disease can lead to heart attacks and strokes. You can do a lot to prevent or slow down diabetes problems.

This text is about the tooth and gum problems caused by diabetes. You will learn what you can do each day and during each year to stay healthy and prevent diabetes problems.

What should I do each day to stay healthy with diabetes?

- Follow the healthy eating plan that you and your doctor or dietitian have worked out.

- Be active a total of 30 minutes most days. Ask your doctor what activities are best for you.

- Take your medicines as directed.

From "Prevent Diabetes Problems: Keep Your Teeth and Gums Healthy," by the National Institute of Diabetes and Digestive and Kidney Diseases (NIDDK, www.niddk.nih.gov), part of the National Institutes of Health, January 2007.

- Check your blood glucose every day. Each time you check your blood glucose, write the number in your record book.

- Check your feet every day for cuts, blisters, sores, swelling, redness, or sore toenails.

- Brush and floss your teeth every day.

- Control your blood pressure and cholesterol.

- Don't smoke.

How can diabetes hurt my teeth and gums?

Tooth and gum problems can happen to anyone. A sticky film full of germs, called plaque, builds up on your teeth. High blood glucose helps germs, also called bacteria, grow. Then you can get red, sore, and swollen gums that bleed when you brush your teeth.

People with diabetes can have tooth and gum problems more often if their blood glucose stays high. High blood glucose can make tooth and gum problems worse. You can even lose your teeth.

Smoking makes it more likely for you to get a bad case of gum disease, especially if you have diabetes and are age 45 or older.

Red, sore, and bleeding gums are the first sign of gum disease. These problems can lead to periodontitis. Periodontitis is an infection in the gums and the bone that holds the teeth in place. If the infection gets worse, your gums may pull away from your teeth, making your teeth look long.

Call your dentist if you think you have problems with your teeth or gums.

How do I know if I have damage to my teeth and gums?

If you have one or more of these problems, you may have tooth and gum damage from diabetes:

- red, sore, swollen gums;

- bleeding gums;

- gums pulling away from your teeth so your teeth look long;

- loose or sensitive teeth;

- bad breath;

- a bite that feels different; and

- dentures—false teeth—that do not fit well.

How can I keep my teeth and gums healthy?

- Keep your blood glucose as close to normal as possible.

- Use dental floss at least once a day. Flossing helps prevent the buildup of plaque on your teeth. Plaque can harden and grow under your gums and cause problems. Using a sawing motion, gently bring the floss between the teeth, scraping from bottom to top several times.

- Brush your teeth after each meal and snack. Use a soft toothbrush.

- Turn the bristles against the gum line and brush gently. Use small, circular motions. Brush the front, back, and top of each tooth.

- If you wear false teeth, keep them clean.

- Ask the person who cleans your teeth to show you the best way to brush and floss your teeth and gums. Ask this person about the best toothbrush and toothpaste to use.

- Call your dentist right away if you have problems with your teeth and gums.

- Call your dentist if you have red, sore, or bleeding gums; gums that are pulling away from your teeth; a sore tooth that could be infected; or soreness from your dentures.

- Get your teeth and gums cleaned and checked by your dentist twice a year.

- If your dentist tells you about a problem, take care of it right away.

- Be sure your dentist knows that you have diabetes.

- If you smoke, talk to your doctor about ways to quit smoking.

How can my dentist take care of my teeth and gums?

Your dentist can help you take care of your teeth and gums by:

- cleaning and checking your teeth and gums twice a year;

- helping you learn the best way to brush and floss your teeth and gums;

- telling you if you have problems with your teeth or gums and what to do about them; and

- making sure your false teeth fit well.

Get your teeth cleaned and checked twice a year. Plan ahead. You may be taking a diabetes medicine that can cause low blood glucose, also called hypoglycemia. Talk to your doctor and dentist before the visit about the best way to take care of your blood glucose during the dental work. You may need to bring some diabetes medicine and food with you to the dentist's office.

If your mouth is sore after the dental work, you might not be able to eat or chew for several hours or days. For guidance on how to adjust your normal routine while your mouth is healing, ask your doctor:

- what foods and drinks you should have;

- how you should change your diabetes medicines; and

- how often you should check your blood glucose.

Chapter 52

Oral Complications in People with Eating Disorders

Chapter Contents

Section 52.1—Oral Signs and Symptoms of Eating
    Disorders 514
Section 52.2—Eating Disorders May Be Detected at the
    Dental Office 515

513

Section 52.1

Oral Signs and Symptoms of Eating Disorders

"Eating Concerns and Oral Health," © 2005 National Eating Disorders Association. Reprinted with permission. For additional information, visit www.NationalEatingDisorders.org, or call the toll-free Information and Referral Helpline at 800-931-2237.

Did You Know?

Dietary habits can and do play a role in oral health. Everyone has heard from their dentist that eating too much sugar can lead to cavities, but did you know that high intake of acidic "diet" foods can have an equally devastating effect on your teeth?

In fact, while up to 89% of bulimic patients show signs of the tooth erosion usually associated with regurgitation, some studies have found similar prevalence rates in patients with highly restrictive dietary habits.

The harmful habits and nutritional deficiencies that often accompany disordered eating can have severe consequences on one's dental health.

It is often the pain and discomfort associated with dental complications that causes individuals with eating disorders to seek treatment.

Signs and Symptoms

- **Loss of tissue and erosive lesions on the surface of teeth due to the effects of acid.** These lesions can appear as early as 6 months from the start of the problem.

- **Changes in the color, shape, and length of teeth.** Teeth can become brittle, translucent, and weak.

- **Increased sensitivity to temperature.** In extreme cases the pulp can be exposed and cause infection, discoloration, or even pulp death.

- **Enlargement** of the salivary glands, dry mouth, and reddened, dry, cracked lips.

514

- **Tooth decay**, which can actually be aggravated by extensive tooth brushing or rinsing following vomiting.

- **Unprovoked, spontaneous pain** within a particular tooth.

Changes in the mouth are oftentimes the first physical signs of an eating disorder. If you are experiencing any of these symptoms, talk with your dentist about ways to care for your teeth and mouth. There are methods for improving your oral health while you are seeking help to change harmful eating habits.

Section 52.2

Eating Disorders May Be Detected at the Dental Office

"Eating Away at Your Oral Health," Word of Mouth, Winter-Spring 2008. © 2008 Massachusetts Dental Society (www.massdental.org). Reprinted with permission.

More than 35 million Americans—both women and men—suffer from eating disorders. And while the long-term physical health implications of eating disorders include heart failure, kidney damage, osteoporosis, and digestive system problems, the frequent vomiting and nutritional deficiencies associated with eating disorders can severely affect oral health, as well.

Changes in the mouth are often the first physical signs of an eating disorder, according to the National Eating Disorders Association (NEDA). That is why dental offices are one of the first places where the physical damages that may accompany such a disorder can be detected. Common oral health issues that result from eating disorders include tooth erosion, tooth sensitivity, dry mouth, and bad breath.

The two most common eating disorders, affecting approximately 11 million sufferers, are bulimia and anorexia nervosa. Both disorders are psychological in nature and are predominant in young women, revolving around body-image issues that result in the sufferer depriving his or her body of essential nutrients—nutrients that are critical to not only a healthy body but also a healthy mouth.

Bulimia is characterized by compulsive overeating ("bingeing") followed by self-induced vomiting ("purging"), whereas anorexia nervosa is marked by extreme weight loss typically achieved through self-starvation. Yet both diseases produce signs and symptoms that can be detected in the mouth during a routine oral exam, such as dry mouth, reddening of the palate, and chapped lips.

In addition to these symptoms, repeated vomiting, a common characteristic of both disorders, exposes teeth to gastric acids which erode tooth enamel, the hard protective covering of the tooth. According to NEDA, studies have indicated that up to 89 percent of bulimic patients show signs of tooth erosion due to the powerful effects of stomach acid. With prolonged exposure to these acids, teeth may change in shape, color, and length, and amalgam fillings may start to protrude above a tooth's surface. Left untreated, extreme cases of eating disorders may expose the innermost layer of the teeth, called the pulp, resulting in infection, discoloration, and, eventually, pulp death. If the latter occurs, the patient may need to have a root canal performed or the tooth extracted.

The oral effects of eating disorders often can be successfully treated when detected early. Dentists may be able to teach patients how to minimize the impact of constant purging, but if the patient has not sought medical or psychological treatment for the eating disorder, any reconstructive efforts may prove ineffective because additional acid will destroy any new restorations.

Although eating disorders are potentially fatal (anorexia nervosa has the highest mortality rate of any mental illness, according to NEDA), they are treatable. And the oral implications, if detected early enough, can be reversed.

If you think you or someone you know may have an eating disorder and are experiencing any of the symptoms described above, please talk with your physician and your dentist.

Chapter 53

Oral-Facial Clefts

Chapter Contents

Section 53.1—All about Cleft Lip and Palate 518
Section 53.2—Scientists Discover How Maternal
　　　　　　　Smoking Causes Cleft Lip and Palate 524

517

Section 53.1

All about Cleft Lip and Palate

Oral-facial clefts are birth defects in which the tissues of the mouth or lip don't form properly during fetal development. In the United States, clefts occur in 1 in 700 to 1,000 births, making it the one of the most common major birth defects. Clefts occur more often in children of Asian, Latino, or Native American descent.

The good news is that both cleft lip and cleft palate are treatable birth defects. Most kids who are born with these conditions can have reconstructive surgery within the first 12 to 18 months of life to correct the defect and significantly improve facial appearance.

What Is Oral Clefting?

Oral clefting occurs when the tissues of the lip and/or palate of a fetus don't grow together early in pregnancy. Children with clefts often don't have enough tissue in their mouths, and the tissue they do have isn't fused together properly to form the roof of their mouths.

A cleft lip appears as a narrow opening or gap in the skin of the upper lip that extends all the way to the base of the nose. A cleft palate is an opening between the roof of the mouth and the nasal cavity. Some children have clefts that extend through both the front and rear part of the palates, while others have only partial clefting.

There are generally three different kinds of clefts:

- cleft lip without a cleft palate
- cleft palate without a cleft lip
- cleft lip and cleft palate together

In addition, clefts can occur on one side of the mouth (unilateral clefting) or on both sides of the mouth (bilateral clefting).

More boys than girls have a cleft lip, while more girls have cleft palate without a cleft lip.

Because clefting causes specific visible symptoms, it's easy to diagnose. It can be detected through a prenatal ultrasound. If the clefting has not been detected prior to the baby's birth, it's identified immediately afterward.

What Causes Oral Clefting?

Doctors don't know exactly why a baby develops cleft lip or cleft palate, but believe it may be a combination of genetic (inherited) and environmental factors (such as certain drugs, illnesses, and the use of alcohol or tobacco while a woman is pregnant). The risk may be higher for kids whose sibling or parents have a cleft or who have a history of clefting in their families. Both mothers and fathers can pass on a gene or genes that cause cleft palate or cleft lip.

Complications Related to Oral Clefting

A child with a cleft lip or palate tends to be more susceptible to colds, hearing loss, and speech defects. Dental problems—such as missing, extra, malformed, or displaced teeth, and cavities—also are common in children born with cleft palate.

Many children with clefts are especially vulnerable to ear infections because their eustachian tubes don't drain fluid properly from the middle ear into the throat. Fluid accumulates, pressure builds in the ears, and infection may set in. For this reason, a child with cleft lip or palate may have special tubes surgically inserted into his or her ears at the time of the first reconstructive surgery.

Feeding can be another complication for an infant with a cleft lip or palate. A cleft lip can make it more difficult for a child to suck on a nipple, while a cleft palate may cause formula or breast milk to be accidentally taken up into the nasal cavity. Special nipples and other devices can help make feeding easier; you will probably be given information on how to use them and where to buy them before you take your baby home from the hospital. And in some cases, a child with a cleft lip or palate may need to wear a prosthetic palate called an obturator to help him or her eat properly.

If you're experiencing problems with feeding, your doctor may be able to offer other suggestions or feeding aids to help you and your baby.

Treating Clefts

The good news is that there have been many medical advancements in the treatment of oral clefting. Reconstructive surgery can repair cleft lips and palates, and in severe cases, plastic surgery can address specific appearance-related concerns.

A child with oral clefting will need to see a variety of specialists who will work together as a team to treat the condition. Treatment usually begins in the first few months of an infant's life, depending on the health of the infant and the extent of the cleft.

Members of a child's cleft lip and palate treatment team usually include:

- a geneticist
- a plastic surgeon
- an ear, nose, and throat physician (otolaryngologist)
- an oral surgeon
- an orthodontist
- a dentist
- a speech pathologist (often called a speech therapist)
- an audiologist
- a nurse coordinator
- a social worker and/or psychologist

The team specialists will evaluate your child's progress regularly, examining your child's hearing, speech, nutrition, teeth, and emotional state. They will share their recommendations with you, and can forward their evaluation to your child's school, and any speech therapists that your child may be working with.

In addition to treating your child's cleft, the specialists will work with your child on any issues related to feeding, social problems, speech, and how you approach the condition with your child. They'll provide feedback and recommendations to help you through the phases of your child's growth and treatment.

Surgery for Oral Clefting

Surgery is usually performed during the first 12 to 18 months to repair cleft lip and/or cleft palate. Both types of surgery are performed in the hospital under general anesthesia.

Cleft lip often requires only one reconstructive surgery, especially if the cleft is unilateral. The surgeon will make an incision on each side of the cleft from the lip to the nostril. The two sides of the lip are then sutured together. Bilateral cleft lips may be repaired in two surgeries, about a month apart, and usually requires a short hospital stay.

Cleft palate surgery involves drawing tissue from either side of the mouth to rebuild the palate. It requires 2 or 3 nights in the hospital, with the first night spent in the intensive care unit. The initial surgery is intended to create a functional palate, reduce the chances that fluid will develop in the middle ears, and help the child's teeth and facial bones develop properly. In addition, this functional palate will help your child's speech development and feeding abilities.

The necessity for more operations depends on the skill of the surgeon as well as the severity of the cleft, its shape, and the thickness of available tissue that can be used to create the palate. Some children with a cleft palate require more surgeries to help improve their speech. Additional surgeries may also improve the appearance of the lip and nose, close openings between the mouth and nose, help breathing, and stabilize and realign the jaw. Subsequent surgeries are usually scheduled at least 6 months apart to allow a child time to heal and to reduce the chances of serious scarring.

It's a good idea to meet regularly with your child's plastic surgeon to determine what's most appropriate in your child's case. Final repairs of the scars left by the initial surgery may not be performed until adolescence, when facial structure is more fully developed. Surgery is designed to aid in normalizing function and cosmetic appearance so that the child will have as few difficulties as possible.

Dental Care and Orthodontia

Children with oral clefting often undergo dental and orthodontic treatment to help align the teeth and take care of any gaps that exist because of the cleft.

Routine dental care may get lost in the midst of these major procedures, but healthy teeth are critical for a child with clefting because they're needed for proper speech.

A child with oral clefting generally needs the same dental care as other children—regular brushing supplemented with flossing once the child's 6-year molars come in. Depending on the shape of your child's mouth and teeth, your child's dentist may recommend a Toothette, a soft sponge that contains mouthwash, rather than a toothbrush. As your child grows, you may be able to switch to a soft children's toothbrush. The key is to make sure that your child brushes regularly and well.

Children with cleft palate often have an alveolar ridge defect. The alveolus is the bony upper gum that contains teeth, and defects can:

- displace, tip, or rotate permanent teeth

- prevent permanent teeth from appearing

- prevent the alveolar ridge from forming

These problems can be fixed by grafting bone matter onto the alveolus, which allows the placement of your child's teeth to be corrected orthodontically.

Orthodontic treatment usually involves a number of phases, with the first phase beginning as the permanent teeth start to come in. In the first phase, which is called an orthopalatal expansion, the upper dental arch is rounded out and the width of the upper jaw is increased. A device called an expander is placed inside the child's mouth. The widening of the jaw may be followed by a bone graft in the alveolus.

Your child's orthodontist may wait until the remainder of your child's permanent teeth come in before beginning the second phase of orthodontic treatment. The second phase may involve removing extra teeth, adding dental implants if teeth are missing, or applying braces to straighten teeth.

In about 25% of children with a unilateral cleft lip and palate, the upper jaw growth does not keep up with the lower jaw growth. If this occurs, your child may need orthognathic surgery to align the teeth and help the upper jaw to develop.

For these children, phase-two orthodontics may include an operation called an osteotomy on the upper jaw that moves the upper jaw both forward and down. This usually requires another bone graft for stability.

Speech Therapy

A child with oral clefting may have trouble speaking—the clefting can make the voice nasal and difficult to understand.

Some will find that surgery fixes the problem completely. Catching speech problems early can be a key part of solving them. It's a good idea to take your child to a speech therapist between the ages of 18 months and 2 years. Many speech therapists like to talk with parents at least once during the child's first 6 months to provide an overview of the treatment and suggest specific language- and speech-stimulation games to play with the baby.

Shortly after the initial surgery is completed, the speech patholo-gist will see your child for a complete assessment. The therapist will evaluate your child's developing communication skills by assessing the number of sounds he or she makes and the actual words your child tries to use, and by observing interaction and play behavior.

This analysis helps determine what, if any, speech exercises your child needs and if further surgery is required. The speech pathologist will often continue to work with your child through additional sur-geries. Many children who have clefts work with a speech therapist throughout their grade-school years.

Dealing with Emotional and Social Issues

Our society often focuses on people's appearances, and this can make childhood—and, especially, the teen years—very difficult for someone with a physical difference. Because a child with oral clefting has a prominent facial difference, your child may experience painful teasing, which can damage self-esteem. Part of the cleft palate and lip treatment team includes psychiatric and emotional support per-sonnel.

Ways that you can support your child include:

• Try not to focus on your child's cleft and do not allow it to define your child as an individual.

• Create a warm and supportive home environment, where each person's individual worth is openly celebrated.

• Let your child know that you feel good about who he or she is by showing acceptance and by not trying to make your child into your idea of who he or she should be.

• Encourage your child to develop friendships with people from diverse backgrounds. The best way to do this is to lead by ex-ample and to be open to all people yourself.

• Point out positive attributes in others that do not involve physi-cal appearance.

• Encourage autonomy by giving your child the freedom to make decisions and take appropriate risks, letting your child's own ac-complishments lead to a sense of personal value. By providing opportunities for your child to make decisions early on—like picking out what clothes to wear—he or she can gain more con-fidence and the ability to make bigger decisions down the road.

You might also consider encouraging your child to present information about clefting to his or her class with a special presentation that you arrange with the teacher. Or perhaps your child would like you to talk to the class. This can be especially effective with young children.

If your child does experience teasing, encourage discussions about it and be a patient listener. Give your child the tools to confront the teasers by asking what he or she would like to say and then practicing those statements.

If your child seems to have ongoing self-esteem problems, you may want to consult with a child psychologist or social worker for support and information. Together with the members of your child's treatment team, you can help your child through tough times.

Also, it's important to keep the lines of communication open as your child approaches adolescence so that you can address any concerns he or she may have about appearance.

Section 53.2

Scientists Discover How Maternal Smoking Causes Cleft Lip and Palate

From "Scientists Discover How Maternal Smoking Can Cause Cleft Lip and Palate," by the National Institute of Dental and Craniofacial Research (NIDCR,www.nidcr.nih.gov), part of the National Institutes of Health, January 3, 2007.

Scientists supported by the National Institute of Dental and Craniofacial Research (NIDCR), part of the National Institutes of Health, report that women who smoke during pregnancy and carry a fetus whose DNA [deoxyribonucleic acid] lacks both copies of a gene involved in detoxifying cigarette smoke substantially increase their baby's chances of being born with a cleft lip and/or palate.

According to the scientists, about a quarter of babies of European ancestry and possibly up to 60 percent of those of Asian ancestry lack both copies of the gene called GSTT1 [glutathione S-transferase theta-1]. Based on their data, published in the January [2007] issue of the *American Journal of Human Genetics*, the scientists calculated that if a pregnant woman smokes 15 cigarettes or more per day, the chances of her GSTT1-lacking fetus developing a cleft increase nearly 20-fold. Globally, about 12 million women each year smoke through their pregnancies.

Dr. Jeff Murray, a scientist at the University of Iowa and senior author of the study, noted that parents who are considering having a child and need added motivation for the mother to quit smoking might one day be tested to determine their GSTT1 status. Because the fetus inherits its genes from both mother and father, the test would determine the likelihood of the baby developing without the GSTT1 gene to detoxify the cigarette smoke.

"A test that indicates the GSTT1 gene is present certainly would not eliminate a baby's risk of a cleft because many other genetic and environmental factors can be involved," said Murray. "But the opposite result would give the mother one more compelling reason to quit smoking for her own health and for the sake of her child."

In the United States, about one in every 750 babies is born with isolated, also called nonsyndromic, cleft lip and/or palate. The condition is correctable but typically requires several surgeries. Families often undergo tremendous emotional and economic hardship during the process, and children frequently require many other services, including complex dental care and speech therapy.

According to Murray, researchers have built a strong statistical case over the past several years that pregnant women who smoke put their unborn babies at greater risk of developing a cleft. The data raised two related questions. "Do genetic variations in the mother influence her own metabolism of the cigarette smoke and its byproducts, thus setting in motion developmental changes that cause the cleft in the fetus? Or do genetic variations in the fetus itself compromise its ability to metabolize the cigarette smoke and cause the cleft?" said Dr. Min Shi, now a scientist at NIH's National Institute of Environmental Health Sciences and a lead author of the paper.

To find the answers, Murray's group teamed with colleagues in Denmark to perform a large, complex, and possibly first-of-its-kind international study. The group first assembled a list of 16 genes of interest, each of which encode proteins that plug into various pathways in the body involved in detoxifying dangerous chemicals. "We picked genes that previous evidence shows either are directly involved in cigarette smoke toxicity or are major players in general toxicity management in people," said Dr. Kaare Christensen, a scientist at the University of Southern Denmark in Odense and an author on the paper.

"These genes tend to be quite variable from person to person in their precise DNA structure, or spelling," Christensen added. "We wanted to see if any of these variations might adversely affect a person's ability to break down the toxic products of cigarette smoke."

Christensen and his colleagues then turned to their existing database of kids with clefts, their parents, and siblings. In all, the scientists analyzed 5,000 DNA samples from both continents—including 1,244 from children born with clefts. Importantly, the families in Denmark and Iowa provided the opportunity to independently confirm the findings in two distinct populations.

In addition, they had free public access to the NIDCR-funded COGENE [Craniofacial and Oral Gene Expression Network] project, a comprehensive online database of genes expressed throughout the various stages of development. Working closely with Dr. Mike Lovett at Washington University in St. Louis, one of COGENE's founders, the database proved especially helpful because cleft lip and/or palate occurs during the first 5-to-12 weeks of development. This meant the scientists had to be sure not only that their genes of interest are expressed during this vital period but are switched on in fetal craniofacial structures. If the genes met both criteria, the investigators said they hoped their subsequent data might point them to a gene-environment interaction.

As reported, the scientists determined from their analyses that the mother provides the toxic environmental exposure, which then can be greatly amplified by the genetics of the fetus to produce the cleft. This marks the first time a gene-environment interaction in clefting has been documented at a molecular level. The data also point the way for future studies to define the specific molecular chain of events that lead to the cleft, vital information to understand and hopefully one day prevent the process.

While sifting through the data, the researchers took particular note of the GSTT gene and its contribution to clefting. The gene encodes one of the body's approximately 20 different glutathione S-transferase enzymes. These enzymes collectively play roles in common detoxification processes, ranging from chemically altering drugs and industrial chemicals to detoxifying polycyclic aromatic hydrocarbons, a key component of cigarette smoke.

The scientists found that pregnant women who smoked and also carried fetuses that lacked the GSTT1 enzyme were much more likely to give birth to a baby with a cleft. This finding was true in Iowa and Denmark, and they noted in the COGENE database that the gene is highly expressed in developing craniofacial structures. "It may be that be that the lip and palate can form normally without GSTT1," said Murray. "But if the chemicals in cigarette smoke challenge the normal development of these structures, fetuses that lack the gene are at a distinct disadvantage."

Murray and his collaborators continue their genetic analyses. "We now have data from about 350 genes on this cohort of families," he said. "It's certainly a more complicated analysis to perform, but we're working our way through it and hope to have some very interesting data in the months ahead."

The article is titled "Orofacial Cleft Risk is Increased with Maternal Smoking and Specific Detoxification-Gene Variants," and is published in the January 2007 issue of the *American Journal of Human Genetics*. The authors are Min Shi, Kaare Christensen, Clarice R. Weinberg, Paul Romitti, Lise Bathum, Anthony Lozada, Richard W. Morris, Michael Lovett, and Jeffrey C. Murray.

The NIDCR is the nation's leading funder of research on oral, dental, and craniofacial health.

Chapter 54

Oral Concerns in People with Heart Problems

Chapter Contents

Section 54.1—New Antibiotic Recommendations for
People with Valve Disease Undergoing
Dental Procedures 530

Section 54.2—Patients with Drug-Eluting Stents Should
Not Discontinue Antiplatelet Therapy Prior
to Dental Procedures 534

Section 54.1

New Antibiotic Recommendations for People with Valve Disease Undergoing Dental Procedures

"Most patients don't need antibiotics before dental procedures to prevent infective endocarditis," reprinted with permission www.americanheart.org. © 2007 American Heart Association, Inc.

Taking a precautionary antibiotic before a trip to the dentist isn't necessary for most people, and in fact, might create more harm than good, according to updated recommendations from the American Heart Association.

The guidelines, published in *Circulation: Journal of the American Heart Association,* are based on a growing body of scientific evidence weighing the effectiveness of antibiotics against possible risks. The updated recommendations say that only people who are at the greatest risk of bad outcomes from infective endocarditis (IE)—an infection of the heart's inner lining or the heart valves—should receive short-term preventive antibiotics before common, routine dental procedures. This includes people with artificial heart valves, a history of previous endocarditis, certain serious congenital heart conditions, and heart transplants patients who develop a problem with a heart valve.

For decades, doctors have given short-term antibiotics prior to a dental procedure to many patients with the belief the drugs would prevent IE. As a result, patients with any kind of heart abnormality from mild, symptomless forms of mitral valve prolapse (MVP) to serious congenital birth defects have been instructed to take an antibiotic prior to dental work, even teeth cleaning.

However, the drugs carry risks, including fatal allergic reactions and possibly making the bacteria that cause IE to become resistant to antibiotics. Although allergic reactions are minimal, new evidence shows the risks outweigh the benefits for most patients receiving these antibiotics.

"We've concluded that if giving prophylactic antibiotics prior to a dental procedure works at all—and there's no evidence that it does work—we should reserve that preventive treatment only for those people who would have the worst outcomes if they get IE. That's a profound change from previous recommendations," said Walter R. Wilson, M.D., a professor of medicine at the Mayo Clinic in Rochester, Minn., and chair of the writing group.

The new recommendations apply to such common dental procedures as teeth cleaning and extractions. They are based on a comprehensive review of published studies that suggests IE is more likely to occur from bacteria that enter the bloodstream as a result of everyday activities than from a dental procedure.

The statement cites a 1999 study estimating that tooth brushing twice a day for a year carried a 154,000 times greater risk of exposure to blood-borne bacteria than a single tooth extraction, the dental procedure reported to be the most likely to cause a bacterial infection. The writing group found no compelling evidence that antibiotic prophylaxis prior to a dental procedure prevents IE in individuals who are at risk of developing this infection.

"In fact, maintaining good oral health and hygiene appears to be more protective than prophylactic antibiotics," Wilson said. "This changes the whole philosophy of how we have constructed these recommendations for the last 50 years. Rather than based on the risk of getting IE, they're based on the risk of which patients would have the worst outcome from the infection."

Wilson said it's difficult to estimate the number of people affected by the new guidelines. Measurements of the prevalence of mitral valve prolapse range from less than 2 percent to almost 20 percent of the population.

According to American College of Cardiology/American Heart Association guidelines for the management of patients with valvular heart disease, when using current echocardiographic criteria for diagnosing MVP, the prevalence is 1 percent to 2.5 percent of the population. Even this estimate means millions of people have been taking antibiotics prior to dental procedures.

Patients at the greatest danger of bad outcomes from IE and for whom preventive antibiotics prior to a dental procedure are worth the risks include those with:

- artificial heart valves

- a history of having had IE

- certain specific, serious congenital (present from birth) heart conditions, including

- unrepaired or incompletely repaired cyanotic congenital heart disease, including those with palliative shunts and conduits

- a completely repaired congenital heart defect with prosthetic material or device, whether placed by surgery or by catheter intervention, during the first 6 months after the procedure

- any repaired congenital heart defect with residual defect at the site or adjacent to the site of a prosthetic patch or a prosthetic device

- a cardiac transplant which develops a problem in a heart valve.

"Except for the conditions listed above, antibiotic prophylaxis is no longer recommended for any other form of congenital heart disease," the statement said.

"These new recommendations are a major change that has evolved over nearly 50 years," said Michael Gewitz, M.D., chair of the AHA Rheumatic Fever, Endocarditis and Kawasaki Disease Committee, a co-author of the guidelines and professor of pediatrics at New York Medical College and Physician-in-Chief for Maria Fareri Children's Hospital at Westchester Medical Center in Valhalla, N.Y. "Over this time, patients with common heart conditions were told they needed to take antibiotics prior to a dental procedure. Now, they'll be told they no longer need them. This will likely cause anxiety and concern in patients and health care providers."

Gewitz says this is especially true for the millions of people, young and old, affected with congenital heart diseases. "There is likely to be some confusion until dentists and primary care doctors, and even specialists, all hear about these changes and get used to them," he said. "Since patients with congenital heart disease can have complicated circumstances, even after surgical or other treatment, families and primary care doctors should check with their cardiologist if there is any question at all as to which category best fits the individual patient."

He added that patients and their families should ask careful questions of their providers any time antibiotics are suggested before a medical or dental procedure. They should also be aware that overuse of antibiotics many times can lead to a worse outcome than if they were not used at all.

Wilson acknowledged that patients and health care professionals may take awhile to get used to the new guidelines. Many dentists and physicians are used to prescribing the drugs to any patient with any possibility of a heart abnormality, no matter how slight. Likewise, many patients are used to taking the antibiotics, which provide a sense of security, he said.

The guidelines say patients who have taken prophylactic antibiotics routinely in the past but no longer need them include people with:

- mitral valve prolapse

- rheumatic heart disease

- bicuspid valve disease

- calcified aortic stenosis

- congenital heart conditions such as ventricular septal defect, atrial septal defect, and hypertrophic cardiomyopathy.

"These patients still have a lifelong risk of IE," Wilson said. "We're just saying that the risk is much greater from a random blood-borne bacterial infection resulting from everyday activities than from a dental or medical procedure."

The guidelines also do not recommend any prophylactic antibiotics to prevent IE for common gastrointestinal procedures or procedures on the urinary tract. This holds true even for patients with the highest risk of bad outcomes from IE.

Wilson said the revised guidelines were prompted in part by the growing body of scientific research that raised questions about the usefulness of widespread prophylactic antibiotic use. The new recommendations are also more in line with international practice.

"Over the years, a number of publications have called into question the rationale and efficacy of prophylaxis," he said. "We did a very thorough search of the literature and assembled the world's experts on endocarditis and we based our conclusions on evidence-based medicine."

The Council on Scientific Affairs of the American Dental Association has approved these guidelines as they relate to dentistry. In addition, the guidelines have been endorsed by the Infectious Diseases Society of America and by the Pediatric Infectious Diseases Society.

Co-authors include: Kathryn A. Taubert, Ph.D.; Peter B. Lockhart, D.D.S.; Larry M. Baddour, M.D.; Matthew Levison, M.D.; Ann Bolger, M.D.; Christopher H. Cabell, M.D., M.H.S.; Masato Takahashi, M.D.; Robert S. Baltimore, M.D.; Jane W. Newburger, M.D., M.P.H.; Brian L. Strom, M.D.; Lloyd Y. Tani, M.D.; Michael Gerber, M.D.; Robert O. Bonow, M.D.; Thomas Pallasch, D.D.S., M.S.; Stanford T. Shulman, M.D.; Anne H. Rowley, M.D.; Jane C. Burns, M.D.; Patricia Ferrieri, M.D.; Timothy Gardner, M.D.; David Goff, M.D., Ph.D. and David T. Durack, M.D., Ph.D.

Section 54.2

Patients with Drug-Eluting Stents Should Not Discontinue Antiplatelet Therapy Prior to Dental Procedures

Excerpted from "Prevention of premature discontinuation of dual antiplatelet therapy in patients with coronary artery stents," National Guideline Clearinghouse (www.guideline.gov), February 2008.

Thienopyridine therapy in combination with aspirin has become the mainstay antiplatelet treatment strategy for the prevention of stent thrombosis. Premature discontinuation of antiplatelet therapy markedly increases the risk of stent thrombosis, a catastrophic event that frequently leads to myocardial infarction (MI) and/or death. Factors contributing to premature cessation of thienopyridine therapy include drug cost, physician/dentist instructions to patients to discontinue therapy before procedures, and inadequate patient education and understanding about the importance of continuing therapy.

To eliminate premature discontinuation of thienopyridine therapy, the advisory group gives the following recommendations:

1. Before implantation of a stent, the physician should discuss the need for dual antiplatelet therapy. In patients not expected to comply with 12 months of thienopyridine therapy, whether for economic or other reasons, strong consideration should be given to avoiding a drug-eluting stent (DES).

2. In patients who are undergoing preparation for percutaneous coronary intervention and are likely to require invasive or surgical procedures within the next 12 months, consideration should be given to implantation of a bare-metal stent or performance of balloon angioplasty with provisional stent implantation instead of the routine use of a DES.

3. A greater effort by health care professionals must be made before patient discharge to ensure patients are properly and thoroughly educated about the reasons they are prescribed

thienopyridines and the significant risks associated with prematurely discontinuing such therapy.

4. Patients should be specifically instructed before hospital discharge to contact their treating cardiologist before stopping any antiplatelet therapy, even if instructed to stop such therapy by another health care provider.

5. Health care providers who perform invasive or surgical procedures and are concerned about periprocedural and post-procedural bleeding must be made aware of the potentially catastrophic risks of premature discontinuation of thienopyridine therapy. Such professionals who perform these procedures should contact the patient's cardiologist if issues regarding the patient's antiplatelet therapy are unclear, to discuss optimal patient management strategy.

6. Elective procedures for which there is significant risk of perioperative or postoperative bleeding should be deferred until patients have completed an appropriate course of thienopyridine therapy (12 months after DES implantation if they are not at high risk of bleeding and a minimum of 1 month for bare-metal stent implantation).

7. For patients treated with DES who are to undergo subsequent procedures that mandate discontinuation of thienopyridine therapy, aspirin should be continued if at all possible and the thienopyridine restarted as soon as possible after the procedure because of concerns about late-stent thrombosis.

8. The health care industry, insurers, the U.S. Congress, and the pharmaceutical industry should ensure that issues such as drug cost do not cause patients to prematurely discontinue thienopyridine therapy and to thus incur catastrophic cardiovascular complications.

Chapter 55

Mouth Problems and Human Immunodeficiency Virus (HIV)

This information is for people who have mouth (oral) problems related to HIV infection. It explains the most common oral problems linked to HIV and shows what they look like. It also describes where in the mouth they occur and how they are treated.

They Are Common

Oral problems are very common in people with HIV. More than a third of people living with HIV have oral conditions that arise because of their weakened immune system. And even though combination antiretroviral therapy has made some oral problems less common, others are occurring more often with this type of treatment.

They Can Be Painful, Annoying, and Lead to Other Problems

You may be told that oral problems are minor compared to other things you have to deal with. But you know that they can cause discomfort and embarrassment and really affect how you feel about yourself. Oral problems can also lead to trouble with eating. If mouth pain or tenderness makes it difficult to chew and swallow, or if you can't taste food as well as you used to, you may not eat enough. And, your

---

From "Mouth Problems and HIV," from the National Institute of Dental and Craniofacial Research (NIDCR, www.nidcr.nih.gov), part of the National Institutes of Health, November 9, 2007.

Table 55.1. Most Common Oral Problems

Description	It could be:	What & where?	Painful?	Contagious?	Treatment
Red sores (ulcers)	Aphthous ulcers. Also known as canker sores	Red sores that might also have a yellow-gray film on top. They are usually on the moveable parts of the mouth such as the tongue or inside of the cheeks and lips.	Yes	No	*Mild cases*—Over-the-counter cream or pre-scription mouthwash that contains corticosteroids; *More severe cases*—cor-ticosteroids in a pill form
	OR				
	Herpes (a viral infection)	Red sores usually on the roof of the mouth. They are sometimes on the outside of the lips, where they are called fever blisters.	Sometimes	Yes	Prescription pill can re-duce healing time and frequency of outbreaks.
White hair-like growth	Hairy leukoplakia caused by the Epstein-Barr virus	White patches that do not wipe away; sometimes very thick and hairlike. Us-ually appear on the side of the tongue or sometimes inside the cheeks and lower lip.	Not usually	No	*Mild cases*—not usually required; *More severe cases*—a prescription pill that may reduce severity of symptoms. In some severe cases, a pain re-liever might also be re quired.

White creamy or bumpy patches like cottage cheese	Candidiasis, a fungal (yeast) infection. Also known as thrush	White or yellowish patches (or can sometimes be red). If wiped away, there will be redness or bleeding underneath. They can appear anywhere in the mouth.	Sometimes, a burning feeling	No	*Mild cases*—prescription antifungal lozenge or mouthwash; *More severe cases*—prescription antifungal pills.
Warts		Small, white, gray, or pinkish rough bumps that look like cauliflower. They can appear inside the lips and on other parts of the mouth.	Not usually	Possibly	Inside the mouth—a doctor can remove them surgically or use cryosurgery, a way of freezing them off; On the lips—a prescription cream that will wear away the wart. Warts can return after treatment.

539

doctor may tell you to eat more than normal so your body has enough energy to deal with HIV.

They Can Be Treated

The most common oral problems linked with HIV can be treated. So talk with your doctor or dentist about what treatment might work for you.

Remember, with the right treatment, your mouth can feel better. And that's an important step toward living well, not just longer, with HIV.

If You Have Dry Mouth

Dry mouth happens when you do not have enough saliva, or spit, to keep your mouth wet. Saliva helps you chew and digest food, protects teeth from decay, and prevents infections by controlling bacteria and fungi in the mouth. Without enough saliva you could develop tooth decay or other infections and might have trouble chewing and swallowing. Your mouth might also feel sticky, dry, and have a burning feeling. And you may have cracked, chapped lips.

To help with a dry mouth, try these things:

- Sip water or sugarless drinks often.
- Chew sugarless gum or suck on sugarless hard candy.
- Avoid tobacco.
- Avoid alcohol.
- Avoid salty foods.
- Use a humidifier at night.
- Talk to your doctor or dentist about prescribing artificial saliva, which may help keep your mouth moist.

Chapter 56

Neurological Disorders That Involve the Tongue and Mouth

Chapter Contents

Section 56.1—Melkersson-Rosenthal Syndrome 542

Section 56.2—Parry-Romberg Syndrome 543

541

Section 56.1

Melkersson-Rosenthal Syndrome

From "Melkersson-Rosenthal Syndrome Information Page," by the National Institute of Neurological Disorders and Stroke (NINDS, www.ninds.nih.gov). part of the National Institutes of Health, February 13, 2007.

What is Melkersson-Rosenthal Syndrome?

Melkersson-Rosenthal syndrome is a rare neurological disorder characterized by recurring facial paralysis, swelling of the face and lips (usually the upper lip), and the development of folds and furrows in the tongue. Onset is in childhood or early adolescence. After recurrent attacks (ranging from days to years in between), swelling may persist and increase, eventually becoming permanent. The lip may become hard, cracked, and fissured with a reddish-brown discoloration. The cause of Melkersson-Rosenthal syndrome is unknown, but there may be a genetic predisposition. It can be symptomatic of Crohn disease or sarcoidosis.

Is there any treatment?

Treatment is symptomatic and may include medication therapies with nonsteroidal anti-inflammatory drugs (NSAIDs) and corticosteroids to reduce swelling, as well as antibiotics and immunosuppressants. Surgery may be recommended to relieve pressure on the facial nerves and to reduce swollen tissue, but its effectiveness has not been established. Massage and electrical stimulation may also be prescribed.

What is the prognosis?

Melkersson-Rosenthal syndrome may recur intermittently after its first appearance. It can become a chronic disorder. Follow-up care should exclude the development of Crohn disease or sarcoidosis.

Section 56.2

Parry-Romberg Syndrome

From "Parry-Romberg Information Page," by the National Institute of Neurological Disorders and Stroke (NINDS, www.ninds.nih.gov), part of the National Institutes of Health, February 14, 2007.

What is Parry-Romberg?

Parry-Romberg syndrome is a rare disorder characterized by slowly progressive deterioration (atrophy) of the skin and soft tissues of half of the face (hemifacial atrophy), usually the left side. It is more common in females than in males. Initial facial changes usually involve the tissues above the upper jaw (maxilla) or between the nose and the upper corner of the lip (nasolabial fold) and subsequently progress to the angle of the mouth, areas around the eye, the brow, the ear, and the neck. The deterioration may also affect the tongue, the soft and fleshy part of the roof of the mouth, and the gums. The eye and cheek of the affected side may become sunken and facial hair may turn white and fall out (alopecia). In addition, the skin overlying affected areas may become darkly pigmented (hyperpigmentation) with, in some cases, areas of hyperpigmentation and patches of unpigmented skin (vitiligo). Parry-Romberg syndrome is also accompanied by neurological abnormalities including seizures and episodes of severe facial pain (trigeminal neuralgia). The onset of the disease usually begins between the ages of 5 and 15 years. The progression of the atrophy often lasts from 2 to 10 years, and then the process seems to enter a stable phase. Muscles in the face may atrophy and there may be bone loss in the facial bones. Problems with the retina and optic nerve may occur when the disease surrounds the eye.

Is there any treatment?

There is no cure and there are no treatments that can stop the progression of Parry-Romberg syndrome. Reconstructive or microvascular surgery may be needed to repair wasted tissue. The timing of surgical intervention is generally agreed to be the best following exhaustion of the disease course and completion of facial growth. Most surgeons will recommend a waiting period of one or two years before proceeding with reconstruction. Muscle or bone grafts may also be helpful. Other treatment is symptomatic and supportive.

What is the prognosis?

The prognosis for individuals with Parry-Romberg syndrome varies. In some cases, the atrophy ends before the entire face is affected. In mild cases, the disorder usually causes no disability other than cosmetic effects.

Chapter 57

Obstructive Sleep Apnea and Snoring: Oral Appliances May Help

Snoring and Sleep Apnea

What Causes Snoring?

Snoring occurs when the soft tissue structures of the upper airway collapse onto themselves and vibrate against each other as we attempt to move air through them. This produces the sound we know as snoring. Large tonsils, a long soft palate, a large tongue, the uvula, and excess fat deposits in the throat all contribute to airway narrowing and snoring. Usually, the more narrow the airway space, the louder or more habitual the snoring.

Obstructive Sleep Apnea

Obstructive sleep apnea (OSA) occurs when the tongue and soft palate collapse onto the back of the throat. This blocks the upper airway, causing air flow to stop. When the oxygen level drops low enough, the brain moves out of deep sleep and the individual partially awakens. The airway then contracts and opens, causing the obstruction in the throat to clear. The flow of air starts again, usually with a loud gasp. When the air flow starts again, you then move back into a deep sleep. The airway muscles collapse, as you awaken with a gasp. The

This chapter includes text from "Snoring & Sleep Apnea," "Oral Appliances," and "Oral Surgery" © 2008 American Academy of Dental Sleep Medicine (AADSM, www.aadsm.org). Reprinted with permission.

airway clears once again as the process repeats itself. This scenario may occur many times during the night. The combination of low oxygen levels and fragmented sleep are the major contributors to most of the ill effects that the sleep apnea patient suffers. In addition to excessive daytime sleepiness, studies show that sleep apnea patients are much more likely to suffer from heart problems (heart attack, congestive heart failure, hypertension), strokes, as well as having a higher incidence of work-related and driving-related accidents.

How Do You Know If You Have OSA?

Take a simple self-test [http://www.aadsm.org/SelfTest.aspx], but be sure to visit your physician if you think you have a problem.

Diagnosis of Obstructive Sleep Apnea

Since OSA is a serious medical condition, it must be diagnosed by a physician. Diagnosis is based on the results of an overnight sleep study, called a polysomnogram (PSG). Other factors of determining OSA are patient evaluation and history.

Treatment Options

Good sleep hygiene, weight loss, and exercise are some helpful OSA treatments a patient can practice on their own. However, medical and dental treatments include continuous positive airway pressure, oral appliance therapy, and surgery.

Continuous positive airway pressure (CPAP): Continuous positive airway pressure (CPAP) is pressurized air generated from a bedside machine. The air is delivered through a tube, connected to a mask, covering the nose. The force of the pressurized air splints the airway open. The CPAP opens the airway like air into a balloon; when air is blown into the balloon, it opens and gets wider. This is exactly how CPAP clears the airway.

Oral appliance therapy: Oral appliances are worn in the mouth to treat snoring and OSA. These devices are similar to orthodontic retainers or sports mouth guards. Oral appliance therapy involves the selection, design, fitting and use of a custom designed oral appliance that is worn during sleep. This appliance then attempts to maintain an opened, unobstructed airway in the throat. There are many different oral appliances available. Approximately 40 appliances have been approved through the U.S. Food and Drug Administration for treatment of snoring and/or sleep apnea. Oral appliances may be used alone or in combination with other means of treating OSA. These means include general health, weight management, surgery, or CPAP. Oral appliances work in several ways:

- repositioning the lower jaw, tongue, soft palate and uvula;
- stabilizing the lower jaw and tongue; and
- increasing the muscle tone of the tongue.

Dentists with training in oral appliance therapy are familiar with the various designs of appliances. They can determine which one is best suited for your specific needs. The dentist will work with your physician as part of the medical team in your diagnosis, treatment, and ongoing care. Determination of proper therapy can only be made by joint consultation of your dentist and physician. Initiation of oral appliance therapy can take from several weeks to several months to complete. Your dentist will continue to monitor your treatment and evaluate the response of your teeth and jaws.

Surgical Procedures

In addition to oral appliance therapy, dentists who are oral and maxillofacial surgeons may consider a variety of methods to evaluate, diagnose, and treat upper airway obstruction. These dental specialists treat upper airway obstructive disorders by utilizing both minimally invasive procedures as well as more complex surgery, including jaw advancement. Additionally, an ENT [ear, nose, and throat] specialist may evaluate you for other types of surgery, mainly the removal of the excess tissues in the throat. It may be necessary to remove tonsils and adenoids (especially in children), the uvula, or even parts of the soft palate and the throat.

Oral Appliances

Snoring and Obstructive Sleep Apnea

Snoring is the sound of partially obstructed breathing during sleep. While snoring can be harmless, it can also be the sign of a more serious medical condition known as obstructive sleep apnea (OSA). When obstructive sleep apnea occurs, the tongue and soft palate collapse onto the back of the throat and completely block the airway, which restricts the flow of oxygen. The condition known as upper airway resistance syndrome (UARS) is midway between primary snoring and true obstructive sleep apnea. People with UARS suffer many of the symptoms of OSA but require special sleep testing techniques.

Standards of Care

Oral appliance therapy is indicated for:

- patients with primary snoring or mild OSA who do not respond to, or are not appropriate candidates for treatment with behavioral measures such as weight loss or sleep-position change;

- patients with moderate to severe OSA should have an initial trial of nasal CPAP, due to greater effectiveness with the use of oral appliances; and

- patients with moderate to severe OSA who are intolerant of or refuse treatment with nasal CPAP. Oral appliances are also indicated for patients who refuse treatment, or are not candidates for tonsillectomy and adenoidectomy, craniofacial operations, or tracheostomy.

Oral Appliances

Oral appliances that treat snoring and obstructive sleep apnea are small plastic devices that are worn in the mouth, similar to orthodontic retainers or sports mouth guards. These appliances help prevent the collapse of the tongue and soft tissues in the back of the throat, keeping the airway open during sleep and promoting adequate air intake. Currently, there are approximately 70 different oral appliances available. Oral appliances may be used alone or in combination with other means of treating OSA, including general health and weight management, surgery, or CPAP.

Types of Oral Appliances

With so many different oral appliances available, selection of a specific appliance may appear somewhat overwhelming. Nearly all appliances fall into one of two categories. The diverse variety is simply a variation of a few major themes. Oral appliances can be classified by mode of action or design variation.

Tongue retaining appliances: Tongue retaining appliances function by holding the tongue in a forward position by means of a suction bulb. When the tongue is in a forward position, it serves to keep the back of the tongue from collapsing during sleep and obstructing the airway in the throat.

Mandibular repositioning appliances: Mandibular repositioning appliances function to reposition and maintain the lower jaw (mandible) in a protruded position during sleep. This serves to open the airway by indirectly pulling the tongue forward, stimulating activity of the muscles in the tongue and making it more rigid. It also holds the lower jaw and other structures in a stable position to prevent opening of the mouth.

Oral appliance therapy: Oral appliance therapy involves the selection, fitting, and use of a specially designed oral appliance worn during sleep that maintains an opened, unobstructed airway in the throat.

Oral appliances work in several ways:

• repositioning the lower jaw, tongue, soft palate, and uvula;

• stabilizing the lower jaw and tongue; and

• increasing the muscle tone of the tongue.

Dentists with training in oral appliance therapy are familiar with the various designs of appliances. They can determine which one is best suited for your specific needs. The dentist will work with your physician as part of the medical team in your diagnosis, treatment, and ongoing care. Determination of effective treatment can only be made by joint consultation of your dentist and physician. The initial evaluation phase of oral appliance therapy can take from several weeks to several months to complete. This includes examination, evaluation to determine the most appropriate oral appliance, fitting, maximizing adaptation of the appliance, and the function.

Other Treatment Options

In addition to lifestyle changes, such as good sleep hygiene, exercise, and weight loss, there are three primary ways to treat snoring and sleep apnea. The most common way is with therapy delivered through a continuous positive air pressure [CPAP] machine. CPAP is usually applied through a tube to a mask that covers the nose. The air pressure that is generated splints the structures in the back of the throat, holding the airway open during sleep. Treatment can also be accomplished with surgery to the soft palate, uvula, and tongue to eliminate the tissue that collapses during sleep. More complex surgery can reposition the anatomic structure of your mouth and facial bones. Many of these procedures can be performed by an AADSM member trained as an oral and maxillofacial surgeon.

Ongoing Care

Ongoing care, including short- and long-term follow-up is an essential step in the treatment of snoring and obstructive sleep apnea with oral appliance therapy. Follow-up care serves to assess the treatment of your sleep disorder, the condition of your appliance, your physical response to your appliance, and to ensure that it is comfortable and effective.

Advantages of Oral Appliance Therapy

Oral appliance therapy has several advantages over other forms of therapy:

- Oral appliances are comfortable and easy to wear. Most people find that it only takes a couple of weeks to become acclimated to wearing the appliance.

- Oral appliances are small and convenient making them easy to carry when traveling.

- Treatment with oral appliances is reversible and noninvasive.

Oral Surgery

Snoring and Obstructive Sleep Apnea

Snoring is the sound of partially obstructed breathing during sleep. While snoring can be harmless, it can also be the sign of a more serious medical condition known as obstructive sleep apnea (OSA). OSA occurs when the tongue and soft palate collapse onto the back of the throat, which completely blocks the airway and restricts the flow of oxygen. The condition known as upper airway resistance syndrome (UARS) is midway between primary snoring and true obstructive sleep apnea. People with UARS suffer many of the symptoms of OSA, but normal sleep testing may be negative.

Treatment Options

In addition to good sleep hygiene, exercise, and weight loss, there are three primary methods to treat snoring and sleep apnea. The most common method is therapy involving a continuous positive air pressure (CPAP) machine. CPAP is usually applied through a tube to a mask that covers the nose. The air pressure that is generated splints the structures in the back of the throat, holding the airway open during sleep. Treatment may also be accomplished through oral appliance therapy. Oral appliances that treat snoring and obstructive sleep apnea are small plastic devices, worn in the mouth, similar to orthodontic retainers or sports mouth guards. These appliances help prevent the collapse of the tongue and soft tissues in the back of the throat, keeping the airway open during sleep and promoting adequate air intake. Treatment can also be accomplished with surgery to the soft palate, uvula, and tongue to eliminate the tissue that collapses during sleep. More complex surgery can reposition the anatomic structure of your mouth and facial bones. Many of these procedures can be performed by an AADSM member trained as an oral and maxillofacial surgeon. There are many surgical procedures available, some of which are detailed in the following text.

Surgical Treatment Options

In general, surgery is indicated when the other therapies are nonapplicable, unsuccessful, or intolerable. Surgery may be an effective treatment for snoring and OSA, but only if performed on the correct portions of the upper airway. Surgery is "site-specific," meaning it requires the identification of specific anatomic areas contributing to airway obstruction. This may vary from patient to patient. A detailed examination of the entire upper airway is necessary before deciding which surgical procedures may be most effective.

Maxillomandibular advancement (MMA): Maxillomandibular advancement involves osteotomies (bony cuts performed via intraoral incisions) to advance the upper and lower jaws to pull forward and tighten the soft palate, tongue, and other attached soft tissues. This process enlarges and stabilizes the entire upper airway. MMA is the most effective and acceptable surgical treatment of OSA. MMA has published success rates ranging from 94 to 100 percent. An overnight hospital stay is required, and the jaws may be wired shut for several weeks, which may result in weight loss.

Anterior inferior mandibular osteotomy (AIMO) with hyoid suspension: The AIMO involves a chin bone osteotomy for advancement of the genial tubercles to pull forward the attached tongue and hyoid (the U-shaped bone in the anterior neck) muscles to enlarge and stabilize the airway behind the tongue base. Although not as effective as MMA, the jaws do not have to be wired shut and there is no change in bite. AIMO may be performed solely as an outpatient procedure or in combination with MMA and other procedures.

Surgery of the soft palate: There are many soft-palatal operations that may be effective for snoring, such as upper airway resistance syndrome (UARS) and obstructive sleep apnea (OSA). Possible adverse side effects of the soft palatal surgery include throat swelling and nasal reflux of air during speech and fluid during drinking. Throat swelling usually occurs immediately after surgery. The most commonly performed procedure is an uvulopalatopharyngoplasty (UPPP), which involves trimming of a bulky soft palate, often performed in combination with removal of enlarged tonsils and/or adenoids. A laser-assisted uvuloplasty (LAUP) is a modified UPPP that involves "scarring" cuts to tighten the soft palate and sequential trimming of the uvula over several appointments. While LAUP is less painful and has fewer side effects, it is less effective than UPPP in the treatment of OSA. Radiofrequency volumetric tissue reduction (RFVTR), sometimes called somnoplasty, attempts to shrink the soft palate and tongue base using energy waves, similar to microwaves.

Nasal surgery: Nasal obstruction may be treated by surgical procedures, including septoplasty, to straighten a deviated septum, and turbinate reduction, to remove or reduce large turbinates and polyps. While these procedures may be performed independently as outpatient procedures, they are often used in combination with other procedures to treat snoring and OSA.

Tongue reduction surgery: This procedure involves a wedge-shaped surgical reduction of the tongue base. It is not typically performed to treat OSA and may have many potentially adverse side effects.

Weight reduction surgery: Bariatric surgery, such as gastric bypass, may be indicated as a last resort treatment of morbidly obese patients with OSA. Cervicofacial liposuction is a relatively safe procedure that selectively removes excessive fatty tissue below the chin and anterior neck to reduce the weight against underlying soft tissues.

It also helps minimize airway collapse behind the tongue base. It is usually used in combination with other surgical procedures.

Tracheostomy: This operation bypasses the entire upper airway by creating an opening in the larynx, or windpipe. Although having the highest therapeutic efficacy for OSA, tracheostomy has many psychosocial problems and is typically reserved as a last resort for the treatment of severe OSA. Tracheostomy is particularly beneficial for patients with complicated medical conditions that prevent other above-listed surgical procedures.

Currently, there is no single universal effective and tolerable treatment for sleep-related breathing disorders. Therefore, sleep medicine requires an interdisciplinary approach partnering physician and dentist for the management of snoring, UARS, and OSA.

Chapter 58

Tobacco and Drug Addiction and Oral Health

Chapter Contents

Section 58.1—Oral Problems in Tobacco Users 556
Section 58.2—Spit Tobacco: A Quitting Guide......................... 559
Section 58.3—Methamphetamine Use Can Leave Users
        Toothless.. 568

Section 58.1

Oral Problems in Tobacco Users

You are probably aware of the devastating effects that smoking and tobacco use can have on the heart, lungs, and other organs. However, you might not be familiar with the whole other "mouthful" of problems caused by tobacco use.

For example, tobacco use is one of the most important risk factors in the development and progression of periodontal diseases, which are the main cause of tooth loss in adults. The sooner you take aim at your tobacco use and quit, the sooner you will hit your target of a healthy smile!

Tobacco users are more likely to have calculus, a hard substance that can only be removed from your teeth during professional cleanings. If this calculus is not removed and it remains below the gum line, the bacteria in the calculus will infect the gums and release toxins that cause redness and swelling (inflammation). The inflammation and toxins cause destruction of the tissues that support the teeth, including the bone. When this happens, the gums separate from the teeth, forming pockets. Smokers and tobacco users have deeper pockets than people who do not use tobacco. These pockets fill with more plaque and bacterial toxins leading to more infection. If these pockets are left untreated, the gums may shrink away from the teeth, making the teeth appear longer and possibly causing them to become loose and fall out.

The detection of periodontal diseases is often more difficult in tobacco users. This is because the nicotine and other chemicals found in tobacco hide the symptoms commonly associated with periodontal diseases, such as bleeding gums. Since the detection of periodontal diseases in tobacco users can be difficult, necessary treatment is sometimes delayed.

Treatment of Periodontal Diseases

Treatment of periodontal diseases in tobacco users can be a difficult task, but not an impossible one. Smoking and tobacco use reduces the delivery of oxygen and nutrients to the gingival tissues weakening the body's defense mechanisms. This can slow down the healing process and make treatment results less predictable following any form of periodontal treatment. As a matter of fact, dental implants that are placed in a tobacco user's mouth fail more often than they would in a patient who does not use tobacco.

The actual treatment of periodontal diseases can vary widely depending on how far the disease has progressed. In fact, if caught in the early stages, simple nonsurgical periodontal therapy, such as scaling and root planing, can be done. If the disease has advanced to the point where the periodontal pockets are deep and bone is lost, surgical therapy may be necessary.

Other Oral Conditions

In addition to causing periodontal diseases, there are many other oral conditions caused by tobacco use. Many of these can affect a person's appearance, health, or self-esteem:

- oral and lip cancer;
- stained teeth;
- bad breath;
- loss of taste and smell;
- mouth sores and spots; and
- black hairy tongue.

Harmful Forms and Tips to Help You Quit

Tobacco's Harmful Forms

All forms of tobacco are harmful, so whether you smoke or dip you are more likely to have severe periodontal diseases and many of the other oral conditions listed above.

- **Cigarettes:** There are more than 4,000 different toxins in cigarette smoke. Toxins impair the body's defense mechanisms, which can leave smokers more susceptible to infections like periodontal diseases. In fact, smokers are about four times more likely than people who have never smoked to have advanced periodontal diseases.

- **Cigars and Pipes:** Despite the glamorous image portrayed with popular culture, cigar and pipe smoking can be very detrimental to your oral health. Recent studies have shown that cigar and pipe smokers experience the same adverse effects on periodontal health and tooth loss as cigarette smokers.

- **Smokeless Tobacco (Chewing Tobacco):** Users of chewing tobacco, spit or dip tobacco, and other forms of smokeless tobacco are not out of harm's way. Smokeless tobacco increases the risk of cancers of the cheek, gums, and lining of the lips by about 50 times. In addition, to hide the unpleasant taste, some brands of smokeless tobacco are heavily sweetened with sugars, which promote tooth decay. The tobacco leaves in the smokeless tobacco contain gritty material which can wear down the surfaces of the teeth and soft tissues of the mouth.

- **Hookah:** In the past it was thought that hookah smoking was a safer alternative to traditional tobacco use because the smoke is filtered out by water. Studies now show that the inhalation of toxic substances through a hookah pipe is similar to or even greater than that of cigarette smoking.

Tips to Help You Quit

Because the treatment of periodontal diseases can be more difficult in tobacco users, your periodontist will urge you to target your tobacco use. Quitting seems to gradually erase the harmful effects of tobacco use on periodontal health. One study showed that 11 years after quitting, a former smoker's likelihood of having periodontal diseases was not much different from one who had never smoked. Smoking cessation takes a huge commitment and it is usually easier if you have help. To begin a tobacco cessation program, ask your periodontist or physician for more information on programs that might fit your needs. Other tips recommended to help you quit include:

- picking a stress-free time to quit;

- asking for support and encouragement from family, friends, and colleagues;

- starting some form of exercise or activity each day to relieve stress and improve your health;

- getting plenty of rest and eating a well-balanced diet;

- joining a stop-smoking program or other support group;

- brushing your teeth often;

- changing your daily routine and spending more time in places where smoking is prohibited; and

- keeping oral substitutes handy such as carrots, apples, and sugarless gum.

Start taking aim at your tobacco use today and move one step closer to a lifetime of periodontal health and happy smiles!

Section 58.2

Spit Tobacco: A Quitting Guide

Excerpted from "Spit Tobacco: A Guide for Quitting," by the National Institute of Dental and Craniofacial Research (NIDCR, www.nidcr.nih .gov), part of the National Institutes of Health, November 19, 2007.

Introduction

So you're a dipper and you'd like to quit. Maybe you've already found that quitting dip or chew is not easy. But you can do it! This information is intended to help you make your own plan for quitting.

Many former dippers have shared advice on quitting that can help you. This information is the result of advice from chewers and dippers who have canned the habit.

Like most dippers, you probably know that the health-related reasons to quit are awesome. But you must find your own personal reasons for quitting. They can motivate you more than the fear of health consequences. It's important to develop your own recipe for willpower.

In this information we refer more to dip than chew, just to keep it simple. Also, note that we call it spit tobacco, not smokeless tobacco. Smokeless tobacco is the term preferred by the tobacco industry. It makes the products sound safe; they aren't.

The Dangers of Dip and Chew

Here's a brief summary of the harm dipping does in the mouth:

- Spit tobacco use may cause cancer of the mouth.
- Sugar in spit tobacco may cause decay in exposed tooth roots.

- Dip and chew can cause your gums to pull away from the teeth in the place where the tobacco is held. The gums do not grow back.

- Leathery white patches and red sores are common in dippers and chewers and can turn into cancer.

Can spit tobacco use cause problems in other parts of the body?

Recent research shows that spit tobacco use might also cause problems beyond the mouth. Some studies have shown that using spit tobacco may cause pancreatic cancer. And scientists are also looking at the possibility that spit tobacco use might play a role in the development of cardiovascular disease—heart disease and stroke.

Need more reasons to quit?

It's expensive! A can of dip costs an average of nearly $3. A two-can-a-week habit costs about $300 per year. A can-a-day habit costs nearly $1,100 per year. Likewise, chewing tobacco costs about $2. A pouch-a-day habit costs over $700 a year. Think of all the things you could do with that money instead of dipping or chewing. It adds up.

It's disgusting! If the health effects don't worry you, think of how other people see your addiction.

The smell of spit tobacco in your mouth is not pleasant. While you may have become used to the odor and don't mind it, others around you notice.

Check out your clothes. Do you have tobacco juice stains on your clothes, your furniture, or on your car's upholstery? Your tobacco spit and drool could be making a mess.

Look at your teeth. Are they stained from tobacco juice? Brushing your teeth won't make this go away.

Understanding Your Addiction

Hard to believe you're a nicotine addict?

Believe it. Nicotine, found in all tobacco products, is a highly addictive drug that acts in the brain and throughout the body.

Dip and chew contain more nicotine than cigarettes. Holding an average-size dip in your mouth for 30 minutes gives you as much nicotine as smoking three cigarettes. A two-can-a-week snuff dipper gets as much nicotine as a 1-1/2 pack-a-day smoker does.

Think about your own habit. Check how many of the following apply to you.

How Addicted Are You?

- I no longer get sick or dizzy when I dip or chew, like I did when I first started.
- I dip more often and in different settings.
- I've switched to stronger products, with more nicotine.
- I swallow juice from my tobacco on a regular basis.
- I sometimes sleep with dip or chew in my mouth.
- I take my first dip or chew first thing in the morning.
- I find it hard to go more than a few hours without dip or chew.
- I have strong cravings when I go without dip or chew.

The more items you check, the more likely that you are addicted.

Myths and Truths

There are several myths about spit tobacco. Sometimes these myths make users feel more comfortable in their habits. Below are some myths and the truths that relate to them.

Myth: Spit tobacco is a harmless alternative to smoking.

Truth: Spit tobacco is still tobacco. In tobacco are nitrosamines, cancer-causing chemicals from the curing process. Note the warnings on the cans.

Myth: Dip (or chew) improves my athletic performance.

Truth: A study of professional baseball players found no connection between spit tobacco use and player performance. Using spit tobacco increases your heart rate and blood pressure within a few minutes. This can cause a buzz or rush, but the rise in pulse and blood pressure places an extra stress on your heart.

Myth: Good gum care can offset the harmful effects of using dip or chew.

Truth: There is no evidence that brushing and flossing will undo the harm that dip and chew are doing to your teeth and gums.

Myth: It's easy to quit using dip or chew when you want to.

Truth: Unfortunately, nicotine addiction makes quitting difficult. But those who have quit successfully are very glad they did.

Quitting Plan

Kicking the spit or chew habit can be tough, but it can be done, and you can do it. The best way to quit spit tobacco is to have a quit date and a quitting plan. These methods make it easier. Try what you think will work best for you.

Decide to Quit

Quitting spit tobacco is not something you do on a whim. You have to want to quit to make it through those first few weeks off tobacco. You know your reasons for stopping. Don't let outside influence—like peer pressure—get in your way. Focus on all you don't like about dipping and chewing.

Reasons to Quit

Here are some reasons given by others. Are any of them important to you?

- To avoid health problems
- To prove I can do it
- I have sores or white patches in my mouth
- To please someone I care about
- To set a good example for my kids or other kids
- To save money
- I don't like the taste
- I have gum or tooth problems
- It's disgusting
- Because it's banned at work or school
- I don't want it to control me
- My girlfriend (or a girl I'd like to date) hates it
- My wife hates it
- My physician or dentist told me to quit

Pick a Quit Date

Pick your quit date. Even if you think you're ready to quit now, take at least a week to get ready. But don't put off setting a date.

Get Psyched up for Quitting

Cut back before you quit by tapering down.

Have your physician or dentist check your mouth. Ask whether you need nicotine replacement therapy (gum, nicotine patches, etc.).

There is no "ideal" time to quit, but low-stress times are best. Having a quit date in mind is important, no matter how far off it is. But it's best to pick a date in the next two weeks, so you don't put it off too long.

Cut Back before You Quit

- Some people are able to quit spit tobacco "cold turkey." Others find that cutting back makes quitting easier. There are many ways to cut back.

- Taper down. Cut back to half of your usual amount before you quit. If you usually carry your tin or pouch with you, try leaving it behind. Carry substitutes instead—sugar-free chewing gum or hard candies or sunflower seeds. During this period, you might also try a mint-leaf snuff.

- Cut back on when and where you dip or chew. First, notice when your cravings are strongest. What events trigger dipping or chewing for you? Do you always reach for a dip after meals? When you work out? In your car or truck? On your job? Don't carry your pouch or tin. Use a substitute instead. Go as long as you possibly can without giving into a craving, at least 10 minutes. Try to go longer and longer as you approach your quit day. Now, pick three of your strongest triggers and stop dipping or chewing at those times. This will be hard at first. The day will come when you are used to going without tobacco at the times you want it most.

- Notice what friends and co-workers who don't dip or chew are doing at these times. This will give you ideas for dip or chew substitutes. It's a good idea to avoid your dipping and chewing pals while you're trying to quit. That will help you avoid the urge to reach for a can or chew.

- Switch to a lower nicotine tobacco product. This way, you cut down your nicotine dose while you're getting ready to quit. This can help to prevent strong withdrawal when you quit.

- Don't switch to other tobacco products like cigarettes or cigars! In fact, if you already smoke, this is a good time to quit smoking. That way you can get over all your nicotine addiction at once.

Right before Your Quit Day, Build a Support Team

Let friends, family, and co-workers know you're quitting. Warn them that you may not be your usual self for a week or two after you quit. Ask them to be patient. Ask them to stand by to listen and encourage you when the going gets rough.

Suggest ways they can help, like joining you for a run or a walk, helping you find ways to keep busy, and telling you they know you can do it. If they've quit, ask them for tips. If they use dip or chew, ask them not to offer you any. They don't have to quit themselves to be support-ive, but maybe someone will want to quit with you.

Quit Day

- Make your quit day special right from the beginning. You're do-ing yourself a huge favor.

- Change daily routines to break away from tobacco triggers. When you eat breakfast, don't sit in the usual place at the kitchen table. Get right up from the table after meals.

- Make an appointment to get your teeth cleaned. You'll enjoy the fresh, clean feeling and a whiter smile.

- Keep busy and active. Start the day with a walk, run, swim, or workout. Aerobic exercise will help you relax. Plus, it boosts energy, stamina, and all-around fitness and curbs your appe-tite.

- Chew substitutes. Try sugar-free hard candies or gum, cinna-mon sticks, mints, beef jerky, or sunflower seeds. Carry them with you and use them whenever you have the urge to dip or chew.

What about Medications?

Nicotine replacement therapy and non-nicotine replacement ther-apy (bupropion) are approved by the U.S. Food and Drug Administration (FDA) for smoking cessation. However, these products have not been approved for spit tobacco cessation. Further research is needed to determine their effectiveness for helping spit tobacco users quit.

Your First Week off Spit Tobacco: Coping with Withdrawal

Withdrawal symptoms don't last long. Symptoms are strongest the first week after you quit. The worst part is over after 2 weeks. As time passes, you'll feel better than when you dipped or chewed. So be patient with yourself.

- **Urges to dip, cravings—especially in the places you used to dip the most:** Wait it out. Deep breathing and exercise help you feel better right away.

- **Feeling irritable, tense, restless, impatient:** Walk away from the situation. Deep breathing and exercise help to blow off steam. Ask others to be patient.

- **Constipation/irregularity:** Add fiber to your diet (whole grain breads and cereals, fresh fruits and vegetables).

- **Hunger and weight gain:** Eat regular meals. Feeling hungry is sometimes mistaken for the desire to dip or chew.

- **Desire for sweets:** Reach for low-calorie sweet snacks (like apples, sugar-free gums, and candies).

About Weight Gain

Nicotine speeds up metabolism, so quitting spit tobacco may result in a slight weight gain. To limit the amount of weight you gain, try the following:

- Eat well-balanced meals and avoid fatty foods. To satisfy your cravings for sweets, eat small pieces of fruit. Keep low-calorie foods handy for snacks. Try popcorn (without butter), sugar-free gums and mints, fresh fruits, and vegetables.

- Drink 6 to 8 glasses of water each day.

- Work about 30 minutes of daily exercise into your routine; try walking or another activity such as running, cycling, or swimming.

Your Second Week: Dealing with Triggers

You've made it through the hardest part—the first week. If you can stay off 1 week, then you can stay off two. Just use the same willpower and strategies that got you this far.

Cravings may be just as strong this week, but they will come less often and go away sooner.

Be Prepared for Temptation

Tobacco thoughts and urges probably still bother you. They will be strongest in the places where you dipped or chewed the most.

The more time you spend in these places without dipping or chewing, the weaker the urges will become. Avoid alcoholic beverages. Drinking them could bust your plan to quit.

Know what events and places will be triggers for you and plan ahead for them.

Write down some of your triggers. And write what you'll do instead of dip or chew. It may be as simple as reaching for gum or seeds, walking away, or thinking about how far you've come.

Tips for Going the Distance

You've broken free of a tough addiction. If you can stay off 2 weeks, then you know you can beat this addiction. It will get easier.

Keep using whatever worked when you first quit. Don't expect new rituals to take the place of spit tobacco right away. It took time to get used to chewing or dipping at first, too.

Keep up your guard. Continue to plan ahead for situations that may tempt you.

What if you should slip?

Try not to slip, not even once. But, if you do slip, get right back on track.

Don't let feelings of guilt lead you back to chewing or dipping. A slip does not mean failure. Figure out why you slipped and how to avoid it next time. Get rid of any leftover tobacco.

Pick up right where you left off before the slip. If slips are frequent, or you are dipping or chewing on a regular basis, make a new quitting plan. Quitting takes practice. The spit tobacco habit can be tough to beat. Most users don't quit for good on the first try. Don't give up!

Figure out what would have helped. Try a new approach next time. Talk to your physician or dentist for extra help.

You may also wish to call one of these services for additional guidance and support:

- The National Cancer Institute (NCI) Cancer Information Service at 800-4-CANCER (1-800-422-6237)

- The National Network of Tobacco Cessation Quitlines at 800-QUIT-NOW (1-800-784-8669)

- The NCI's Smoking Cessation Quitline at 877-44U-QUIT (1-877-448-7848)

Celebrate Your Success

Congratulations! You've done it. You've beaten the spit tobacco habit.

You're improving your health and your future. Celebrate with the people on your support team. Offer your support to friends and co-workers who are trying to quit using tobacco. Pledge to yourself never to take another dip or chew.

Section 58.3

Methamphetamine Use Can Leave Users Toothless

"Brush Up on the Facts about Meth Mouth," © 2007 Partnership for a Drug-Free America (www.drugfree.org). Reprinted with permission.

"Meth mouth" is one of the most notorious physical effects found among meth users. Poor hygiene and the consumption of sugary food and drinks can rapidly turn pearly-whites into a yellow, decaying, stomach-turning mess that often leaves meth users with enormous dental bills and gaping holes in their mouths.

To fully investigate this phenomenon, the Partnership interviewed Dr. Robert Brandjord, former President of the American Dental Association (ADA).

What exactly is meth mouth?

"Meth mouth" occurs when a person has a rapid onset of dental decay. Often, their teeth become blackened and stained and appear to be rotting away and falling apart. What makes it different from normal dental decay is the rapid rate at which it occurs.

The difference between meth mouth and other types of decay can be pretty clear. Most of the time when people have tooth decay, it happens in the back of the mouth, in the grooves of the teeth because that area is the hardest to clean. When a person has tooth decay as a result of meth use, the decay occurs on the front teeth, along the surfaces of the gumline—which, ironically, is the easiest area to get clean.

Can someone get meth mouth even if they don't smoke meth—but, say, uses the drug intravenously?

You can get any of the effects of meth mouth without actually smoking meth. Contrary to popular belief, meth mouth is not a result of the toxic chemicals of the drug itself.

Meth mouth can occur for a number of reasons. First, meth users often become less and less concerned with their personal hygiene and sometimes stop taking care of their teeth altogether. Second, meth users crave sugary drinks, like sodas, when they're high on meth. Having a high intake of these beverages can help to cause tooth decay. The sugar combined with poor oral hygiene is a terrible combination for the mouth. Third, the use of meth slows down saliva production in the mouth—which is a natural cleanser of the oral cavity. Also, meth stimulates the grinding and clenching of teeth—this is how the teeth break apart while they are decaying.

So, do all meth users get meth mouth?

No, not all meth users get meth mouth, since it's brought on more by personal hygiene than the actual drug itself. If a meth user can still remember to brush his or her teeth and refrains from drinking sugary beverages, the risk of getting meth mouth will decrease. However, as stated before, chronic methamphetamine use can cause dry mouth (xerostomia), which significantly increases the risk of dental decay, enamel erosion, and periodontal disease.

How many dental treatments can it take to cure meth mouth?

This can vary—some teeth can be restored quickly, but so many people come in to see dentists in such a severe state that their teeth can't be saved. Many people have no choice but to have dentures and partial dentures put in. Meth mouth robs people, especially young people, of their teeth.

What are typical treatments for meth mouth?

Frequent professional dental hygiene visits with the application of concentrated fluoride to prevent rapid progression of the tooth decay. After this, the teeth would be restored or removed (depending on the damage). The appropriate treatment is dependent on the extent of damage done to the teeth.

Are these treatments expensive? Up to how much can they cost?

The cost of the treatments depends on the amount of damage to the teeth that has occurred and the treatment needed to restore the teeth. If the damage is to the extent you have seen in some of the pictures [See http://www.drugfree.org/Portal/DrugIssue/MethResources/meth_mouth.html] the costs can be in the thousands of dollars.

What have you done to prepare American dentists to fix this type of tooth decay?

We've put together brochures and information that's available on our website and we encourage all dentists to share any experience they have had treating meth mouth with the ADA [American Dental Association] and their colleagues.

What do you suggest for a meth user who is concerned about the condition of his or her mouth?

First, I would hope that if they are concerned about the condition of their mouth, they would seek professional help to treat the overall methamphetamine addiction. Cessation of the meth use would be the most desirable first step to stop the progression of meth mouth.

If a person is still using, the dry mouth (xerostomia) induced by meth will cause an individual to want to drink plenty of liquids—I would recommend drinking water and not sugary carbonated beverages. As stated earlier, the rate of progression of meth mouth can be reduced by practicing good oral hygiene, which includes brushing, flossing, and rinsing with fluoridated mouthwash and getting frequent professional dental cleanings.

Part Eight

Additional Help
and Information

Chapter 59

Glossary of Terms Related to Dental and Oral Health

air abrasion: The application of a mixture of small abrasive particles by air blast to prepare a cavity in a tooth or remove deposits from teeth.

allergic contact dermatitis: A type IV or delayed-hypersensitivity reaction resulting from contact with a chemical allergen (e.g., poison ivy, certain components of patient care gloves), generally localized to the contact area. Reactions occur slowly over 12–48 hours.

antiseptic: A germicide that is used on skin or living tissue for the purpose of inhibiting or destroying microorganisms. Examples include alcohols, chlorhexidine, chlorine, hexachlorophene, iodine, chloroxylenol (PCMX), quaternary ammonium compounds, and triclosan.

baby bottle tooth decay: Also known as severe early childhood caries. A severe pattern of dental caries in infants and young children that first attacks the upper front teeth.

bicuspid (premolar): One of the two permanent teeth located in front of the molars and behind each cuspid. These teeth have two cusps (points) and are used to tear and grind food.

bolus: A chewed, soft mass of food.

This glossary contains terms excerpted from publications by the Centers for Disease Control and Prevention (CDC), Department of Health and Human Services (HHS), National Institute of Dental and Craniofacial Research (NIDCR), National Institutes of Health (NIH), and U.S. Food and Drug Administration, June 2008.

braces: Braces put pressure against the teeth. Most of the pressure comes from a metal wire that goes across the outside of the teeth. Very slowly this pressure makes the teeth move and become straight.

bruxism: Habitual grinding of teeth. In extreme cases, bruxism leads to tooth abrasion and flat biting surfaces.

caries (dental caries): The bacterial disease known as tooth decay or cavities that causes demineralization of teeth through frequent exposure to sugars and starches.

cavity (carious lesion): An area of the tooth affected by dental caries.

cementum: A layer of bone-like mineralized tissue that covers the roots of a tooth.

cleft lip and/or palate: A malformation present at birth where the lip or palate fails to fuse. A cleft lip and/or palate require surgical correction.

complete tooth loss: Complete tooth loss (edentulism) is the loss of all natural teeth. It can substantially reduce quality of life, self-image, and daily functioning.

craniofacial: That which is involved or related to the skull and the face.

crown: The part of the tooth covered with enamel and protruding above the gum line. Also, a restoration of a major part or entire clinical crown of a tooth. It may be made of cast metal, cast metal with a veneer of tooth-colored porcelain baked onto its surface, or a "jacket crown" composed entirely of porcelain or ceramic.

cuspid (canine): A sharp, pointed tooth used for tearing food; located between the first bicuspid and the lateral incisor.

deciduous teeth: See primary teeth.

demineralization: Process of mineral loss from the enamel during the early stages of dental caries. The mineral loss results in chalky white or opaque patches on the tooth surface.

dental hygienist: A person who cleans teeth and examines the mouth, head, and neck for signs of oral disease. May educate patients on oral hygiene, take and develop x-rays, or apply fluoride or sealants.

dental visits: Regular use of the oral health care delivery system leads to better oral health by providing an opportunity for clinical preventive services and early detection of oral diseases. Infrequent users of dental services have more decayed teeth, more severe periodontal diseases, and are more likely to lose all of their teeth.

dentin: A tissue, hard and bone-like, that forms most of the tooth.

dentist: A person who diagnoses and treats diseases, injuries, and malformations of teeth and gums and related oral structures. May also treat diseases of nerve, pulp, and other dental tissues.

dextran: An oral bacteria waste product that is sticky and adheres to the tooth, creating a film called plaque.

digestive enzymes: Enzymes that speed the process of breaking large food molecules into smaller units that are absorbed into the cells.

enamel: The visible outer layer of the tooth.

enamel fluorosis: Enamel fluorosis is a hypomineralization of the enamel surface of the tooth that develops during tooth formation. Clinically this appears as a range of cosmetic changes varying from barely noticeable white spots to pitting and staining. Severe forms can occur when young children consume excess fluoride, from any source, during critical periods of tooth development.

enzyme: A catalyst produced by an organism and used to speed up a specific kind of chemical reaction.

esophagus: The tubular portion of the digestive tract that leads from the pharynx to the stomach.

facial nerve (cranial nerve VII): Nerve that supplies sensory and parasympathetic fibers to the tongue, palate, and the narrow passage from the mouth, and motor fibers to the muscles of the face and jaw.

fluoride: A mineral that is effective in preventing and reversing the early signs of dental caries. Fluoride occurs naturally and contains the element fluorine.

frenulum: A small fold of tissue that connects a more fixed part, such as the floor of the mouth, to a movable part, like the tongue.

fructose: Known as fruit sugar; a member of the simple sugars carbohydrate group found in fruits, honey and syrups, and certain vegetables.

gingiva (gums): The tissue that surrounds the neck of the tooth and covers the alveolar bone.

gingivitis: Gum inflammation caused by the buildup of plaque along the gum line.

glucose: A member of the simple sugar carbohydrate group that is found in fruits and honey. Glucose is the most common free sugar that circulates in the blood of higher animals.

halitosis: Bad breath odor.

herpes simplex virus (HSV): Herpes is a common and usually mild infection. It can cause cold sores (fever blisters) on the mouth or face (known as oral herpes) and similar symptoms in the genital area (genital herpes).

incisor: One of the four front teeth on the upper and lower jaw.

inlay: A restoration that fits into a prepared cavity in a tooth and is secured in place by cementation. The inlay usually is cast in gold alloy, but newer techniques allow for fabrication of composite and ceramic inlays.

latex allergy: A type I or immediate anaphylactic hypersensitivity reaction to the proteins found in natural rubber latex.

malocclusion: Teeth that are misaligned or fit together poorly when the jaws are closed. Teeth that are crowded or out of alignment are more difficult to keep clean, contributing to periodontal disease and dental caries.

mamelon: A small bump on the biting surface of an incisor tooth when it first appears in the mouth. Normal chewing and biting usually wear down mamelons to leave a smooth tooth edge.

molar: A tooth located in the back of the mouth used for crushing and grinding food. There are usually three permanent molars on each side of the jaws. There are two primary molars on each side of the jaw.

olfactory system: Anything connected with or relating to the sense of smell.

onlay: A restoration that restores one or more complete cusps of a tooth and is cemented onto the prepared surface of the tooth. It can be constructed of the same materials as the inlay. It is used generally for coverage of extensively damaged posterior teeth.

oral cavity: The inside of the mouth, bounded by the palate, teeth, and tongue.

oral hygiene: Activities that promote good health of the mouth.

oral mucositis/stomatitis: Inflammation and ulceration of the mucous membranes; can increase the risk for pain, oral and systemic infection, and nutritional compromise.

oropharyngeal candidiasis: Candidiasis of the mouth and throat, also known as a thrush or oropharyngeal candidiasis (OPC), is a fungal infection that occurs when there is overgrowth of fungus called *Candida.*

orthodontist: An orthodontist specializes in correcting teeth or jaw problems.

osteonecrosis: Blood vessel compromise and necrosis of bone exposed to high-dose radiation therapy, resulting in decreased ability to heal if traumatized and in extreme susceptibility to infection.

palate: The roof of the mouth; the partition between the oral and nasal cavities that is formed by the hard palate and the soft palate.

papilla: One of the small bumps on the upper surface of the tongue.

pemphigus: A group of rare autoimmune diseases that cause blistering of the skin and mucous membranes (mouth, nose, throat, eyes, and genitals).

periodontal diseases: Periodontal diseases include gingivitis and periodontitis. Both are inflammatory conditions of the gingival tissues (gum tissues around the teeth). In more severe forms, periodontitis includes loss of supporting bone tissue which can lead to tooth loss.

permanent teeth: The second and final set of teeth to appear in the mouth, consisting of 32 teeth.

pharynx: The area where the air and food passages cross; found in the throat of vertebrates.

pits and fissures: Dimples (pits) and creases (fissures) found on 6- and 12-year molars, and premolar teeth. Pits also may be found on the back surfaces of upper front teeth.

plaque: A sticky, thin film that is made up of a protein substance and microorganisms that adhere to the tooth.

primary teeth: The first set of teeth. This set of 20 teeth is also known as baby, deciduous, or milk teeth.

prosthodontist: A specialist who makes oral prostheses to replace missing teeth and other oral structures to correct natural and acquired deformations of mouth and jaws, to restore and maintain oral function (such as chewing and speaking), and to improve appearance.

pulp chamber: The tooth's innermost part containing blood vessels, cells, and nerves.

remineralization: The reversal of demineralization of tooth enamel.

root: The part of the tooth that anchors it to the bone and is normally beneath the gum.

saliva: The watery liquid secreted into the mouth from the salivary glands.

salivary gland: An organ that secretes saliva.

sealants: Thin coatings made of plastic applied to the chewing surfaces of back teeth to prevent decay.

sensory organs: Organs that are capable of receiving and responding to outside information (stimulus).

six-year molars: The first permanent molar teeth to come into the mouth.

Sjögren syndrome: Sjögren syndrome is an autoimmune disease—that is, a disease in which the immune system turns against the body's own cells. This results in symptoms that include dry eyes and dry mouth.

sucrose: Also known as white or table sugar. Sucrose is made up of two simple sugar units: glucose and fructose. Sucrose occurs naturally in many green plants as a product of photosynthesis.

taste bud: A sense organ found primarily on the tongue's upper surface consisting of small flask-shaped groups of cells.

teeth cleaning: A dentist or dental hygienist removes soft debris, stain, and hard deposits (calculus or tartar) on the teeth that cannot be removed by brushing and flossing. Regular teeth cleaning by a dentist or dental hygienist helps prevent periodontal diseases.

temporomandibular joint and muscle disorders: A group of conditions that cause pain and dysfunction in the jaw joint and muscles that control jaw movement.

Tongue: Movable organ on the floor of the mouth.

tooth decay: Tooth decay is the commonly known term for dental caries, an infectious, transmissible, disease caused by bacteria. The damage done to teeth by this disease is commonly known as cavities. Tooth decay can cause pain and lead to infections in surrounding tissues and tooth loss if not treated properly.

trismus/tissue fibrosis: Loss of elasticity of masticatory muscles that restricts normal ability to open the mouth.

uvula: The fleshy structure hanging from the center of the soft palate.

white spot: A chalky or opaque patch on the tooth surface resulting from early loss of minerals from the tooth enamel. White spots can be precursors to cavities if proper oral hygiene and diet are not followed.

wisdom tooth: The third molar found in each jaw.

xerostomia/salivary gland dysfunction: Dryness of the mouth because of thickened, reduced, or absent salivary flow; increases the risk for infection and compromises speaking, chewing, and swallowing. Persistent dry mouth increases the risk of dental cavities.

x-ray: A photograph that reveals details not normally visible.

Chapter 60

Directory of Agencies That Provide Information about Dental and Oral Health

Government Agencies That Provide Information about Dental and Oral Health

Administration on Aging
Washington, DC 20201
Toll-Free: 800-677-1116
(Eldercare Locator)
Phone: 202-619-0724
Website: www.aoa.gov
E-mail: aoainfo@aoa.hhs.gov

Agency for Healthcare Research and Quality
Office of Communications and Knowledge Transfer
540 Gaither Road, Suite 2000
Rockville, MD 20850
Phone: 301-427-1364
Website: www.ahrq.gov

Centers for Disease Control and Prevention
1600 Clifton Road
Atlanta, GA 30333
Toll-Free: 800-311-3435
Phone: 404-639-3311
Website: www.cdc.gov
E-mail: cdcinfo@cdc.gov

Healthfinder®
National Health Information Center
P.O. Box 1133
Washington, DC 20013-1133
Toll-Free: 800-336-4797
Phone: 301-565-4167
Fax: 301-984-4256
Website: www.healthfinder.gov
E-mail: healthfinder@nhic.org

Resources in this chapter were compiled from several sources deemed reliable; all contact information was verified and updated in June 2008.

National Cancer Institute
Cancer Information Service
6116 Executive Boulevard
Room 3036A
Bethesda, MD 20892-8322
Toll-Free: 800-4-CANCER
(422-6237)
TTY Toll-Free: 800-332-8615
Website: www.cancer.gov
E-mail:
cancergovstaff@mail.nih.gov

National Institute of Arthri-tis and Musculoskeletal and Skin Diseases
National Institutes of Health
1 AMS Circle
Bethesda, MD 20892-3675
Toll-Free: 877-22-NIAMS
(226-4267)
Phone: 301-495-4484
TTY: 301-565-2966
Fax: 301-718-6366
Website: www.niams.nih.gov
E-mail:
NIAMSinfo@mail.nih.gov

National Institute of Child Health and Human Development
P.O. Box 3006
Rockville, MD 20847
Phone: 800-370-2943
TTY: 888-320-6942
Fax: 301-984-1473
Website: www.nichd.nih.gov
E-mail:
NICHDInformationResourceCenter
@mail.nih.gov

National Institute of Dental and Craniofacial Research
National Institutes of Health
Bethesda, MD 20892-2190
Phone: 301-402-7364;
301-496-4261
Fax: 301-480-4098
Website: www.nidcr.nih.gov
E-mail: nidcrinfo@mail.nih.gov

National Institute of Neurological Disorders and Stroke
NIH Neurological Institute
P.O. Box 5801
Bethesda, MD 20824
Toll-Free: 800-352-9424
Phone: 301-496-5751
TTY: 301-468-5981
Website: www.ninds.nih.gov
E-mail: braininfo@ninds.nih.gov

National Institute on Aging
Building 31, Room 5C27
31 Center Drive, MSC 2292
Bethesda, MD 20892
Publications Toll-Free:
800-222-2225
Phone: 301-496-1752
TTY: 800-222-4225
Fax: 301-496-1072
Website: www.nia.nih.gov
Publications Website:
www.niapublications.org
E-mail: niainfo@nia.nih.gov

National Institutes of Health

9000 Rockville Pike
Bethesda, MD 20892
Phone: 301-496-4000
TTY: 301-402-9612
Website: www.nih.gov
E-mail: NIHinfo@od.nih.gov

National Women's Health Information Center

8270 Willow Oaks
Corporate Drive
Fairfax, VA 22031
Toll-Free: 800-994-9662
TDD: 888-220-5446
Website: www.4women.gov

U.S. Department of Health and Human Services

200 Independent Avenue, SW
Washington, DC 20201
Toll-Free: 877-696-6775
Phone: 202-619-0257
Website: www.hhs.gov

U.S. Food and Drug Administration

5600 Fishers Lane
Rockville, MD 20857-0001
Toll-Free: 888-463-6332
Phone: 301-827-4420
Fax: 301-443-9767
Website: www.fda.gov

U.S. National Library of Medicine

8600 Rockville Pike
Bethesda, MD 20894
Toll-Free: 888-346-3656
Phone: 301-594-5983
TDD: 800-735-2258
Website: www.nlm.nih.gov
E-mail: custserv@nlm.nih.gov

Private Agencies That Provide Information about Dental and Oral Health

Academy of General Dentistry

211 East Chicago Avenue
Suite 900
Chicago, IL 60611-1999
Phone: 888-AGD-DENT
(243-3368)
Fax: 312-440-0559
Website: www.agd.org

Academy of Laser Dentistry

P.O. Box 8667
Coral Springs, FL 33075
Toll-Free: 877-LASERS6
(527-3776)
Phone: 954-346-3776
Fax: 954-757-2598
Website: www.laserdentistry.org
E-mail: MemberServices
@LaserDentistry.org

American Academy of Cosmetic Dentistry

Toll-Free: 800-543-9220
Fax: 608-222-9540
Website: www.aacd.com
E-mail: info@aacd.com

American Academy of Dental Sleep Medicine
One Westbrook Corporate Center
Suite 920
Westchester, IL 60154
Phone: 708-273-9366
Fax: 708-492-0943
Website: www.aadsm.org
E-mail: info@aadsm.org

American Academy of Family Physicians
11400 Tomahawk Creek Parkway
Shawnee Mission, KS
66207-1210
Toll-Free: 800-274-2237
Phone: 913-906-6000
Website: www.aafp.org
E-mail: fp@aafp.org

American Academy of Pediatric Dentistry
211 East Chicago Avenue
Suite 1700
Chicago, IL 60611-2637
Phone: 312-337-2169
Fax: 312-337-6329
Website: www.aapd.org

American Academy of Pediatrics
141 Northwest Point Boulevard
Elk Grove Village, IL, 60007
Phone: 847-434-4000
Fax: 847-434-8000
Website: www.aap.org
E-mail: kidsdocs@aap.org

American Academy of Periodontology
737 N. Michigan Avenue
Suite 800
Chicago, IL 60611-6660
Phone: 312-787-5518
Fax: 312-787-3670
Website: www.perio.org

American Association of Endodontists
211 E. Chicago Avenue
Suite 1100
Chicago, IL 60611-2691
Toll-Free: 800-872-3636
Phone: 312-266-7255
Fax: 866-451-9020
Website: www.aae.org
E-mail: info@aae.org

American Association of Oral and Maxillofacial Surgeons
9700 West Bryn Mawr Avenue
Rosemont, IL 60018-5701
Toll-Free: 800-822-6637
Phone: 847-678-6200
Fax: 847-678-6286
Website: www.aaoms.org

American Association of Orthodontists
401 North Lindbergh Boulevard
St. Louis, MO 63141-7816
Phone: 314-993-1700
Fax: 314-997-1745
Website: www.braces.org
E-mail: info@aaortho.org

American Chronic Pain Association

P.O. Box 850
Rocklin, CA 95677
Toll-Free: 800-533-3231
Fax: 916-632-3208
Website: www.theacpa.org
E-mail: ACPA@pacbell.net

American Dental Assistants Association

35 East Wacker Drive, Suite 1730
Chicago, IL 60601-2211
Phone: 312-541-1550
Fax: 312-541-1496
Website: www.dentalassistant.org

American Dental Association

211 East Chicago Avenue
Chicago, IL 60611-2678
Phone: 312-440-2500
Website: www.ada.org

American Dental Hygienists Association

444 North Michigan Avenue
Suite 3400
Chicago, IL 60611
Phone: 312-440-8900
Website: www.adha.org
E-mail: mail@adha.net

American Dental Society of Anesthesiology

211 East Chicago Ave
Suite 780
Chicago, IL 60611
Toll-Free: 877-255-3742
Phone: 312-664-8270
Fax: 312-224-8624
Website: www.adsahome.org
E-mail: adsahome@mac.com

American Heart Association

National Center
7272 Greenville Avenue
Dallas, TX 75231
Toll-Free: 800-AHA-USA-1
(242-8721)
Website: www.americanheart.org

American Medical Association/Medem

100 Pine Street, 3rd Floor
San Francisco, CA 94111
Toll-Free: 877-926-3336
Phone: 415-644-3800
Fax: 415-644-3950
Website: www.medem.com
E-mail: info@medem.com

Association of State and Territorial Dental Directors

105 Westerly Road
New Bern, NC 28560
Phone: 252-637-6333
Fax: 252-637-3343
Website: www.astdd.org

Canadian Dental Association

1815 Alta Vista Drive
Ottawa, Ontario K1G 3Y6
CANADA
Phone: 613-523-1770
Website: www.cda-adc.ca
E-mail: reception@cda-adc.ca

Children's Dental Health Project

2001 L Street, NW
Suite 400
Washington, DC 20036
Phone: 202-833-8288
Fax: 202-318-0667
Website: www.cdhp.org

Cleft Palate Foundation
1504 East Franklin Street
Suite 102
Chapel Hill, NC 27514-2820
Phone: 919-933-9044
Fax: 919-933-9604
Website: www.cleftline.org
E-mail: info@cleftline.org

Cleveland Clinic
9500 Euclid Avenue
Cleveland, OH 44195
Toll-Free: 800-223-2273
Phone: 216-444-2200
TTY: 216-444-0261
Website:
www.clevelandclinic.org

FACES: The National Craniofacial Association
P.O. Box 11082
Chattanooga, TN 37401
Toll-Free: 800-3FACES3
(332-2373)
Website: www.faces-cranio.org
E-mail: faces@faces-cranio.org

Hispanic Dental Association
3085 Stevenson Drive
Suite 200
Springfield, IL 62703
Phone: 800-852-7921
Phone: 217-529-6517
Fax: 217-529-9120
Website: www.hdassoc.org
E-mail:
HispanicDental@hdassoc.org

Johns Hopkins Center for Craniofacial Development and Disorders
Website:
www.hopkinsmedicine.org/
craniofacial

Let's Face It
University of Michigan
School of Dentistry/Dentistry
Library
1011 N. University
Ann Arbor, MI 48109-1078
Website: www.dent.umich.edu/
faceit
E-mail: faceit@umich.edu

National Dental Association
3517 16th Street, NW
Washington, DC 20010
Phone: 202-588-1697
Fax: 202-588-1244
Website: www.ndaonline.org
E-mail: admin@ndaonline.org

National Eating Disorders Association
603 Stewart Street
Suite 803
Seattle, WA 98101
Phone: 206-382-3587
Fax: 206-829-8501
Website:
www.nationaleatingdisorders.org
E-mail:
info@NationalEatingDisorders.org

National Maternal & Child Oral Health Resource Center
Georgetown University
P.O. Box 571272
Washington, DC 20057-1272
Phone: 202-784-9771
Fax: 202-784-9777
Website: www.mchoralhealth.org
E-mail: info@mchoralhealth.org

National Museum of Dentistry
University of Maryland
31 South Greene Street
Baltimore, MD 21201-1504
Phone: 410-706-0600
Fax: 410-706-8313
Websites:
www.dentalmuseum.org;
www.mouthpower.org

Nemours Foundation Center for Children's Health Media
1600 Rockland Road
Wilmington, DE 19803
Phone: 302-651-4000
Fax: 302-651-4055
Website: www.kidshealth.org
E-mail: info@kidshealth.org

Oral Cancer Foundation
3419 Via Lido # 205
Newport Beach, CA 92663
Phone: 949-646-8000
Fax: 949-496-3331
Website:
www.oralcancerfoundation.org
E-mail:
info@oralcancerfoundation.org

Oral Health America
410 N. Michigan Avenue
Suite 352
Chicago, IL 60611
Phone: 312-836-9900
Fax: 312-836-9986
Website:
www.oralhealthamerica.org
E-mail:
liz@oralhealthamerica.org

Science News for Kids
Website:
www.sciencenewsforkids.org
E-mail: editor@snkids.com

Simple Steps to Better Dental Health
Columbia University College of
Dental Medicine
Website:
www.simplestepsdental.com

Sjögren's Syndrome Foundation
6707 Democracy Blvd.
Suite 325
Bethesda, MD 20817
Toll-Free: 800-475-6473
Fax: 301-530-4415
Website: www.sjogrens.org

Special Care Dentistry Association
401 North Michigan Avenue
Suite 2200
Chicago, IL 60611
Phone: 312-527-6764
Fax: 312-673-6663
Website: www.scdonline.org
E-mail: scda@scdaonline.org

Support for People with Oral and Head and Neck Cancer
Website: www.spohnc.org
E-mail: info@spohnc.org

Trigeminal Neuralgia Association
925 Northwest 56th Terrace
Suite C
Gainesville, FL 32605-6402
Toll-Free: 800-923-3608
Phone: 352-331-7009
Fax: 352-331-7078
Website: www.fpa-support.org

Chapter 61

Sources for Charitable and Accessible Dental Care

The National Institute of Dental and Craniofacial Research (NIDCR), one of the federal government's National Institutes of Health, leads the nation in conducting and supporting research to improve oral health. As a research organization, NIDCR does not provide financial assistance for dental treatment. The following resources, however, may help you find the dental care you need.

Clinical Trials

NIDCR sometimes seeks volunteers with specific dental, oral, and craniofacial conditions to participate in research studies, also known as clinical trials. Researchers may provide study participants with limited free or low-cost dental treatment for the particular condition they are studying. To find out if there are any NIDCR clinical trials that you might fit into, visit the NIDCR web site at http://www.nidcr.nih.gov and click on "NIDCR Studies Seeking Patients." For a complete list of all federally funded clinical trials, visit http://clinicaltrials.gov. If you do not have access to the Internet, you may need to visit your local library or ask a friend or family member for assistance.

To see if you qualify for any clinical trials being conducted at our Bethesda, Maryland, campus, you can call the Clinical Center's Patient Recruitment and Public Liaison Office at 800-411-1222.

From "Finding Low Cost Dental Care," by the National Institute of Dental and Craniofacial Research (NIDCR, www.nidcr.nih.gov), part of the National Institutes of Health, November 19, 2007.

Dental Schools

Dental schools can be a good source of quality, reduced-cost dental treatment. Most of these teaching facilities have clinics that allow dental students to gain experience treating patients while providing care at a reduced cost. Experienced, licensed dentists closely supervise the students. Postgraduate and faculty clinics are also available at most schools.

To find out if there is a dental school in your area, call your state dental society or association. These organizations are listed in your telephone book. For a complete list of dental schools, visit the NIDCR website at http://www.nidcr.nih.gov and click on "Finding Dental Care," or contact the National Oral Health Information Clearinghouse at:

National Institute of Dental and Craniofacial Research
National Institutes of Health
Bethesda, MD 20892-2190
Phone: 301-402-7364; 301-496-4261
Fax: 301-480-4098
Website: www.nidcr.nih.gov
E-mail: nidcrinfo@mail.nih.gov

Bureau of Primary Health Care

The Bureau of Primary Health Care, a service of the Health Resources and Services Administration (HRSA), supports federally funded community health centers across the country that provide free or reduced-cost health services, including dental care. To obtain a list of centers in your area, contact the HRSA Information Center toll-free at 888-ASK-HRSA (888-275-4772) or visit their web site at http://ask.hrsa.gov/pc.

Centers for Medicare & Medicaid Services

The Centers for Medicare & Medicaid Services (CMS) administers three important federally funded programs: Medicare, Medicaid, and the State Children's Health Insurance Program (SCHIP).

Medicare is a health insurance program for people who are 65 years and older or for people with specific disabilities. Medicare does not cover most routine dental care or dentures. Visit http://www.cms.hhs.gov/MedicareDentalCoverage.

Medicaid is a state-run program that provides medical benefits, and in some cases dental benefits, to eligible individuals and families. States set their own guidelines regarding who is eligible and what services are covered. Most states provide limited emergency dental services for people age 21 or over, while some offer comprehensive services. For most individuals under the age of 21, dental services are provided under Medicaid. Visit http://www.cms.hhs.gov/MedicaidDentalCoverage.

SCHIP helps children up to age 19 who are without health insurance. SCHIP provides medical coverage and, in most cases, dental services to children who qualify. Dental services covered under this program vary from state to state. Visit http://www.cms.hhs.gov/SCHIP DentalCoverage.

CMS can provide detailed information about each of these programs and refer you to state programs where applicable. If you currently have Medicare, call 800-MEDICARE (800-633-4227). Others may call 877-267-2323 or visit the CMS web site at http://www.cms .hhs.gov. You can also write to them at the address below:

Centers for Medicare & Medicaid Services
7500 Security Boulevard
Baltimore, MD 21244

State and Local Resources

Your state or local health department may know of programs in your area that offer free or reduced-cost dental care. Call your local or state health department to learn more about their financial assistance programs. Check your local telephone book for the number to call.

United Way

The United Way may be able to direct you to free or reduced-cost dental services in your community. Check your telephone book for the number of your local United Way chapter.

Index

Index

Page numbers followed by 'n' indicate a footnote. Page numbers in *italics* indicate a table or illustration.

A

AADSM *see* American Academy of Dental Sleep Medicine
AAPD *see* American Academy of Pediatric Dentistry
ABOMS *see* American Board of Oral and Maxillofacial Surgery
"Abscessed Teeth" (A.D.A.M., Inc.) 236n
abscessed teeth, pain management 235, 236–38
Academy of General Dentistry
  contact information 583
  publications
    air abrasion 211n
    crowns 337n
    dental implants 331n
    laser dentistry 215n
    men, dental care 60n
    minimally invasive dentistry 213n
    smile improvements 382n
    toothpaste 102n
Academy of Laser Dentistry, contact information 583

accreditation *see* certification
acid reflux, dental erosion 230–31
Actisite *286*
Actonel (risedronate) 481
ADA *see* American Dental Association
A.D.A.M., Inc., publications
  abscessed teeth 236n
  facial trauma 292n
adjuvant therapy, oral cavity cancer 424
Administration on Aging, contact information 581
adolescents
  oral health advice 44–48
  orthodontic treatment 371–75
  pediatric dentists 163
  wisdom teeth 314–16
adults
  braces 376–80
  dental anxiety 181–82
  health issues 52–54
  orthodontic appliances 349
  see also older adults
"Advice for Patients: Denture Cleansers" (FDA) 115n
age factor
  adult orthodontic treatments 376
  canker sores 448
  early childhood caries 29

age factor, continued
  primary teeth 5–6
  Sjögren syndrome 469
  teething 22
  trigeminal neuralgia 394
Agency for Healthcare Research
  and Quality (AHRQ),
  contact information 581
AHRQ *see* Agency for Healthcare
  Research and Quality
AIMO *see* anterior inferior
  mandibular osteotomy
air abrasion
  defined 573
  described 213–14
  overview 211–12
alcohol use
  dry mouth 437
  older adults 66
  oral cavity cancer 419–20
  oral health 53
alendronate 481
alginate, retainers 358
"All About Orthodontia"
  (Nemours Foundation) 342n
allergic contact dermatitis,
  defined 573
allergies
  braces 352–53
  dental materials 252
  dentist offices 194–98
  denture cleansers 115–16
  orthodontic treatment 352–53,
    370
amalgam fillings 187–88, 246–47,
  255–64
American Academy of Cosmetic
  Dentistry, contact information
  583
American Academy of Dental
  Sleep Medicine (AADSM)
  contact information 584
  sleep apnea publication 545n
American Academy of Family
  Physicians (AAFP), contact
  information 584
American Academy of Pediatric
  Dentistry (AAPD)
  contact information 584

American Academy of Pediatric
  Dentistry (AAPD), continued
  publications
    dental anxiety 180n
    enamel microabrasion 387n
    nutrition, oral health 40n
    pacifiers 33n
    pediatric dentists 161n
    space maintenance 362n
    tooth-colored fillings 254n
    x-ray safety 203n
American Academy of Pediatrics,
  contact information 584
American Academy of
  Periodontology
  contact information 584
  publications
    menstrual cycle 57n
    periodontal disease 266n,
      269n
    pregnancy 58n
    tobacco use 556n
    women, oral health 54n
American Association of
  Endodontists
  contact information 584
  publications
    cracked teeth 239n
    endodontic retreatment 324n
    endodontic surgery 321n
    root canals 318n
American Association of Oral
  and Maxillofacial Surgeons,
  contact information 584
American Association of
  Orthodontists
  contact information 584
  publications
    adolescents orthodontics
      371n
    adult orthodontics 376n
    braces 347n
    pediatric orthodontics 363n
American Board of Oral and
  Maxillofacial Surgery (ABOMS),
  surgical procedures publication
  304n
American Chronic Pain Association,
  contact information 585

American College of Prosthodontists, prosthodontic procedures publication 328n
American Dental Assistants Association, contact information 585
American Dental Association (ADA) contact information 585
publications
  dental fillings 244n
  dental grills 389n
  dental tourism 88n
  dentists, choices 164n
  dentures 333n
  tooth whitening 384n
American Dental Hygienists Association
contact information 585
infectious diseases publication 192n
American Dental Society of Anesthesiology
contact information 585
dental anesthesia publication 209n
American Heart Association
contact information 585
prophylactic antibiotics publication 530n
American Medical Association/ Medem, contact information 585
American Student Dental Association, contact information 160
amitriptyline 395
amylase, described 4
anesthesia, dental procedures 209–11
see also conscious sedation
anorexia nervosa, oral care 515–16
anosmia 461
anterior inferior mandibular osteotomy (AIMO) 552
antibacterial mouth rinses *114*
antibiotic medications
gum disease *276*, 283–84
heart valve disease 530–33
oral contraceptives 56
pemphigus 480
tooth discoloration 37

anticavity mouth rinses *114*
anticonvulsant medications, trigeminal neuralgia 395
antimicrobials
bottled water 147
gum disease *276*
oral irrigation devices 107–11
peptides 80–82
antiseptic
defined 573
halitosis 445
antiseptic chip, gum disease *276*
aphthous stomatitis *see* canker sores
aphthous ulcers 447
appliances
obstructive sleep apnea 546–50
orthodontic treatment 367–68
overview 347–49
archwire, described 351–52
Arestin 111, *286*
"Are You at Risk for Dental Erosion?" (US Army Center for health Promotion and Preventive Medicine) 230n
arthritis, temporomandibular joint disorders 405
artificial salivary gland, described 438
Association of State and Territorial Dental Directors, contact information 585
Atridox 111, *286*
auriculotherapy 187
azathioprine 480

B

baby bottle tooth decay
defined 573
overview 25–32
prevention 21
baby teeth
dental sealants 227
described 5
orthodontic treatment 363–67
see also primary teeth
baclofen 395
bad breath *see* halitosis

balloon compression,
  trigeminal neuralgia 396
barium swallow, oral cavity
  cancer 421
Barrett, Stephen 183n
"Best to Have Wisdom Teeth
  Removed as a Teenager"
  (Medical College of
  Wisconsin) 314n
bicuspid, defined 573
biofilms, described 80–81
biological dentists, described 185
biopsy
  oral cavity cancer 421
  salivary gland cancer 429
  Sjögren syndrome 471
birth defects
  oral and maxillofacial surgery 306
  prosthodontists 328
"Bisphosphonate-Associated
  Osteonecrosis of the Jaw:
  Pathophysiology and
  Epidemiology" (NIDCR) 486n
bite splints, minimally invasive
  dentistry 214
blood tests, Sjögren syndrome
  471–72
board certification
  oral and maxillofacial
    surgery 304–5
  orthodontists 370
bolus, defined 573
bonding, described 382–83
bone grafts, gum disease 284–85
bone surgery, gum disease 285
bottled water
  classifications 148
  fluoride requirements 141
  overview 145–51
"Bottled Water: Better Than
  the Tap?" (Bullers) 145n
bottle mouth, described 25, 36
braces
  adolescents 371–75
  age factor 38
  defined 574
  malocclusion 8
  overview 342–46, 347–56
  see also orthodontic treatment

Brandjord, Robert 568
Bren, Linda 349n
bridges
  overview 339–40
  prosthodontists 328
"Bridging the Gap with a Dental
  Bridge" (Ceatus Media Group)
  339n
brushing teeth
  adolescents 45
  arthritis 68
  caregivers 75–76
  depicted *122–23*
  men 62
  overview 121–23
  plaque removal 221
  women 57
"Brush Up on the Facts about
  Meth Mouth" (Partnership for
  a Drug-Free America) 568n
bruxism
  adult orthodontic treatments 378
  defined 574
  minimally invasive dentistry 214
  overview 399–402
  prosthodontists 329
  retainers 358
  temporomandibular joint
    disorder 235
"Bruxism (Teeth Grinding or
  Clenching)" (Nemours
  Foundation) 399n
bulimia nervosa, oral care 515–16
Bullers, Anne Christiansen 145n
Bureau of Primary Health Care,
  contact information 590
"Burning Mouth Syndrome"
  (NIDCR) 439n
burning mouth syndrome,
  overview 439–41

C

Cain, Lee 90
calcium, oral health 128
calculus, tobacco use 556
California Dental Association,
  dental insurance publication 169n

"Calming the Anxious Child"
(AAPD) 180n
Canadian Dental Association
contact information 585
flossing, brushing publication
119n
cancer treatment
dry mouth 437
older adults 66
oral cavity cancer 423–26
oral complications overview 490–96
oral health checkup 54, 492–95
oral problems 52
supplemental fluoride 495
Candida 455–56, 475
Canfield, Gayl 131
canines
age factor 5–6
chewing process 6
defined 574
described 4, 5
canker sores (aphthous stomatitis)
described 7
overview 447–49
"Canker Sores" (Nemours
Foundation) 447n
capitation insurance plans,
described 172–73
carbamazepine 395
carbamide peroxide 448
carbohydrates
adolescents 47
cavities 8
chewing process 6
infants 25, 31
cardiovascular disease,
periodontal disease 14–15
caregivers
dental care 73–78
older adults 66
caries *see* cavities; dental caries;
tooth decay
carious lesion *see* cavity
CAT scan *see* computed axial
tomography scan
cavitations 188
cavities
defined 574
described 8, 67, 244, 579

cavities, continued
overview 221–24
see also dental caries;
tooth decay
cavity prevention
adolescents 47–48
children 37–38
described 244–45
pediatric dentists 161–62
research 80–82
CDC *see* Centers for Disease
Control and Prevention
Ceatus Media Group, dental
bridges publication 339n
Ceja, Frank 89–90
CellCept (mycophenolate
mofetil) 480
cementum
defined 574
described 5
Centers for Disease Control
and Prevention (CDC)
contact information 581
publications
contact dermatitis 194n
enamel fluorosis 152n
latex allergy 194n
oral health 52n
oral health, elders 64n
oral thrush 455n
teeth cleaning 175n
toothbrushes 99n
Centers for Medicare and
Medicaid Services
contact information 591
described 590
central incisors, described 22
certification
dental specialties 158–60
oral and maxillofacial
surgery 304–5
cevimeline 474
chemosenses 457
chemotherapy
dry mouth 437
oral care 496, 504–7
oral cavity cancer 425
oral complications 491
salivary gland cancer 432–33

"Chemotherapy and Your Mouth"
(NIDCR) 504n
"Chew for Health" (Science
News for Kids) 129n
chewing, described 3–4, 6
chewing tobacco, oral problems 558
chi 187
children
amalgam fillings 257–60
appliances 354–56
bruxism 399–402
chemotherapy 507
composite resin fillings 254–55
dental anxiety 180–81
dental sealants 228
dental x-rays 203–4
dentist visits 177
enamel fluorosis 152–53
fluoride requirements 140–44
orthodontic treatment 363–70
pediatric dentists 162
radiation therapy 502–3
space maintainers 362–63
tooth formation 5–6
see also infants
Children's Dental Health Project,
contact information 585
chlorhexidine 110, *276*, *286*
"Choose Your Weapon: Mouth
Rinses" (US Army Center for
health Promotion and
Preventive Medicine)
113n
"Choosing Dental Care Products"
(Cleveland Clinic) 96n
Christensen, Kaare 525–26
cleft lip
defined 574
dental care 72
described 7
overview 518–24
"Cleft Lip and Palate"
(Nemours Foundation) 518n
cleft palate
defined 574
dental care 72
described 7
overview 518–24
prosthodontists 328

Cleft Palate Foundation,
contact information 586
Cleveland Clinic
contact information 586
dental care products publication
96n
clinical trials
described 589
gum disease 277–78
mouth rinses 288
oral cavity cancer 426
periodontal disease 13–17
clonazepam 395
cold sores
described 448
overview 452–54
"Cold Sores (HSV-1)"
(Nemours Foundation) 452n
common chemical sense 458
complete tooth loss, defined 574
composite resins, tooth fillings 38,
248–49, 254–55, 256
comprehensive orthodontic
treatment, described 366
computed axial tomography scan
(CAT scan; CT scan)
oral cavity cancer 421
salivary gland cancer 429, 430
condyle, temporomandibular joint
disorders 405
Connecticut Department of Health,
early childhood caries publication
29n
conscious sedation, overview 206–9
"Conscious (moderate) sedation for
Adults" (NIH) 206n
"Contact Dermatitis and Latex
Allergy" (CDC) 194n
contact dermatitis described 194, *196*
continuous positive airway pressure
(CPAP) 546, 548, 549, 551
contouring, described 383–84
conventional dentures, described 333
Cooke, David A. 145n, 199n, 220n,
278n, 295n, 307n, 310n, 457n
corrective appliances, age factor 39
corticosteroids
pemphigus 480
Sjögren syndrome 473

600

cosmetic dentistry, overview 382–90
cosmetic surgery
  oral and maxillofacial surgery 306
  prosthodontists 329
counterfeit toothpaste 105–6
coxsackie virus, described 7
CPAP *see* continuous positive
  airway pressure
cracked teeth
  overview 239–42
  toothache 235–36
"Cracked Teeth" (American
  Association of Endodontists) 239n
cranial nerve VII, defined 575
craniofacial, defined 574
Craven, Kent 90
craze lines, described 236, 240
crowns
  defined 574
  described 5, 383
  overview 337–38
  prosthodontists 328–29
CT scan *see* computed axial
  tomography scan
curettage, gum disease 284
cuspid, defined 574
cyclophosphamide 473, 480
Cytoxan (cyclophosphamide) 473,
  480

D

dapsone 480
DDS (Doctor of Dental Surgery),
  described 166–67, 370
Decapinol Oral Rinse 287–88
deciduous teeth, described 5–6
  see also primary teeth
DEG *see* diethylene glycol
demineralization, defined 574
dental amalgam *see* amalgam fillings
dental anxiety
  adults 181–82
  children 180–81
"Dental Benefit Coverage"
  (California Dental Association)
  169n
dental bonding, described 382–83

dental bridges
  overview 339–40
  prosthodontists 328
"Dental Care Every Day: A
  Caregiver's Guide" (NIDCR) 73n
dental caries
  adolescents 48
  defined 574
  described 579
  infants 25–28
  see also tooth decay
"Dental Emergency Tips"
  (New York State Dental
  Association) 290n
dental erosion, overview 230–31
dental examinations
  adolescents 47–48
  described 176–77
  health issues 10–12
  see also dentist visits
"Dental Filling Facts" (ADA) 244n
"Dental Grills (Grillz or Fronts)"
  (American Dental Association)
  389n
dental grills, described 389–90
Dental Health Maintenance
  Organization (DHMO),
  described 172–73
dental hygienists
  chemotherapy 505
  defined 574
  dental care devices 96
  described 47–48
dental implants
  appliances 355
  oral and maxillofacial surgery 305
  overview 331–32
  prosthodontists 329
dental injuries, overview 290–94
dental insurance *see* insurance
  coverage
dental public health specialty,
  described 159
dental records, described 168
dental schools, described 590
dental sealants
  children 38
  defined 578
  depicted *226*

dental sealants, continued
  minimally invasive dentistry
    214
  overview 225–28
"Dental Symptoms Can Expose
  Health Issues" (Medical College
  of Wisconsin) 10n
dental tourism, overview 88–91
"Dental Treatment Anxiety"
  (US Army Center for health
  Promotion and Preventive
  Medicine) 181n
dentin
  cavities 8
  cracked teeth 239
  defined 575
  described 5
"Dentist & dental specialties"
  (Wisconsin Dental Association)
  158n
dentists
  choices 164–69
  defined 575
  specialties 158–60
dentist visits
  adolescents 47–48
  cancer treatment 497–99
  caregivers 77–78
  chemotherapy 504–5
  children 36–39
  defined 575
  dentures 336
  eating disorders 515–16
  infants 1
  infection prevention 192–93
  older adults 65
  oral health 53–54
  overview 175–77
  women 56–57
  see also dental examinations;
    dental hygienists
dentures
  cleansers 115–17
  older adults 68–69
  overview 333–36
  prosthodontists 329
"Dentures: Frequently Asked
  Questions" (American Dental
  Association) 333n

Department of Health and Human
  Services (DHHS) see US
  Department of Health and
  Human Services
DeRouen, Tim 259
dextran, defined 575
DHHS see US Department of
  Health and Human Services
DHMO see Dental Health
  Maintenance Organization
diabetes mellitus
  gum disease 273
  oral health 54, 509–12
  periodontal disease 15–16,
    270
diet and nutrition
  adolescents 46–47
  canker sores 448
  children 40–42
  conscious sedation 207
  dental erosion 230–31
  early childhood caries 31–32
  impacted tooth surgery 312
  oral health 126–36
  Streptococcus mutans 222–23
"Diet and Snacking" (AAPD) 40n
diethylene glycol (DEG),
  toothpaste 104–5
digestion, mouth 3
digestive enzymes, defined 575
diphyodont, described 5
diplomate, described 305
DipOrtho, described 370
direct reimbursement (DR),
  dental insurance 173–74
disabilities
  dental care 72–78
  pediatric dentists 163
DMD (Doctor of Dental Medicine),
  described 166–67, 370
Dodes, John E. 183
"Don't Be So Sensitive"
  (Massachusetts Dental Society)
  231n
doxycycline *276, 286*
DR see direct reimbursement
drug-eluting stents, dental
  procedures 534–35
dry eyes, Sjögren syndrome 469

dry mouth
halitosis 444
HIV infection 540
older adults 69
overview 436–38
Sjögren syndrome 469, 474–75
"Dry Mouth" (NIA) 436n
dry socket, described 310

E

"Early Childhood Caries"
(Connecticut Department
of Health) 29n
early childhood caries (ECC) 25–32
see also baby bottle tooth decay
"Eating Away at Your Oral Health"
(Massachusetts Dental Society)
515n
"Eating Concerns and Oral Health"
(National Eating Disorders
Association) 514n
eating disorders
dental erosion 230
oral care 514–16
ECC *see* early childhood caries
Eckert, Randal 82
ectodermal dysplasia, dental
care 72
edentulism, defined 574
electroacupuncture 187
electrodermal testing 187
Employee Retirement and Income
Security Act (ERISA)
dental insurance 172
direct reimbursement plans 174
enamel
cavities 8
defined 575
described 5
enamel fluorosis
defined 575
described 152–53
"Enamel Fluorosis" (CDC) 152n
"Enamel Microabrasion" (AAPD)
387n
enamel microabrasion,
described 387–88

enamel stripping, described 380
"Endodontic Retreatment"
(American Association of
Endodontists) 324n
endodontics specialty, described 159
"Endodontic Surgery"
(American Association of
Endodontists) 321n
endodontic treatment
overview 318–23
retreatment procedure 324–26
see also root canal therapy
endoscopy
oral cavity cancer 421
salivary gland cancer 429
enteroviral stomatitis, described 7
enzyme, defined 575
enzyme suppressants, gum
disease 276
EPO *see* Exclusive Provider
Organization
ERISA *see* Employee Retirement
and Income Security Act
erupt, described 6
esophagus, defined 575
ethical considerations, dentists 165,
168
Evoxac (cevimeline) 474
Exclusive Provider Organization
(EPO), described 172
exfoliative cytology, oral cavity
cancer 421
eye teeth, age factor 22

F

FACES: The National Craniofacial
Association, contact information
586
facial nerve, defined 575
facial trauma
oral and maxillofacial surgery 306
overview 292–94
"Facial Trauma" (A.D.A.M., Inc.) 292n
"Facts and Fallacies About
Periodontal Disease" (American
Academy of Periodontology) 266n
falling-off teeth, described 5

FDA *see* US Food and Drug
Administration
"FDA Approves New Oral Rinse to
Help Treat Gingivitis" (FDA) 287n
fee for service plans, dental
insurance 173
Ferguson, John B. 151
"Fighting Gum Disease: How
to Keep Your Teeth" (Lewis) 278n
fillings
composite resins 38, 248–49,
254–55, 256
mercury 187–88, 246–47, 252–53
overview 244–54
silver amalgam 38, 246–47
filtered water, described 151
financial considerations
adult orthodontic treatments 379
dental bridges 340
dental care 164, 167
dental tourism 88–91
early childhood caries 26
endodontic retreatment 325
halitosis 443
older adults 70
orthodontists 370
root canal therapy 320
"Finding Low Cost Dental Care"
(NIDCR) 589n
Findley, John S. 89
fine needle aspiration, salivary
gland cancer 429
first aid, knocked-out tooth 291–92
fissures, defined 577
fixed functional appliance,
orthodontic treatment 367–68
flap surgery, gum disease 284
flossing
adolescents 45–46
caregivers 76–77
children 38
depicted *120–21*
infants 37
men 62
overview 119–20
plaque removal 220–21
women 57
"Flossing and Brushing" (Canadian
Dental Association) 119n

fluoridated water
cancer risk 139–40
cavity prevention 228
children 37
overview 138–42
"Fluoridated Water: Questions
and Answers" (NCI) 138n
fluoride
bottled water 150
children 37
defined 575
described 138, 140–41
early childhood caries 26
infants 20, 24
mouthwashes 99
older adults 65, 67
oral health 53
overexposure 143–44
"Fluoride and Water"
(Nemours Foundation) 140n
Food and Drug Administration
(FDA) *see* US Food and Drug
Administration
Fosamax (alendronate) 481
fractured cusp, described 240
frenulum, defined 575
"Frequently Asked Questions"
(ABOMS) 304n
"Frequently Asked Questions
About Periodontal (Gum) Disease
and General Health" (American
Academy of Periodontology) 269n
"Frequently Asked Questions:
Teeth Cleaning" (CDC) 175n
fructose, defined 575
Fuller, Janie 353–55

G

gabapentin 395
galvanic testing 187
gastroesophageal reflux disease
(GERD), dental erosion 230–31
Genco, Robert 283
gender factor
canker sores 7
dental concerns 54–62
genes, clefts 524–27

gene therapy, dry mouth
   437
GERD *see* gastroesophageal
   reflux disease
Gewitz, Michael 532
Giannobile, William 85
gingiva, defined 576
gingivitis
   adolescents 48
   adult orthodontic
      treatments 377–78
   defined 576
   described 7–8, 272–73, 279
   menstrual cycle 55, 57–58
   pregnancy 55
gingivostomatitis, described 56
glass ionomer, tooth fillings 249,
   256
glucose, defined 576
glycerol injection, trigeminal
   neuralgia 396
gold alloy fillings, described 251–52,
   256
Golski, John J. 281, 283
Gordon, Jerry 283
Goss, Lisa A. 3n, 22n, 36n, 44n,
   140n, 342n, 399n, 447n
grinding teeth *see* bruxism
group fully-insured indemnity plan,
   described 173
group self-funded indemnity plan,
   described 173
Guay, Albert 91
guided tissue regeneration,
   gum disease 285
Guideline Clearinghouse,
   drug-eluting stents publication
   534n
gum chewing, benefits 129–31
gum disease
   approved treatments *286*
   described 235
   general health 269–70
   halitosis 444–45
   older adults 67–68
   overview 272–78
   prevention 274, 278–88
   see also gingivitis; periodontal
      disease

gums
   adult orthodontic treatments
      377–78
   defined 576
gustatory cells 457
gutta-percha 320
Guyer, Ruth Levy 295n

H

halitosis
   defined 576
   overview 443–45
hard palate, described 4
"Head and Neck Radiation
   Treatment and Your Mouth"
   (NIDCR) 499n
headgear, orthodontic treatment
   367
Healthfinder, contact information
   581
Health Insurance Portability
   and Accountability Act (HIPAA),
   dental records 168
health issues
   adults 52–54
   dental symptoms 10–12
   gum disease 273, 284
"A Healthy Mouth for Your Baby"
   (NIDCR) 20n
heart disease
   antibiotic medications 530–33
   periodontal disease 269
heredity
   crooked teeth 350
   gum disease 273, 280
   orthodontic problems 363
   orthodontic treatment 371
   pemphigus 477
   Sjögren syndrome 469–70
   trigeminal neuralgia 394
herpes simplex virus (HSV)
   defined 576
   overview 452–54
Herr, Amy 84
Hill, Brian 86–87
HIPAA *see* Health Insurance
   Portability and Accountability Act

Hirsch, Larissa 291n, 357n, 452n
Hispanic Dental Association,
   contact information 586
HIV *see* human immunodeficiency
   virus
holistic dentistry, overview 183–89
"Home Care Instructions After
   Oral or Maxillofacial Surgery"
   (UPMC) 307n
Homeier, Barbara P. 518n
homeopathy, described 186–87
hookah smoking, oral problems 558
Horanic, Dennis R. 234n, 236
hormonal changes, gum disease 273,
   285
hormone replacement therapy
   (HRT), periodontal disease 56
"How Can My Dentist Improve
   My Smile?" (Academy of General
   Dentistry) 382n
"How Do X-rays work?"
   (Massachusetts Dental
   Society) 202n
"How to Recognize Potentially
   Unsafe Imported Toothpastes"
   (FDA) 104n
HPV *see* human papillomavirus
HSV *see* herpes simplex virus
Huggins, Hal A. 188
human immunodeficiency virus (HIV)
   mouth problems 537–40
   oral problems 53, *538–39*
human papillomavirus (HPV),
   oral cancers 86–88
hydrogen peroxide 449
hydroxychloroquine 473
Hyman, Frederick N. 279
hyperfractionated radiation therapy,
   oral cavity cancer 425
hyperthermia therapy, oral cavity
   cancer 425–26
hypogeusia 458
hyposmia 461

I

immediate dentures, described 333
immune system, oral problems 53

impacted teeth
   described 8
   oral and maxillofacial
      surgery 305
   overview 310–16
"Implants" (Academy of
   General Dentistry) 331n
IMPOD (Integrated Microfluidic
   Platform for Oral Diagnostics)
   83–85
Imuran (azathioprine) 480
incisors
   age factor 5–6, 22
   chewing process 6
   defined 576
   described 4
indemnity plans,
   dental insurance 171,
   173
infants
   mouth health 20–21
   pediatric dentists 162
   see also children
infections
   abscessed teeth 238
   dentist offices 192–93
   periodontal disease 269–70
Inga, Charlie J. 342n, 399n
inlays
   defined 576
   minimally invasive
      dentistry 214
insurance coverage
   dental sealants 227
   dental tourism 88–91
   older adults 64
   oral problems 53
   overview 169–74
Integrated Microfluidic Platform
   for Oral Diagnostics (IMPOD)
   83–85
interceptive orthodontic
   treatment, described
   365–66
interceptive treatment therapy,
   described 343
interproximal reduction 380
Invisalign 353–54
ionomer fillings 249–50, 256

J

jaw disease, described 235
Johns Hopkins Center for
    Craniofacial Development and
    Disorders, contact information 586
Joondeph, Donald 349, 353–56

K

Kamimori, Gary 131
Kay, Stephen 149–50
"Keeping Your Child's Teeth
    Healthy" (Nemours
    Foundation) 36n
Kelsey, John V. 283
Kim, Henry 147
knocked-out tooth,
    treatment 290, 291–92
"Knocked-out Tooth Instruction
    Sheet" (Nemours Foundation)
    291n

L

labels
    snacks 134
    toothpaste 106–7
lamotrigine 395
"Laser Dentistry" (Academy
    of General Dentistry) 215n
lasers, dentistry 215–16
latex allergy
    defined 576
    described 194–98, *196*
lead exposure, dentist offices
    199–200
Let's Face It, contact
    information 586
Leveille, Gil 130
Lewis, Carol 278n
lingual braces
    adolescents 372
    described 352
"Lip and Oral Cavity Cancer"
    (NCI) 419n
lip biopsy, Sjögren syndrome 471

lip cancer, overview 419–26
lips, described 3, 4
Listerine antiseptic 110
"Looking at the Periodontal-Systemic
    Disease Connection" (NIDCR)
    13n
Lyons, Garrett B., Jr. 3n
Lyons, Garrett B., Sr. 22n, 36n,
    44n, 140n, 447n

M

MacAulay, Calum 416
McConnachie, Ian 298–99
Machtei, Eli E. 57–58
McKinlay, Sonja 259–60
magnetic resonance imaging
    (MRI)
    oral cavity cancer 421
    salivary gland cancer 428–29,
    430
Warren Grant Magnuson
    Clinical Center, impacted
    teeth publication 310n
malocclusion
    children 364
    defined 576
    described 8, 343
    orthodontic treatment 371
    retainers 358
mamelon, defined 576
managed care plans, dental
    insurance 171–72
mandibular orthopedic
    repositioning devices (MORA) 18
Massachusetts Dental Society,
    publications
    bad breath 443n
    dental x-rays 202n
    eating disorders 515n
    sensitive teeth 231n
    veneers 386n
maxillomandibular advancement
    (MMA) 551–52
Medicaid
    dental care 64
    described 591
    early childhood caries 27

Medical College of Wisconsin,
  publications
  health issues 10n
  wisdom teeth 314n
Medicare
  dental care 64
  described 590
medications
  canker sores 448–49
  conscious sedation 207
  dry mouth 65, 66, 436
  gum disease 273, 275, 285
  halitosis 444
  oral health 54
  Sjögren syndrome 473–74
  smell disorders 462
  taste disorders 459
  trigeminal neuralgia 395
Meinig, George A. 188
Melkersson-Rosenthal
  syndrome 542
"Melkersson-Rosenthal
  Syndrome Information Page"
  (NINDS) 542n
men, oral health 60–62
menopause, oral health 56
"Menstrual Cycle Affects
  Periodontal Health" (American
  Academy of Periodontology) 57n
menstrual gingivitis
  described 55
  overview 57–58
mercury, amalgam fillings 187–88,
  246–47, 252–53, 255–64
"Mercury Exposure" (NIEHS) 260n
meridians 187
meth mouth, described 568–70
methotrexate 473, 480
microabrasion, described 387–88
microdentistry, overview 213–14
microvascular decompression,
  trigeminal neuralgia 397
milk bottle mouth, described 8
  see also baby bottle tooth decay
milk teeth, described 5
minerals, oral health 126–27
"Minimally Invasive Dentistry"
  (Academy of General Dentistry)
  213n

minimally invasive dentistry,
  overview 213–14
minocycline *276, 286*
Mississippi State Department of
  Health, soft drinks publication
  135n
MMA *see* maxillomandibular
  advancement
molars
  age factor 5–6, 22
  chewing process 6
  defined 576
  described 4–5
  impacted teeth 310
MORA *see* mandibular orthopedic
  repositioning devices
"Most patients don't need
  antibiotics before dental
  procedures to prevent infective
  endocarditis" (American
  Heart Association)
  530n
mouth
  health issues 10–12
  overview 3–8
"Mouth and Teeth" (Nemours
  Foundation) 3n
mouth examination, Sjögren
  syndrome 471
mouth guards
  bruxism 401
  sports injuries 298–300
"Mouth Problems and HIV"
  (NIDCR) 537n
mouthwashes
  described 98–99
  gum disease 287–88
  halitosis 445
  overview 113–15
MRI *see* magnetic resonance imaging
MS (Masters of Science), described
  370
mucous membranes, mouth 4
Murray, Jeff 525, 527
musical instruments, orthodontic
  treatment 368
mycophenolate mofetil 480
myofascial pain, temporomandibular
  joint disorders 405

N

nasal surgery, obstructive sleep
apnea 552
National Cancer Institute (NCI)
contact information 582
publications
fluoridated water 138n
oral cavity cancer 419n
salivary gland cancer 427n
National Dental Association,
contact information 586
National Eating Disorders
Association
contact information 586
eating disorders publication
514n
National Institute of Arthritis
and Musculoskeletal and Skin
Diseases (NIAMS)
contact information 582
publications
osteoporosis 484n
pemphigus 476n
Sjögren syndrome 468n
National Institute of Child
Health and Human Development
(NICHD)
calcium publication 128n
contact information 582
National Institute of Dental and
Craniofacial Research (NIDCR)
contact information 582, 590
publications
burning mouth syndrome 439n
cancer treatment
complications 490n
cancer treatment
preparations 497n
caregivers, dental care 73n
chemotherapy 504n
dental amalgam, children 257n
dental sealants 225n
head and neck radiation 499n
human immunodeficiency virus
537n
infant oral care 20n
low cost dental care 589n
oral cancer 412n

National Institute of Dental and
Craniofacial Research (NIDCR)
publications, continued
oral cancer detection 415n
oral cancer examination 414n
osteonecrosis 486n
periodontal disease 272n
periodontal/systemic disease
connection 13n
plaque 220n
salivary diagnostic device 83n
snacks 132n
special dental care 72n
spit tobacco 559n
temporomandibular joint
disorders 403n
tobacco use, clefts 524n
tooth decay prevention 80n
National Institute of Diabetes
and Digestive and Kidney
Diseases (NIDDK), diabetes
mellitus publication 509n
National Institute of Environmental
Health Sciences (NIEHS), mercury
exposure publication 260n
National Institute of Neurological
Disorders and Stroke (NINDS)
contact information 582
publications
Melkersson-Rosenthal
syndrome 542n
Parry-Romberg syndrome 543n
trigeminal neuralgia 393n
National Institute on Aging (NIA)
contact information 582
publications
dry mouth 436n
oral health 67n
National Institute on Deafness and
Other Communication Disorders
(NIDCD), publications
smell disorders 457n
taste disorders 457n
National Institutes of Health (NIH)
conscious sedation publication
206n
contact information 583
National Library of Medicine (NLM),
contact information 583

National Maternal and Child
Oral Health Resource Center
contact information 587
publications
baby bottle tooth decay 25n
cavities 221n
National Museum of Dentistry,
contact information 587
National Women's Health
Information Center, contact
information 583
NCI *see* National Cancer Institute
Nemours Foundation
contact information 587
publications
bruxism 399n
canker sores 447n
children, oral health 36n
clefts 518n
cold sores 452n
fluoride 140n
knocked-out tooth 291n
mouth structure 3n
oral care, adolescents 44n
orthodontia 342n
retainers 357n
teething process 22n
neuralgia-inducing cavitational
osteonecrosis (NICO) 188
neurectomy, trigeminal neuralgia
397
New York State Dental Association,
dental emergencies publication
290n
NIA *see* National Institute on Aging
NIAMS *see* National Institute of
Arthritis and Musculoskeletal
and Skin Diseases
NICHD *see* National Institute
of Child Health and Human
Development
nickel allergies 353, 370
NICO *see* neuralgia-inducing
cavitational osteonecrosis
NIDCR *see* National Institute of
Dental and Craniofacial Research
NIEHS *see* National Institute of
Environmental Health Sciences
NIH *see* National Institutes of Health

NINDS *see* National Institute of
Neurological Disorders and Stroke
NLM *see* National Library of
Medicine
nortriptyline 395
"Novel Device Shows Potential in
Better Detecting Oral Cancer"
(NIDCR) 415n
Nowjack-Raymer, Ruth 295–97
nursing decay, described 25, 30
"Nutrition and Oral Health" (US
Army Center for health Promotion
and Preventive Medicine) 126n

O

obstructive sleep apnea
overview 545–53
prosthodontists 330
obturator, prosthodontists 328
older adults, oral health 64–66
olfactory system, defined 576
onlays
defined 576
minimally invasive dentistry 214
Ontario Dental Association, mouth
guards publication 298n
OPC *see* oropharyngeal candidiasis
Open Wide: Oral Health Training
for Health Professionals" (National
Maternal and Child Oral Health
Resource Center) 221n
Ophaug, Robert 150
oral and maxillofacial pathology
specialty, described 159
oral and maxillofacial radiology
specialty, described 159
oral and maxillofacial surgery
home care 307–8
overview 304–6
oral and maxillofacial surgery
specialty, described 159
"Oral Appliances" (AADSM) 545n
"Oral Cancer" (NIDCR) 412n
"Oral Cancer Exam" (NIDCR) 414n
Oral Cancer Foundation
contact information 587
HPV vaccine publication 86n

"The Oral Cancer Foundation Urges
HPV Vaccination for Males" (Oral
Cancer Foundation) 86n
oral cancers
  age factor 65
  examinations 414
  overview 412–13
  vaccine 86–88
  VELscope 415–17
oral cavity, defined 577
oral cavity cancer, overview 419–26
"Oral Complications of Cancer
Treatment: What the Oral
Health Team Can Do" (NIDCR)
490n
oral contraceptives, periodontal
disease 56, 59
Oral Health America, contact
information 587
"Oral Health and Bone Health"
(NIAMS) 484n
"Oral Health and Calcium"
(NICHD) 128n
"Oral Health for Adults"
(CDC) 52n
"Oral Health for Older Americans"
(CDC) 64n
oral herpes (herpetic stomatitis),
described 7
oral hygiene, defined 577
"Oral Irrigation" (Parker) 107n
oral irrigation devices
  described 98
  overview 107–12
oral mucositis, defined 577
"Oral Piercing and Soldiers"
(US Army Center for health
Promotion and Preventive
Medicine) 49n
oral piercings 49–50
oral stomatitis, defined 577
"Oral Surgery" (AADSM) 545n
oral thrush 455–56
orbicularis oris, described 4
"Oropharyngeal Candidiasis"
(CDC) 455n
oropharyngeal candidiasis (OPC)
  defined 577
  described 455–56

orthodontic appliances *see*
  appliances; braces; retainers
orthodontics and dentofacial
  orthopedics specialty, described
  159
orthodontic treatment
  adolescents 371–75
  age factor 38–39
  children 363–70
  clefts 521–22
  overview 342–46
orthodontists
  appliances 347–49
  defined 577
  described 343
  retainers 358–59
  space maintenance 369–70
osteogenesis imperfecta,
  dental care 72
osteonecrosis
  bisphosphonate associated 486–88
  defined 577
  described 485
osteoporosis
  oral health 484–86
  periodontal disease 56
overbite, described 8, 343
overdenture, described 333
oxcarbazepine 395
OxyJet 109

P

pacifier use, described 33–34
Page, Melvin 184
pain management
  abscessed teeth 235, 236–38
  endodontic treatment 319
  impacted tooth surgery 312
  temporomandibular joint
    disorders 408
  toothaches 234–36
palatal expansion appliance,
  orthodontic treatment 368
palate
  defined 577
  described 4
papilla, defined 577

papillae, described 4
paraneoplastic pemphigus,
 described 478
Parker, Denise 107n
parotid glands, described 427
"Parry-Romberg Information
 Page" (NINDS) 543n
Parry-Romberg syndrome 543–44
Partnership for a Drug-Free
 America, methamphetamine
 publication 568n
patient cooperation
 adolescents 373
 orthodontic treatment 369
"Patient Information" (American
 Dental Society of Anesthesiology)
 209n
"The Pediatric Dentist" (AAPD)
 161n
pediatric dentists
 described 37, 159
 diet and nutrition 41
 overview 161–63
pemphigoid 478–79
pemphigus
 defined 577
 overview 476–82
"Pemphigus" (NIAMS) 476n
pemphigus foliaceus, described
 477–78
pemphigus vegetans, described 478
pemphigus vulgaris, described
 477–78
pericoronitis, wisdom teeth 315
PerioChip 286
periodontal, defined 279
periodontal disease
 adult orthodontic treatments
  377–78
 age factor 65
 bone health 484–85
 cardiovascular disease 14–15
 defined 577
 described 7–8
 diabetes mellitus 15–16
 halitosis 444–45
 men 60–62
 myths 266–68
 oral contraceptives 56

periodontal disease, continued
 overview 272–78
 pregnancy 13–14, 55–56, 58–59
 preterm birth 13–14
 respiratory infection 16–17
 tobacco use 556–57
 wisdom teeth 315
"Periodontal (Gum) Disease:
 Causes, Symptoms, and
 Treatments" (NIDCR)
 272n
periodontists
 described 159
 gum disease 280
periodontitis
 described 8, 273, 279–80
 women 54–55
Periostat 286
permanent teeth
 defined 577
 described 6
persulfates, denture
 cleansers 115–16
PET scan see positron
 emission tomography
phantom taste perception 458
pharyngeal cancers, age factor 65
pharynx
 chewing process 6
 defined 577
 described 4
"The phenomenon of dental
 tourism" (ADA) 88n
phenytoin 395
pheromones, research 80–82
piercings
 orthodontic treatment 375
 tooth damage 49–50
Pik Pocket 109
pilocarpine 474
pits, defined 577
plaque
 adolescents 44–45
 defined 577
 dental hygienists 47–48
 described 8, 575
 overview 220–21
 snacks 132
"Plaque" (NIDCR) 220n

Plaquenil (hydroxychloroquine) 473
plastic surgery, oral cavity cancer 424
"Play safe when going back to school: Mouthguards Protect More than Your Teeth" (Ontario Dental Association) 298n
pontic, described 339
porcelain fillings, described 250–51
positron emission tomography (PET scan)
    oral cavity cancer 421–22
    salivary gland cancer 429
PPO *see* preferred provider organizations
Pracht, Terry 350–51, 353, 355–56
preferred provider organizations (PPO), dental insurance 171–72
pregnancy
    adult orthodontic treatments 379
    amalgam fillings 256–57
    clefts 524–27
    oral health 55–56
    periodontal disease 13–14, 55–56, 58–59, 269–70
    tooth formation 36
premolars
    age factor 6
    chewing process 6
    defined 573
"Preparing for Third Molar Removal" (Magnuson Clinical Center) 310n
preterm birth, periodontal disease 13–14
"Prevent Diabetes Problems: Keep Your Teeth and Gums Healthy" (NIDDK) 509n
"Prevention of premature discontinuation of dual antiplatelet therapy in patients with coronary artery stents" (National Guideline Clearinghouse) 534n
preventive orthodontic treatment, described 365
Price, Weston A. 183–85
primary teeth
    defined 578
    dental sealants 227

primary teeth, continued
    described 5–6
    early childhood caries 30–31
    pediatric dentists 162
"Promoting Awareness, Preventing Pain: Facts on Early Childhood Caries (ECC)" (National Maternal and Child Oral Health Resource Center) 25n
prostaglandin, periodontal disease 58–59
"Prosthodontic Procedures" (American College of Prosthodontics) 328n
prosthodontic procedures, overview 328–30
prosthodontics specialty, described 159
prosthodontists, defined 578
"Protecting Against Disease Transmission" (American Dental Hygienists Association) 192n
"Protecting Oral Health Throughout Your Life" (American Academy of Periodontology) 54n
puberty, swollen gums 55
"Public Health Dispatch: Potential Risk for Lead Exposure in Dental Offices" (CDC) 199n
pulp
    abscessed teeth 237–38
    cracked teeth 239–40
    described 5
pulp chamber
    defined 578
    described 5

Q

"Questions and Answers on Dental Amalgam" (FDA) 255n

R

radiation therapy
    chemosensory disorders 458
    dry mouth 437

radiation therapy, continued
  oral care 496, 499–503
  oral cavity cancer 424–25
  oral complications 491–92
  osteonecrosis 577
  salivary gland cancer 432
radiofrequency thermal lesioning,
  trigeminal neuralgia 396
radiograph, described 202
radiosensitizers, salivary gland
  cancer 433
Radke, Lee M. 10–12
"The Reality of Retainers"
  (Nemours Foundation) 357n
reconstructive surgery, oral and
  maxillofacial surgery 306
remineralization
  defined 578
  described 213
removable functional appliance,
  orthodontic treatment 368
reproximation 380
"Researchers Report Initial
  Success in Promising Approach to
  Prevent Tooth Decay" (NIDCR)
  80n
reshaping, described 383–84
resin *see* dental sealants
resin ionomer, tooth fillings
  249–50
respiratory infections,
  periodontal disease 16–17
retainers
  adolescents 374
  orthodontic treatment 344
  overview 357–59
Rethman, Michael P. 58
Rheumatrex (methotrexate) 473
risedronate 481
rituximab 481
Rodriguez, Ivan E. 89
root, defined 578
root canal, described 5
root canal therapy
  abscessed teeth 237–38
  described 8
  overview 318–26
"Root Canal Treatment" (American
  Association of Endodontists) 318n

root planing
  described 282
  oral irrigation devices 112
  periodontal disease 59
  see also scaling
Rosin, Miriam 415–17
Roth, Kathleen 91
Runner, Susan 282, 350, 352, 354

S

Sabino, Mary Lou 314–16
safety considerations
  amalgam fillings 255–57
  laser dentistry 216
Salagen (pilocarpine) 474
saliva
  chewing process 6
  defined 578
  described 4
  disease diagnosis 83–85
  gum chewing 130–31
"Salivary Diagnostic Device
  Shows Promise" (NIDCR) 83n
"Salivary Gland Cancer" (NCI)
  427n
salivary gland cancer,
  overview 427–33
salivary gland dysfunction,
  defined 579
salivary glands
  chewing process 6
  defined 578
  described 4
scaling
  described 282
  oral irrigation devices 112
  periodontal disease 59
  see also root planing
SCHIP, described 591
Schirmer test, Sjögren
  syndrome 470–71
Schripsema, Thomas J. 91
Schultz, Daniel 287
Science News for Kids
  contact information 587
  gum chewing publication
  129n

"Scientists Discover How Maternal Smoking Can Cause Cleft Lip and Palate" (NIDCR) 524n

sealants *see* dental sealants

"Seal Out Tooth Decay" (NIDCR) 225n

second opinions
dentists 167–68
gum disease treatment 277

sedation
adults 206–9
children 181
dental procedures 209–11

selective reduction 380

sensitive teeth
adolescents 44–45
overview 231–32

sensory organs, defined 578

severe early childhood caries
defined 573

Shi, Wenyuan 81–82

silver amalgam
cavities 8
tooth fillings 38, 246–47

Simple Steps to Better Dental Health, contact information 587

Singh, Anup 83–84

six-year molars, defined 578

"Sjögren's Syndrome" (NIAMS) 468n

Sjögren's Syndrome Foundation, contact information 587

Sjögren syndrome
defined 578
dry mouth 437
overview 468–76

sleep apnea
overview 545–53
prosthodontists 330

slenderizing 380

slit lamp examination, Sjögren syndrome 471

"Smell Disorders" (NIDCD) 457n

smell disorders, overview 460–64

smokeless tobacco, oral problems 558

snacks, oral health 132–35

"Snack Smart for Healthy Teeth" (NIDCR) 132n

snoring, described 545, 547–48

"Snoring & Sleep Apnea" (AADSM) 545n

sodium laurel sulfate 448

soft drinks, oral health 135–36

"Soft Drinks and Oral Health" (Mississippi State Department of Health) 135n

soft palate
chewing process 6
described 4

soft palate surgery, obstructive sleep apnea 552

space maintainers
described 362–63, 366
preventive orthodontic treatment 365

"Space Maintenance" (AAPD) 362n

Special Care Dentistry Association, contact information 587

"Special Care in Oral Health" (NIDCR) 72n

special needs
dental care 72–78, 164–65
pediatric dentists 163

speech, mouth 3

speech therapy, clefts 522–23

spit tobacco, oral problems 559–67

"Spit Tobacco: A Guide for Quitting" (NIDCR) 559n

split tooth, described 241

sports activities
adolescents 373
orthodontic treatment 368

sports injuries
mouth guards 298–300
prevention 295–98
protective gear 292, 296–98

"Sports Injuries: In Your Face" (Guyer) 295n

squamous cell carcinoma, described 419

stabilization splints, temporomandibular joint disorders 408

STAMP (specifically targeted antimicrobial peptides) 80–82

615

statistics
  adult orthodontic treatments 376
  early childhood caries 25–26, 31
  eating disorders 515
  gum disease 278
  halitosis 443
  periodontitis 54–55
"Stay Away from 'Holistic' and
  'Biological' Dentists" (Barrett) 183n
stereotactic radiosurgery, trigeminal
  neuralgia 396–97
"Straight Talk on Braces" (Bren)
  349n
Streptococcus mutans 80–82, 222
stress, gum disease 273, 285
"Studies Evaluate Health Effects of
  Dental Amalgam Fillings in
  Children" (NIDCR) 257n
sublingual glands, described 427
submandibular glands, described 427
sucrose, defined 578
Support for People with Oral and
  Head and Neck Cancer,
  contact information 588
surgical procedures
  abscessed teeth 238
  clefts 520–21
  endodontics 321–23
  facial trauma 293
  gum disease 275–77, 284–85
  impacted teeth 310–16
  obstructive sleep apnea 547, 550–53
  oral and maxillofacial surgery
    304–6
  oral cavity cancer 424
  salivary gland cancer 431–32
  temporomandibular joint disorders
    408–9
  trigeminal neuralgia 395–97
systemic disease, oral health 12,
  13–17, 52–54

T

Tabak, Lawrence 258
"Take Your Bad Breath Away"
  (Massachusetts Dental Society)
  443n

"Taking Care of Your Teeth"
  (Nemours Foundation) 44n
"Taking Care of Your Teeth
  and Mouth" (NIA) 67n
"Targeting Tobacco" (American
  Academy of Periodontology) 556n
tartar
  adolescents 44
  gingivitis 7–8
taste buds
  defined 578
  described 4
"Taste Disorders" (NIDCD) 457n
taste disorders, overview 457–60
teenagers *see* adolescents
teeth, overview 3–8
teeth cleaning
  defined 578
  overview 175–77
teeth grinding *see* bruxism
teething process, overview 22–24
"Teething Tots" (Nemours
  Foundation) 22n
temporary teeth, described 5
temporomandibular joint and
  muscle disorders, defined 579
temporomandibular joint disorders
  (TMJ)
  adult orthodontic treatments 378
  described 235
  oral and maxillofacial surgery 306
  overview 403–9
  prosthodontists 330
  retainers 358
tests
  maternal tobacco use 524–27
  pemphigus 479
  Sjögren syndrome 470–72
  smell disorders 462
tetracycline *286*
Thornley, Stew 146, 149, 151
"Three Good Reasons to See a
  Dentist before Cancer Treatment"
  (NIDCR) 497n
thrush
  defined 577
  described 455–56
"Thumb, Finger and Pacifier Habits"
  (AAPD) 33n

thumbsucking
  described 33–34
  interceptive orthodontic
    treatment 365
tic douloureux 393
tissue fibrosis, defined 579
TMJ *see* temporomandibular
  joint disorders
"TMJ Disorders" (NIDCR) 403n
TN *see* trigeminal neuralgia
tobacco use
  cessation guide 559–67
  clefts 524–27
  dry mouth 437
  gum disease 285
  older adults 66
  oral cavity cancer 419–20
  oral health 53, 61
  oral problems 556–67
tongue
  chewing process 6
  defined 579
  described 3
tongue piercing, orthodontic
  treatment 375
tongue reduction surgery,
  obstructive sleep apnea 552
tonsils, described 4
toothaches
  adults 52
  dental emergency 290
  pain management 234–36
toothbrushes
  described 97–98
  older adults 68
  overview 99–101
"Tooth-Colored Fillings" (AAPD)
  254n
tooth-colored fillings, overview
  254–55
tooth decay
  defined 574, 579
  described 8, 234–35, 244
  fluoride 141
  older adults 67
  overview 221–24
  wisdom teeth 315
  see also cavities; dental caries
toothlessness, statistics 64

toothpaste
  age factor 24
  children 38
  described 86–87
  fluoride 44, 106, 142–43
  imported 104–7
  older adults 65, 67
  oral health 62
  overview 102–3
  whitening 385–86
tooth root sensitivities,
  described 234
tooth whitening
  adolescents 46
  bleach 382, 385
  overview 384–86
  prosthodontists 330
"Tooth Whitening Treatments"
  (American Dental Association)
  384n
topiramate 395
tracheostomy, obstructive
  sleep apnea 553
traditional Chinese
  medicine, described 187
triclosan *286*
tricyclic antidepressants,
  trigeminal neuralgia 395
trigeminal neuralgia (TN),
  overview 393–97
Trigeminal Neuralgia Association,
  contact information 588
"Trigeminal Neuralgia Fact Sheet"
  (NINDS) 393n
trismus fibrosis, defined 579
"The truth about toothaches"
  (Horanic) 234n
two-phase orthodontic treatment,
  described 369
"Types of Braces and Appliances"
  (American Association of
  Orthodontists) 347n

U

ultrasound, salivary gland
  cancer 429
underbite, described 8, 343

University of Pittsburgh Medical Center (UPMC), surgical procedures publication 307n
upper airway resistance syndrome (UARS) 548, 550
US Army Center for health Promotion and Preventive Medicine, publications
dental anxiety 181n
dental erosion 230n
mouth rinses 113n
nutrition 126n
oral piercings 49n
US Department of Health and Human Services (DHHS), contact information 583
"The Use and Handling of Toothbrushes" (CDC) 99n
US Food and Drug Administration (FDA)
contact information 583
publications
dental amalgam 255n
denture cleansers 115n
imported toothpaste 104n
oral rinse, gum disease 287n
uvula
defined 579
described 4

V

vaccines, oral cancers 86–88
valproic acid 395
veneers
described 383
overview 386–87
prosthodontists 330
"Veneers: A Facelift for Your Teeth" (Massachusetts Dental Society) 386n
vertical root fracture, described 241
Via-Jet 109, 111
Visually Enhanced Lesion Scope (VELscope) 415–17
vitamins, oral health 126–27
Volunteers in Health Care, contact information 165

W

"Want information about orthodontic treatment?" (American Association of Orthodontists) 376n
"Want information about orthodontic treatment for children? (Through age 12)" (American Association of Orthodontists) 363n
"Want information about orthodontic treatment for teenagers?" (American Association of Orthodontists) 371n
water *see* bottled water; fluoridated water
Waterpik 107
water treatments, described 149
weight reduction surgery obstructive sleep apnea 552–53
"What are Crowns?" (Academy of General Dentistry) 337n
"What is Air Abrasion?" (Academy of General Dentistry) 211n
"What Your Gums Can Expect When You Are Expecting" (American Academy of Periodontology) 58n
white spot, defined 579
"Why is Brushing with Toothpaste Important?" (Academy of General Dentistry) 102n
"Why is Oral Health Important for Men?" (Academy of General Dentistry) 60n
Wilson, Walter R. 531, 533
Wisconsin Dental Association, dental specialties publication 158n
wisdom teeth
adolescents 314–16
age factor 6
defined 579
described 4–5
impaction 8
orthodontic treatment 346, 374
women
dental concerns 54–59
gum disease 273

X

xerostomia, defined 579
x-rays
defined 579
dentist offices 202–4
impacted wisdom teeth 8
oral cavity cancer 421
orthodontic treatment 343–44

x-rays, continued
Sjögren syndrome 472
"X-Ray Use and Safety" (AAPD)
203n

Y

"You & Your Dentist: Frequently
Asked Questions" (ADA) 164n

Health Reference Series
COMPLETE CATALOG

List price $87 per volume. School and library price $78 per volume.

Adolescent Health Sourcebook, 2nd Edition

Basic Consumer Health Information about the Physical, Mental, and Emotional Growth and Development of Adolescents, Including Medical Care, Nutritional and Physical Activity Requirements, Puberty, Sexual Activity, Acne, Tanning, Body Piercing, Common Physical Illnesses and Disorders, Eating Disorders, Attention Deficit Hyperactivity Disorder, Depression, Bullying, Hazing, and Adolescent Injuries Related to Sports, Driving, and Work

Along with Substance Abuse Information about Nicotine, Alcohol, and Drug Use, a Glossary, and Directory of Additional Resources

Edited by Joyce Brennfleck Shannon. 683 pages. 2006. 978-0-7808-0943-7.

"It is written in clear, nontechnical language aimed at general readers. . . . Recommended for public libraries, community colleges, and other agencies serving health care consumers."
—American Reference Books Annual, 2003

"Recommended for school and public libraries. Parents and professionals dealing with teens will appreciate the easy-to-follow format and the clearly written text. This could become a 'must have' for every high school teacher." —E-Streams, Jan '03

"A good starting point for information related to common medical, mental, and emotional concerns of adolescents." —School Library Journal, Nov '02

"This book provides accurate information in an easy to access format. It addresses topics that parents and caregivers might not be aware of and provides practical, useable information."
—Doody's Health Sciences Book Review Journal, Sep-Oct '02

"Recommended reference source."
—Booklist, American Library Association, Sep '02

AIDS Sourcebook, 3rd Edition

Basic Consumer Health Information about Acquired Immune Deficiency Syndrome (AIDS) and Human Immunodeficiency Virus (HIV) Infection, Including Facts about Transmission, Prevention, Diagnosis, Treatment, Opportunistic Infections, and Other Complications, with a Section for Women and Children, Including Details about Associated Gynecological Concerns, Pregnancy, and Pediatric Care

Along with Updated Statistical Information, Reports on Current Research Initiatives, a Glossary, and Directories of Internet, Hotline, and Other Resources

Edited by Dawn D. Matthews. 664 pages. 2003. 978-0-7808-0631-3.

"The 3rd edition of the AIDS Sourcebook, part of Omnigraphics' Health Reference Series, is a welcome update. . . . This resource is highly recommended for academic and public libraries."
—American Reference Books Annual, 2004

"Excellent sourcebook. This continues to be a highly recommended book. There is no other book that provides as much information as this book provides."
—AIDS Book Review Journal, Dec-Jan '00

"Recommended reference source."
—Booklist, American Library Association, Dec '99

Alcoholism Sourcebook, 2nd Edition

Basic Consumer Health Information about Alcohol Use, Abuse, and Dependence, Featuring Facts about the Physical, Mental, and Social Health Effects of Alcohol Addiction, Including Alcoholic Liver Disease, Pancreatic Disease, Cardiovascular Disease, Neurological Disorders, and the Effects of Drinking during Pregnancy

Along with Information about Alcohol Treatment, Medications, and Recovery Programs, in Addition to Tips for Reducing the Prevalence of Underage Drinking, Statistics about Alcohol Use, a Glossary of Related Terms, and Directories of Resources for More Help and Information

Edited by Amy L. Sutton. 653 pages. 2006. 978-0-7808-0942-0.

"This title is one of the few reference works on alcoholism for general readers. For some readers this will be a welcome complement to the many self-help books on the market. Recommended for collections serving general readers and consumer health collections."
—E-Streams, Mar '01

"This book is an excellent choice for public and academic libraries."
—American Reference Books Annual, 2001

"Recommended reference source."
—Booklist, American Library Association, Dec '00

"Presents a wealth of information on alcohol use and abuse and its effects on the body and mind, treatment, and prevention." —SciTech Book News, Dec '00

"Important new health guide which packs in the latest consumer information about the problems of alcoholism." —Reviewer's Bookwatch, Nov '00

SEE ALSO Drug Abuse Sourcebook

Allergies Sourcebook, 3rd Edition

Basic Consumer Health Information about Allergic Disorders, Such as Anaphylaxis, Hives, Eczema, Rhinitis, Sinusitis, and Conjunctivitis, and Their Triggers, Including Pollen, Mold, Dust Mites, Animal Dander, Insects, Chemicals, Food, Food Additives, and Medications;

Along with Advice about the Diagnosis and Treatment of Allergy Symptoms, a Glossary of Related Terms, a Directory of Resources for Help and Information, and Suggestions for Additional Reading

Edited by Amy L. Sutton. 598 pages. 2007. 978-0-7808-0950-5.

"This book brings a great deal of useful material together. . . . This is an excellent addition to public and consumer health library collections."
—*American Reference Books Annual, 2003*

"This second edition would be useful to laypersons with little or advanced knowledge of the subject matter. This book would also serve as a resource for nursing and other health care professions students. It would be useful in public, academic, and hospital libraries with consumer health collections." —*E-Streams, Jul '02*

■

Alternative Medicine Sourcebook

SEE Complementary & Alternative Medicine Sourcebook

■

Alzheimer's Disease Sourcebook, 3rd Edition

Basic Consumer Health Information about Alzheimer's Disease, Other Dementias, and Related Disorders, Including Multi-Infarct Dementia, AIDS Dementia Complex, Dementia with Lewy Bodies, Huntington's Disease, Wernicke-Korsakoff Syndrome (Alcohol-Related Dementia), Delirium, and Confusional States

Along with Information for People Newly Diagnosed with Alzheimer's Disease and Caregivers, Reports Detailing Current Research Efforts in Prevention, Diagnosis, and Treatment, Facts about Long-Term Care Issues, and Listings of Sources for Additional Information

Edited by Karen Bellenir. 645 pages. 2003. 978-0-7808-0666-5.

"This very informative and valuable tool will be a great addition to any library serving consumers, students and health care workers."
—*American Reference Books Annual, 2004*

"This is a valuable resource for people affected by dementias such as Alzheimer's. It is easy to navigate and includes important information and resources."
—*Doody's Review Service, Feb '04*

"Recommended reference source."
—*Booklist, American Library Association, Oct '99*

SEE ALSO Brain Disorders Sourcebook

Arthritis Sourcebook, 2nd Edition

Basic Consumer Health Information about Osteoarthritis, Rheumatoid Arthritis, Other Rheumatic Disorders, Infectious Forms of Arthritis, and Diseases with Symptoms Linked to Arthritis, Featuring Facts about Diagnosis, Pain Management, and Surgical Therapies

Along with Coping Strategies, Research Updates, a Glossary, and Resources for Additional Help and Information

Edited by Amy L. Sutton. 593 pages. 2004. 978-0-7808-0667-2.

"This easy-to-read volume is recommended for consumer health collections within public or academic libraries." —*E-Streams, May '05*

"As expected, this updated edition continues the excellent reputation of this series in providing sound, usable health information. . . . Highly recommended."
—*American Reference Books Annual, 2005*

"Excellent reference." —*The Bookwatch, Jan '05*

■

Asthma Sourcebook, 2nd Edition

Basic Consumer Health Information about the Causes, Symptoms, Diagnosis, and Treatment of Asthma in Infants, Children, Teenagers, and Adults, Including Facts about Different Types of Asthma, Common Co-Occurring Conditions, Asthma Management Plans, Triggers, Medications, and Medication Delivery Devices

Along with Asthma Statistics, Research Updates, a Glossary, a Directory of Asthma-Related Resources, and More

Edited by Karen Bellenir. 609 pages. 2006. 978-0-7808-0866-9.

"A worthwhile reference acquisition for public libraries and academic medical libraries whose readers desire a quick introduction to the wide range of asthma information." —*Choice, Association of College & Research Libraries, Jun '01*

"Recommended reference source."
—*Booklist, American Library Association, Feb '01*

"Highly recommended." —*The Bookwatch, Jan '01*

"There is much good information for patients and their families who deal with asthma daily."
—*American Medical Writers Association Journal, Winter '01*

"This informative text is recommended for consumer health collections in public, secondary school, and community college libraries and the libraries of universities with a large undergraduate population."
—*American Reference Books Annual, 2001*

■

Attention Deficit Disorder Sourcebook

Basic Consumer Health Information about Attention Deficit/Hyperactivity Disorder in Children and Adults,

622

Including *Facts about Causes, Symptoms, Diagnostic Criteria, and Treatment Options Such as Medications, Behavior Therapy, Coaching, and Homeopathy*

Along with Reports on Current Research Initiatives, Legal Issues, and Government Regulations, and Featuring a Glossary of Related Terms, Internet Resources, and a List of Additional Reading Material

Edited by Dawn D. Matthews. 470 pages. 2002. 978-0-7808-0624-5.

"Recommended reference source."
—*Booklist, American Library Association, Jan '03*

"This book is recommended for all school libraries and the reference or consumer health sections of public libraries." —*American Reference Books Annual, 2003*

■

Back & Neck Sourcebook, 2nd Edition

Basic Consumer Health Information about Spinal Pain, Spinal Cord Injuries, and Related Disorders, Such as Degenerative Disk Disease, Osteoarthritis, Scoliosis, Sciatica, Spina Bifida, and Spinal Stenosis, and Featuring Facts about Maintaining Spinal Health, Self-Care, Pain Management, Rehabilitative Care, Chiropractic Care, Spinal Surgeries, and Complementary Therapies

Along with Suggestions for Preventing Back and Neck Pain, a Glossary of Related Terms, and a Directory of Resources

Edited by Amy L. Sutton. 633 pages. 2004. 978-0-7808-0738-9.

"Recommended . . . an easy to use, comprehensive medical reference book." —*E-Streams, Sep '05*

"The strength of this work is its basic, easy-to-read format. Recommended." —*Reference and User Services Quarterly, American Library Association, Winter '97*

■

Blood & Circulatory Disorders Sourcebook, 2nd Edition

Basic Consumer Health Information about the Blood and Circulatory System and Related Disorders, Such as Anemia and Other Hemoglobin Diseases, Cancer of the Blood and Associated Bone Marrow Disorders, Clotting and Bleeding Problems, and Conditions That Affect the Veins, Blood Vessels, and Arteries, Including Facts about the Donation and Transplantation of Bone Marrow, Stem Cells, and Blood and Tips for Keeping the Blood and Circulatory System Healthy

Along with a Glossary of Related Terms and Resources for Additional Help and Information

Edited by Amy L. Sutton. 659 pages. 2005. 978-0-7808-0746-4.

"Highly recommended pick for basic consumer health reference holdings at all levels."
—*The Bookwatch, Aug '05*

"Recommended reference source."
—*Booklist, American Library Association, Feb '99*

"An important reference sourcebook written in simple language for everyday, non-technical users. "
—*Reviewer's Bookwatch, Jan '99*

■

Brain Disorders Sourcebook, 2nd Edition

Basic Consumer Health Information about Acquired and Traumatic Brain Injuries, Infections of the Brain, Epilepsy and Seizure Disorders, Cerebral Palsy, and Degenerative Neurological Disorders, Including Amyotrophic Lateral Sclerosis (ALS), Dementias, Multiple Sclerosis, and More

Along with Information on the Brain's Structure and Function, Treatment and Rehabilitation Options, Reports on Current Research Initiatives, a Glossary of Terms Related to Brain Disorders and Injuries, and a Directory of Sources for Further Help and Information

Edited by Sandra J. Judd. 625 pages. 2005. 978-0-7808-0744-0.

"Highly recommended pick for basic consumer health reference holdings at all levels."
—*The Bookwatch, Aug '05*

"Belongs on the shelves of any library with a consumer health collection." —*E-Streams, Mar '00*

"Recommended reference source."
—*Booklist, American Library Association, Oct '99*

SEE ALSO *Alzheimer's Disease Sourcebook*

■

Breast Cancer Sourcebook, 2nd Edition

Basic Consumer Health Information about Breast Cancer, Including Facts about Risk Factors, Prevention, Screening and Diagnostic Methods, Treatment Options, Complementary and Alternative Therapies, Post-Treatment Concerns, Clinical Trials, Special Risk Populations, and New Developments in Breast Cancer Research

Along with Breast Cancer Statistics, a Glossary of Related Terms, and a Directory of Resources for Additional Help and Information

Edited by Sandra J. Judd. 595 pages. 2004. 978-0-7808-0668-9.

"This book will be an excellent addition to public, community college, medical, and academic libraries."
—*American Reference Books Annual, 2006*

"It would be a useful reference book in a library or on loan to women in a support group."
—*Cancer Forum, Mar '03*

"Recommended reference source."
—*Booklist, American Library Association, Jan '02*

"This reference source is highly recommended. It is quite informative, comprehensive and detailed in nature, and yet it offers practical advice in easy-to-read language. It could be thought of as the 'bible' of breast cancer for the consumer." —*E-Streams, Jan '02*

"From the pros and cons of different screening methods and results to treatment options, *Breast Cancer Sourcebook* provides the latest information on the subject." —*Library Bookwatch, Dec '01*

"This thoroughgoing, very readable reference covers all aspects of breast health and cancer.... Readers will find much to consider here. Recommended for all public and patient health collections." —*Library Journal, Sep '01*

SEE ALSO *Cancer Sourcebook for Women, Women's Health Concerns Sourcebook*

■

Breastfeeding Sourcebook

Basic Consumer Health Information about the Benefits of Breastmilk, Preparing to Breastfeed, Breastfeeding as a Baby Grows, Nutrition, and More, Including Information on Special Situations and Concerns Such as Mastitis, Illness, Medications, Allergies, Multiple Births, Prematurity, Special Needs, and Adoption

Along with a Glossary and Resources for Additional Help and Information

Edited by Jenni Lynn Colson. 388 pages. 2002. 978-0-7808-0332-9.

"Particularly useful is the information about professional lactation services and chapters on breastfeeding when returning to work.... *Breastfeeding Sourcebook* will be useful for public libraries, consumer health libraries, and technical schools offering nurse assistant training, especially in areas where Internet access is problematic." —*American Reference Books Annual, 2003*

SEE ALSO *Pregnancy & Birth Sourcebook*

■

Burns Sourcebook

Basic Consumer Health Information about Various Types of Burns and Scalds, Including Flame, Heat, Cold, Electrical, Chemical, and Sun Burns

Along with Information on Short-Term and Long-Term Treatments, Tissue Reconstruction, Plastic Surgery, Prevention Suggestions, and First Aid

Edited by Allan R. Cook. 604 pages. 1999. 978-0-7808-0204-9.

"This is an exceptional addition to the series and is highly recommended for all consumer health collections, hospital libraries, and academic medical centers." —*E-Streams, Mar '00*

"This key reference guide is an invaluable addition to all health care and public libraries in confronting this ongoing health issue." —*American Reference Books Annual, 2000*

"Recommended reference source." —*Booklist, American Library Association, Dec '99*

SEE ALSO *Dermatological Disorders Sourcebook*

Cancer Sourcebook, 5th Edition

Basic Consumer Health Information about Major Forms and Stages of Cancer, Featuring Facts about Head and Neck Cancers, Lung Cancers, Gastrointestinal Cancers, Genitourinary Cancers, Lymphomas, Blood Cell Cancers, Endocrine Cancers, Skin Cancers, Bone Cancers, Metastatic Cancers, and More

Along with Facts about Cancer Treatments, Cancer Risks and Prevention, a Glossary of Related Terms, Statistical Data, and a Directory of Resources for Additional Information

Edited by Karen Bellenir. 1,133 pages. 2007. 978-0-7808-0947-5.

"With cancer being the second leading cause of death for Americans, a prodigious work such as this one, which locates centrally so much cancer-related information, is clearly an asset to this nation's citizens and others." —*Journal of the National Medical Association, 2004*

"This title is recommended for health sciences and public libraries with consumer health collections." —*E-Streams, Feb '01*

"... can be effectively used by cancer patients and their families who are looking for answers in a language they can understand. Public and hospital libraries should have it on their shelves." —*American Reference Books Annual, 2001*

"Recommended reference source." —*Booklist, American Library Association, Dec '00*

SEE ALSO *Breast Cancer Sourcebook, Cancer Sourcebook for Women, Pediatric Cancer Sourcebook, Prostate Cancer Sourcebook*

■

Cancer Sourcebook for Women, 3rd Edition

Basic Consumer Health Information about Leading Causes of Cancer in Women, Featuring Facts about Gynecologic Cancers and Related Concerns, Such as Breast Cancer, Cervical Cancer, Endometrial Cancer, Uterine Sarcoma, Vaginal Cancer, Vulvar Cancer, and Common Non-Cancerous Gynecologic Conditions, in Addition to Facts about Lung Cancer, Colorectal Cancer, and Thyroid Cancer in Women

Along with Information about Cancer Risk Factors, Screening and Prevention, Treatment Options, and Tips on Coping with Life after Cancer Treatment, a Glossary of Cancer Terms, and a Directory of Resources for Additional Help and Information

Edited by Amy L. Sutton. 715 pages. 2006. 978-0-7808-0867-6.

"An excellent addition to collections in public, consumer health, and women's health libraries." —*American Reference Books Annual, 2003*

"Overall, the information is excellent, and complex topics are clearly explained. As a reference book for the consumer it is a valuable resource to assist them to make informed decisions about cancer and its treatments." —*Cancer Forum, Nov '02*

"Highly recommended for academic and medical reference collections." — *Library Bookwatch, Sep '02*

"This is a highly recommended book for any public or consumer library, being reader friendly and containing accurate and helpful information." — *E-Streams, Aug '02*

"Recommended reference source." — *Booklist, American Library Association, Jul '02*

SEE ALSO *Breast Cancer Sourcebook, Women's Health Concerns Sourcebook*

◼

Cancer Survivorship Sourcebook

Basic Consumer Health Information about the Physical, Educational, Emotional, Social, and Financial Needs of Cancer Patients from Diagnosis, through Cancer Treatment, and Beyond, Including Facts about Researching Specific Types of Cancer and Learning about Clinical Trials and Treatment Options, and Featuring Tips for Coping with the Side Effects of Cancer Treatments and Adjusting to Life after Cancer Treatment Concludes

Along with Suggestions for Caregivers, Friends, and Family Members of Cancer Patients, a Glossary of Cancer Care Terms, and Directories of Related Resources

Edited by Karen Bellenir. 6561 pages. 2007. 978-0-7808-0985-7.

◼

Cardiovascular Diseases & Disorders Sourcebook, 3rd Edition

Basic Consumer Health Information about Heart and Vascular Diseases and Disorders, Such as Angina, Heart Attacks, Arrhythmias, Cardiomyopathy, Valve Disease, Atherosclerosis, and Aneurysms, with Information about Managing Cardiovascular Risk Factors and Maintaining Heart Health, Medications and Procedures Used to Treat Cardiovascular Disorders, and Concerns of Special Significance to Women

Along with Reports on Current Research Initiatives, a Glossary of Related Medical Terms, and a Directory of Sources for Further Help and Information

Edited by Sandra J. Judd. 713 pages. 2005. 978-0-7808-0739-6.

"This updated sourcebook is still the best first stop for comprehensive introductory information on cardiovascular diseases." — *American Reference Books Annual, 2006*

"Recommended for public libraries and libraries supporting health care professionals." — *E-Streams, Sep '05*

"This should be a standard health library reference." — *The Bookwatch, Jun '05*

"Recommended reference source." — *Booklist, American Library Association, Dec '00*

". . . comprehensive format provides an extensive overview on this subject." — *Choice, Association of College & Research Libraries*

◼

Caregiving Sourcebook

Basic Consumer Health Information for Caregivers, Including a Profile of Caregivers, Caregiving Responsibilities and Concerns, Tips for Specific Conditions, Care Environments, and the Effects of Caregiving

Along with Facts about Legal Issues, Financial Information, and Future Planning, a Glossary, and a Listing of Additional Resources

Edited by Joyce Brennfleck Shannon. 600 pages. 2001. 978-0-7808-0331-2.

"Essential for most collections." — *Library Journal, Apr 1, 2002*

"An ideal addition to the reference collection of any public library. Health sciences information professionals may also want to acquire the *Caregiving Sourcebook* for their hospital or academic library for use as a ready reference tool by health care workers interested in aging and caregiving." — *E-Streams, Jan '02*

"Recommended reference source." — *Booklist, American Library Association, Oct '01*

◼

Child Abuse Sourcebook

Basic Consumer Health Information about the Physical, Sexual, and Emotional Abuse of Children, with Additional Facts about Neglect, Munchausen Syndrome by Proxy (MSBP), Shaken Baby Syndrome, and Controversial Issues Related to Child Abuse, Such as Withholding Medical Care, Corporal Punishment, and Child Maltreatment in Youth Sports, and Featuring Facts about Child Protective Services, Foster Care, Adoption, Parenting Challenges, and Other Abuse Prevention Efforts

Along with a Glossary of Related Terms and Resources for Additional Help and Information

Edited by Dawn D. Matthews. 620 pages. 2004. 978-0-7808-0705-1.

"A valuable and highly recommended resource for school, academic and public libraries whether used on its own or as a starting point for more in-depth research." — *E-Streams, Apr '05*

"Every week the news brings cases of child abuse or neglect, so it is useful to have a source that supplies so much helpful information. . . . Recommended. Public and academic libraries, and child welfare offices." — *Choice, Association of College & Research Libraries, Mar '05*

"Packed with insights on all kinds of issues, from foster care and adoption to parenting and abuse prevention." — *The Bookwatch, Nov '04*

SEE ALSO: *Domestic Violence Sourcebook*

Childhood Diseases & Disorders Sourcebook

Basic Consumer Health Information about Medical Problems Often Encountered in Pre-Adolescent Children, Including Respiratory Tract Ailments, Ear Infections, Sore Throats, Disorders of the Skin and Scalp, Digestive and Genitourinary Diseases, Infectious Diseases, Inflammatory Disorders, Chronic Physical and Developmental Disorders, Allergies, and More

Along with Information about Diagnostic Tests, Common Childhood Surgeries, and Frequently Used Medications, with a Glossary of Important Terms and Resource Directory

Edited by Chad T. Kimball. 662 pages. 2003. 978-0-7808-0458-6.

"This is an excellent book for new parents and should be included in all health care and public libraries."
—*American Reference Books Annual, 2004*

SEE ALSO: *Healthy Children Sourcebook*

■

Colds, Flu & Other Common Ailments Sourcebook

Basic Consumer Health Information about Common Ailments and Injuries, Including Colds, Coughs, the Flu, Sinus Problems, Headaches, Fever, Nausea and Vomiting, Menstrual Cramps, Diarrhea, Constipation, Hemorrhoids, Back Pain, Dandruff, Dry and Itchy Skin, Cuts, Scrapes, Sprains, Bruises, and More

Along with Information about Prevention, Self-Care, Choosing a Doctor, Over-the-Counter Medications, Folk Remedies, and Alternative Therapies, and Including a Glossary of Important Terms and a Directory of Resources for Further Help and Information

Edited by Chad T. Kimball. 638 pages. 2001. 978-0-7808-0435-7.

"A good starting point for research on common illnesses. It will be a useful addition to public and consumer health library collections."
—*American Reference Books Annual, 2002*

"Will prove valuable to any library seeking to maintain a current, comprehensive reference collection of health resources. . . . Excellent reference."
—*The Bookwatch, Aug '01*

"Recommended reference source."
—*Booklist, American Library Association, Jul '01*

■

Communication Disorders Sourcebook

Basic Information about Deafness and Hearing Loss, Speech and Language Disorders, Voice Disorders, Balance and Vestibular Disorders, and Disorders of Smell, Taste, and Touch

Edited by Linda M. Ross. 533 pages. 1996. 978-0-7808-0077-9.

"This is skillfully edited and is a welcome resource for the layperson. It should be found in every public and medical library." —*Booklist Health Sciences Supplement, American Library Association, Oct '97*

■

Complementary & Alternative Medicine Sourcebook, 3rd Edition

Basic Consumer Health Information about Complementary and Alternative Medical Therapies, Including Acupuncture, Ayurveda, Traditional Chinese Medicine, Herbal Medicine, Homeopathy, Naturopathy, Biofeedback, Hypnotherapy, Yoga, Art Therapy, Aromatherapy, Clinical Nutrition, Vitamin and Mineral Supplements, Chiropractic, Massage, Reflexology, Crystal Therapy, Therapeutic Touch, and More

Along with Facts about Alternative and Complementary Treatments for Specific Conditions Such as Cancer, Diabetes, Osteoarthritis, Chronic Pain, Menopause, Gastrointestinal Disorders, Headaches, and Mental Illness, a Glossary, and a Resource List for Additional Help and Information

Edited by Sandra J. Judd. 657 pages. 2006. 978-0-7808-0864-5.

"Recommended for public, high school, and academic libraries that have consumer health collections. Hospital libraries that also serve the public will find this to be a useful resource." —*E-Streams, Feb '03*

"Recommended reference source."
—*Booklist, American Library Association, Jan '03*

"An important alternate health reference."
—*MBR Bookwatch, Oct '02*

"A great addition to the reference collection of every type of library." —*American Reference Books Annual, 2000*

■

Congenital Disorders Sourcebook, 2nd Edition

Basic Consumer Health Information about Nonhereditary Birth Defects and Disorders Related to Prematurity, Gestational Injuries, Congenital Infections, and Birth Complications, Including Heart Defects, Hydrocephalus, Spina Bifida, Cleft Lip and Palate, Cerebral Palsy, and More

Along with Facts about the Prevention of Birth Defects, Fetal Surgery and Other Treatment Options, Research Initiatives, a Glossary of Related Terms, and Resources for Additional Information and Support

Edited by Sandra J. Judd. 647 pages. 2006. 978-0-7808-0945-1.

"Recommended reference source."
—*Booklist, American Library Association, Oct '97*

SEE ALSO *Pregnancy & Birth Sourcebook*

■

Contagious Diseases Sourcebook

Basic Consumer Health Information about Infectious Diseases Spread by Person-to-Person Contact through

Direct Touch, Airborne Transmission, Sexual Contact, or Contact with Blood or Other Body Fluids, Including Hepatitis, Herpes, Influenza, Lice, Measles, Mumps, Pinworm, Ringworm, Severe Acute Respiratory Syndrome (SARS), Streptococcal Infections, Tuberculosis, and Others

Along with Facts about Disease Transmission, Antimicrobial Resistance, and Vaccines, with a Glossary and Directories of Resources for More Information

Edited by Karen Bellenir. 643 pages. 2004. 978-0-7808-0736-5.

"This easy-to-read volume is recommended for consumer health collections within public or academic libraries." — E-Streams, May '05

"This informative book is highly recommended for public libraries, consumer health collections, and secondary schools and undergraduate libraries." — American Reference Books Annual, 2005

"Excellent reference." — The Bookwatch, Jan '05

■

Death & Dying Sourcebook, 2nd Edition

Basic Consumer Health Information about End-of-Life Care and Related Perspectives and Ethical Issues, Including End-of-Life Symptoms and Treatments, Pain Management, Quality-of-Life Concerns, the Use of Life Support, Patients' Rights and Privacy Issues, Advance Directives, Physician-Assisted Suicide, Caregiving, Organ and Tissue Donation, Autopsies, Funeral Arrangements, and Grief

Along with Statistical Data, Information about the Leading Causes of Death, a Glossary, and Directories of Support Groups and Other Resources

Edited by Joyce Brennfleck Shannon. 653 pages. 2006. 978-0-7808-0871-3.

"Public libraries, medical libraries, and academic libraries will all find this sourcebook a useful addition to their collections." — American Reference Books Annual, 2001

"An extremely useful resource for those concerned with death and dying in the United States." — Respiratory Care, Nov '00

"Recommended reference source." — Booklist, American Library Association, Aug '00

"This book is a definite must for all those involved in end-of-life care." — Doody's Review Service, 2000

■

Dental Care & Oral Health Sourcebook, 2nd Edition

Basic Consumer Health Information about Dental Care, Including Oral Hygiene, Dental Visits, Pain Management, Cavities, Crowns, Bridges, Dental Implants, and Fillings, and Other Oral Health Concerns, Such as Gum Disease, Bad Breath, Dry Mouth, Genetic and Developmental Abnormalities, Oral Cancers, Orthodontics, and Temporomandibular Disorders

Along with Updates on Current Research in Oral Health, a Glossary, a Directory of Dental and Oral Health Organizations, and Resources for People with Dental and Oral Health Disorders

Edited by Amy L. Sutton. 609 pages. 2003. 978-0-7808-0634-4.

"This book could serve as a turning point in the battle to educate consumers in issues concerning oral health." — American Reference Books Annual, 2004

"Unique source which will fill a gap in dental sources for patients and the lay public. A valuable reference tool even in a library with thousands of books on dentistry. Comprehensive, clear, inexpensive, and easy to read and use. It fills an enormous gap in the health care literature." — Reference & User Services Quarterly, American Library Association, Summer '98

"Recommended reference source." — Booklist, American Library Association, Dec '97

■

Depression Sourcebook

Basic Consumer Health Information about Unipolar Depression, Bipolar Disorder, Postpartum Depression, Seasonal Affective Disorder, and Other Types of Depression in Children, Adolescents, Women, Men, the Elderly, and Other Selected Populations

Along with Facts about Causes, Risk Factors, Diagnostic Criteria, Treatment Options, Coping Strategies, Suicide Prevention, a Glossary, and a Directory of Sources for Additional Help and Information

Edited by Karen Bellenir. 602 pages. 2002. 978-0-7808-0611-5.

"Depression Sourcebook is of a very high standard. Its purpose, which is to serve as a reference source to the lay reader, is very well served." — Journal of the National Medical Association, 2004

"Invaluable reference for public and school library collections alike." — Library Bookwatch, Apr '03

"Recommended for purchase." — American Reference Books Annual, 2003

■

Dermatological Disorders Sourcebook, 2nd Edition

Basic Consumer Health Information about Conditions and Disorders Affecting the Skin, Hair, and Nails, Such as Acne, Rosacea, Rashes, Dermatitis, Pigmentation Disorders, Birthmarks, Skin Cancer, Skin Injuries, Psoriasis, Scleroderma, and Hair Loss, Including Facts about Medications and Treatments for Dermatological Disorders and Tips for Maintaining Healthy Skin, Hair, and Nails

Along with Information about How Aging Affects the Skin, a Glossary of Related Terms, and a Directory of Resources for Additional Help and Information

Edited by Amy L. Sutton. 645 pages. 2005. 978-0-7808-0795-2.

"... comprehensive, easily read reference book."
—*Doody's Health Sciences Book Reviews, Oct '97*

SEE ALSO *Burns Sourcebook*

Diabetes Sourcebook, 3rd Edition

Basic Consumer Health Information about Type 1 Diabetes (Insulin-Dependent or Juvenile-Onset Diabetes), Type 2 Diabetes (Noninsulin-Dependent or Adult-Onset Diabetes), Gestational Diabetes, Impaired Glucose Tolerance (IGT), and Related Complications, Such as Amputation, Eye Disease, Gum Disease, Nerve Damage, and End-Stage Renal Disease, Including Facts about Insulin, Oral Diabetes Medications, Blood Sugar Testing, and the Role of Exercise and Nutrition in the Control of Diabetes

Along with a Glossary and Resources for Further Help and Information

Edited by Dawn D. Matthews. 622 pages. 2003. 978-0-7808-0629-0.

"This edition is even more helpful than earlier versions. . . . It is a truly valuable tool for anyone seeking readable and authoritative information on diabetes."
—*American Reference Books Annual, 2004*

"An invaluable reference." —*Library Journal, May '00*

Selected as one of the 250 "Best Health Sciences Books of 1999." —*Doody's Rating Service, Mar-Apr '00*

"Provides useful information for the general public."
—*Healthlines, University of Michigan Health Management Research Center, Sep/Oct '99*

". . . provides reliable mainstream medical information . . . belongs on the shelves of any library with a consumer health collection." —*E-Streams, Sep '99*

"Recommended reference source."
—*Booklist, American Library Association, Feb '99*

Diet & Nutrition Sourcebook, 3rd Edition

Basic Consumer Health Information about Dietary Guidelines and the Food Guidance System, Recommended Daily Nutrient Intakes, Serving Proportions, Weight Control, Vitamins and Supplements, Nutrition Issues for Different Life Stages and Lifestyles, and the Needs of People with Specific Medical Concerns, Including Cancer, Celiac Disease, Diabetes, Eating Disorders, Food Allergies, and Cardiovascular Disease

Along with Facts about Federal Nutrition Support Programs, a Glossary of Nutrition and Dietary Terms, and Directories of Additional Resources for More Information about Nutrition

Edited by Joyce Brennfleck Shannon. 633 pages. 2006. 978-0-7808-0800-3.

"This book is an excellent source of basic diet and nutrition information." —*Booklist Health Sciences Supplement, American Library Association, Dec '00*

"This reference document should be in any public library, but it would be a very good guide for beginning students in the health sciences. If the other books in this publisher's series are as good as this, they should all be in the health sciences collections."
—*American Reference Books Annual, 2000*

"This book is an excellent general nutrition reference for consumers who desire to take an active role in their health care for prevention. Consumers of all ages who select this book can feel confident they are receiving current and accurate information." —*Journal of Nutrition for the Elderly, Vol. 19, No. 4, 2000*

SEE ALSO *Digestive Diseases & Disorders Sourcebook, Eating Disorders Sourcebook, Gastrointestinal Diseases & Disorders Sourcebook, Vegetarian Sourcebook*

Digestive Diseases & Disorders Sourcebook

Basic Consumer Health Information about Diseases and Disorders that Impact the Upper and Lower Digestive System, Including Celiac Disease, Constipation, Crohn's Disease, Cyclic Vomiting Syndrome, Diarrhea, Diverticulosis and Diverticulitis, Gallstones, Heartburn, Hemorrhoids, Hernias, Indigestion (Dyspepsia), Irritable Bowel Syndrome, Lactose Intolerance, Ulcers, and More

Along with Information about Medications and Other Treatments, Tips for Maintaining a Healthy Digestive Tract, a Glossary, and Directory of Digestive Diseases Organizations

Edited by Karen Bellenir. 335 pages. 2000. 978-0-7808-0327-5.

"This title would be an excellent addition to all public or patient-research libraries."
—*American Reference Books Annual, 2001*

"This title is recommended for public, hospital, and health sciences libraries with consumer health collections." —*E-Streams, Jul-Aug '00*

"Recommended reference source."
—*Booklist, American Library Association, May '00*

SEE ALSO *Eating Disorders Sourcebook, Gastrointestinal Diseases & Disorders Sourcebook*

Disabilities Sourcebook

Basic Consumer Health Information about Physical and Psychiatric Disabilities, Including Descriptions of Major Causes of Disability, Assistive and Adaptive Aids, Workplace Issues, and Accessibility Concerns

Along with Information about the Americans with Disabilities Act, a Glossary, and Resources for Additional Help and Information

Edited by Dawn D. Matthews. 616 pages. 2000. 978-0-7808-0389-3.

"It is a must for libraries with a consumer health section." —*American Reference Books Annual, 2002*

"A much needed addition to the Omnigraphics *Health Reference Series*. A current reference work to provide people with disabilities, their families, caregivers or those who work with them, a broad range of information in one volume, has not been available until now. . . . It is recommended for all public and academic library reference collections." —*E-Streams, May '01*

"An excellent source book in easy-to-read format covering many current topics; highly recommended for all libraries." —*Choice, Association of College & Research Libraries, Jan '01*

"Recommended reference source." —*Booklist, American Library Association, Jul '00*

■

Domestic Violence Sourcebook, 2nd Edition

Basic Consumer Health Information about the Causes and Consequences of Abusive Relationships, Including Physical Violence, Sexual Assault, Battery, Stalking, and Emotional Abuse, and Facts about the Effects of Violence on Women, Men, Young Adults, and the Elderly, with Reports about Domestic Violence in Selected Populations, and Featuring Facts about Medical Care, Victim Assistance and Protection, Prevention Strategies, Mental Health Services, and Legal Issues

Along with a Glossary of Related Terms and Resources for Additional Help and Information

Edited by Dawn D. Matthews. 628 pages. 2004. 978-0-7808-0669-6.

"Educators, clergy, medical professionals, police, and victims and their families will benefit from this realistic and easy-to-understand resource." —*American Reference Books Annual, 2005*

"Recommended for all collections supporting consumer health information. It should also be considered for any collection needing general, readable information on domestic violence." —*E-Streams, Jan '05*

"This sourcebook complements other books in its field, providing a one-stop resource . . . Recommended." —*Choice, Association of College & Research Libraries, Jan '05*

"Interested lay persons should find the book extremely beneficial. . . . A copy of *Domestic Violence and Child Abuse Sourcebook* should be in every public library in the United States." —*Social Science & Medicine, No. 56, 2003*

"This is important information. The Web has many resources but this sourcebook fills an important societal need. I am not aware of any other resources of this type." —*Doody's Review Service, Sep '01*

"Recommended reference source." —*Booklist, American Library Association, Apr '01*

"Important pick for college-level health reference libraries." —*The Bookwatch, Mar '01*

"Because this problem is so widespread and because this book includes a lot of issues within one volume, this work is recommended for all public libraries." —*American Reference Books Annual, 2001*

SEE ALSO Child Abuse Sourcebook

■

Drug Abuse Sourcebook, 2nd Edition

Basic Consumer Health Information about Illicit Substances of Abuse and the Misuse of Prescription and Over-the-Counter Medications, Including Depressants, Hallucinogens, Inhalants, Marijuana, Stimulants, and Anabolic Steroids

Along with Facts about Related Health Risks, Treatment Programs, Prevention Programs, a Glossary of Abuse and Addiction Terms, a Glossary of Drug-Related Street Terms, and a Directory of Resources for More Information

Edited by Catherine Ginther. 607 pages. 2004. 978-0-7808-0740-2.

"Commendable for organizing useful, normally scattered government and association-produced data into a logical sequence." —*American Reference Books Annual, 2006*

"This easy-to-read volume is recommended for consumer health collections within public or academic libraries." —*E-Streams, Sep '05*

"An excellent library reference." —*The Bookwatch, May '05*

"Containing a wealth of information, this book will be useful to the college student just beginning to explore the topic of substance abuse. This resource belongs in libraries that serve a lower-division undergraduate or community college clientele as well as the general public." —*Choice, Association of College & Research Libraries, Jun '01*

"Recommended reference source." —*Booklist, American Library Association, Feb '01*

SEE ALSO Alcoholism Sourcebook

■

Ear, Nose & Throat Disorders Sourcebook, 2nd Edition

Basic Consumer Health Information about Disorders of the Ears, Hearing Loss, Vestibular Disorders, Nasal and Sinus Problems, Throat and Vocal Cord Disorders, and Otolaryngologic Cancers, Including Facts about Ear Infections and Injuries, Genetic and Congenital Deafness, Sensorineural Hearing Disorders, Tinnitus, Vertigo, Ménière Disease, Rhinitis, Sinusitis, Snoring, Sore Throats, Hoarseness, and More

Along with Reports on Current Research Initiatives, a Glossary of Related Medical Terms, and a Directory of Sources for Further Help and Information

Edited by Sandra J. Judd. 659 pages. 2006. 978-0-7808-0872-0.

"Overall, this sourcebook is helpful for the consumer seeking information on ENT issues. It is recommended for public libraries."
—*American Reference Books Annual, 1999*

"Recommended reference source."
—*Booklist, American Library Association, Dec '98*

■

Eating Disorders Sourcebook, 2nd Edition

Basic Consumer Health Information about Anorexia Nervosa, Bulimia Nervosa, Binge Eating, Compulsive Exercise, Female Athlete Triad, and Other Eating Disorders, Including Facts about Body Image and Other Cultural and Age-Related Risk Factors, Prevention Efforts, Adverse Health Effects, Treatment Options, and the Recovery Process

Along with Guidelines for Healthy Weight Control, a Glossary, and Directories of Additional Resources

Edited by Joyce Brennfleck Shannon. 585 pages. 2007. 978-0-7808-0948-2.

"Recommended for health science libraries that are open to the public, as well as hospital libraries. This book is a good resource for the consumer who is concerned about eating disorders." —*E-Streams, Mar '02*

"This volume is another convenient collection of excerpted articles. Recommended for school and public library patrons; lower-division undergraduates; and two-year technical program students."
—*Choice, Association of College & Research Libraries, Jan '02*

"Recommended reference source."
—*Booklist, American Library Association, Oct '01*

SEE ALSO *Diet & Nutrition Sourcebook, Digestive Diseases & Disorders Sourcebook, Gastrointestinal Diseases & Disorders Sourcebook*

■

Emergency Medical Services Sourcebook

Basic Consumer Health Information about Preventing, Preparing for, and Managing Emergency Situations, When and Who to Call for Help, What to Expect in the Emergency Room, the Emergency Medical Team, Patient Issues, and Current Topics in Emergency Medicine

Along with Statistical Data, a Glossary, and Sources of Additional Help and Information

Edited by Jenni Lynn Colson. 494 pages. 2002. 978-0-7808-0420-3.

"Handy and convenient for home, public, school, and college libraries. Recommended."
— *Choice, Association of College & Research Libraries, Apr '03*

"This reference can provide the consumer with answers to most questions about emergency care in the United States, or it will direct them to a resource where the answer can be found."
—*American Reference Books Annual, 2003*

"Recommended reference source."
— *Booklist, American Library Association, Feb '03*

■

Endocrine & Metabolic Disorders Sourcebook

Basic Information for the Layperson about Pancreatic and Insulin-Related Disorders Such as Pancreatitis, Diabetes, and Hypoglycemia; Adrenal Gland Disorders Such as Cushing's Syndrome, Addison's Disease, and Congenital Adrenal Hyperplasia; Pituitary Gland Disorders Such as Growth Hormone Deficiency, Acromegaly, and Pituitary Tumors; Thyroid Disorders Such as Hypothyroidism, Graves' Disease, Hashimoto's Disease, and Goiter; Hyperparathyroidism; and Other Diseases and Syndromes of Hormone Imbalance or Metabolic Dysfunction

Along with Reports on Current Research Initiatives

Edited by Linda M. Shin. 574 pages. 1998. 978-0-7808-0207-0.

"Omnigraphics has produced another needed resource for health information consumers."
—*American Reference Books Annual, 2000*

"Recommended reference source."
— *Booklist, American Library Association, Dec '98*

■

Environmental Health Sourcebook, 2nd Edition

Basic Consumer Health Information about the Environment and Its Effect on Human Health, Including the Effects of Air Pollution, Water Pollution, Hazardous Chemicals, Food Hazards, Radiation Hazards, Biological Agents, Household Hazards, Such as Radon, Asbestos, Carbon Monoxide, and Mold, and Information about Associated Diseases and Disorders, Including Cancer, Allergies, Respiratory Problems, and Skin Disorders

Along with Information about Environmental Concerns for Specific Populations, a Glossary of Related Terms, and Resources for Further Help and Information

Edited by Dawn D. Matthews. 673 pages. 2003. 978-0-7808-0632-0.

"This recently updated edition continues the level of quality and the reputation of the numerous other volumes in Omnigraphics' *Health Reference Series*."
—*American Reference Books Annual, 2004*

"An excellent updated edition."
— *The Bookwatch, Oct '03*

"Recommended reference source."
— *Booklist, American Library Association, Sep '98*

"This book will be a useful addition to anyone's library." —*Choice Health Sciences Supplement, Association of College & Research Libraries, May '98*

". . . a good survey of numerous environmentally induced physical disorders . . . a useful addition to anyone's library."
— *Doody's Health Sciences Book Reviews, Jan '98*

Ethnic Diseases Sourcebook

Basic Consumer Health Information for Ethnic and Racial Minority Groups in the United States, Including General Health Indicators and Behaviors, Ethnic Diseases, Genetic Testing, the Impact of Chronic Diseases, Women's Health, Mental Health Issues, and Preventive Health Care Services

Along with a Glossary and a Listing of Additional Resources

Edited by Joyce Brennfleck Shannon. 664 pages. 2001. 978-0-7808-0336-7.

"Recommended for health sciences libraries where public health programs are a priority."
— E-Streams, Jan '02

"Not many books have been written on this topic to date, and the *Ethnic Diseases Sourcebook* is a strong addition to the list. It will be an important introductory resource for health consumers, students, health care personnel, and social scientists. It is recommended for public, academic, and large hospital libraries."
— American Reference Books Annual, 2002

"Recommended reference source."
— Booklist, American Library Association, Oct '01

"Will prove valuable to any library seeking to maintain a current, comprehensive reference collection of health resources.... An excellent source of health information about genetic disorders which affect particular ethnic and racial minorities in the U.S."
— The Bookwatch, Aug '01

■

Eye Care Sourcebook, 2nd Edition

Basic Consumer Health Information about Eye Care and Eye Disorders, Including Facts about the Diagnosis, Prevention, and Treatment of Common Refractive Problems Such as Myopia, Hyperopia, Astigmatism, and Presbyopia, and Eye Diseases, Including Glaucoma, Cataract, Age-Related Macular Degeneration, and Diabetic Retinopathy

Along with a Section on Vision Correction and Refractive Surgeries, Including LASIK and LASEK, a Glossary, and Directories of Resources for Additional Help and Information

Edited by Amy L. Sutton. 543 pages. 2003. 978-0-7808-0635-1.

". . . a solid reference tool for eye care and a valuable addition to a collection."
— American Reference Books Annual, 2004

■

Family Planning Sourcebook

Basic Consumer Health Information about Planning for Pregnancy and Contraception, Including Traditional Methods, Barrier Methods, Hormonal Methods, Permanent Methods, Future Methods, Emergency Contraception, and Birth Control Choices for Women at Each Stage of Life

Along with Statistics, a Glossary, and Sources of Additional Information

Edited by Amy Marcaccio Keyzer. 520 pages. 2001. 978-0-7808-0379-4.

"Recommended for public, health, and undergraduate libraries as part of the circulating collection."
— E-Streams, Mar '02

"Information is presented in an unbiased, readable manner, and the sourcebook will certainly be a necessary addition to those public and high school libraries where Internet access is restricted or otherwise problematic." — American Reference Books Annual, 2002

"Recommended reference source."
— Booklist, American Library Association, Oct '01

"Will prove valuable to any library seeking to maintain a current, comprehensive reference collection of health resources. . . . Excellent reference."
— The Bookwatch, Aug '01

SEE ALSO Pregnancy & Birth Sourcebook

■

Fitness & Exercise Sourcebook, 3rd Edition

Basic Consumer Health Information about the Physical and Mental Benefits of Fitness, Including Cardiorespiratory Endurance, Muscular Strength, Muscular Endurance, and Flexibility, with Facts about Sports Nutrition and Exercise-Related Injuries and Tips about Physical Activity and Exercises for People of All Ages and for People with Health Concerns

Along with Advice on Selecting and Using Exercise Equipment, Maintaining Exercise Motivation, a Glossary of Related Terms, and a Directory of Resources for More Help and Information

Edited by Amy L. Sutton. 663 pages. 2007. 978-0-7808-0946-8.

"This work is recommended for all general reference collections."
— American Reference Books Annual, 2002

"Highly recommended for public, consumer, and school grades fourth through college." — E-Streams, Nov '01

"Recommended reference source."
— Booklist, American Library Association, Oct '01

"The information appears quite comprehensive and is considered reliable. . . . This second edition is a welcomed addition to the series."
— Doody's Review Service, Sep '01

■

Food Safety Sourcebook

Basic Consumer Health Information about the Safe Handling of Meat, Poultry, Seafood, Eggs, Fruit Juices, and Other Food Items, and Facts about Pesticides, Drinking Water, Food Safety Overseas, and the Onset, Duration, and Symptoms of Foodborne Illnesses, Including Types of Pathogenic Bacteria, Parasitic Protozoa, Worms, Viruses, and Natural Toxins

Forensic Medicine Sourcebook

Basic Consumer Information for the Layperson about Forensic Medicine, Including Crime Scene Investigation, Evidence Collection and Analysis, Expert Testimony, Computer-Aided Criminal Identification, Digital Imaging in the Courtroom, DNA Profiling, Accident Reconstruction, Autopsies, Ballistics, Drugs and Explosives Detection, Latent Fingerprints, Product Tampering, and Questioned Document Examination

Along with Statistical Data, a Glossary of Forensics Terminology, and Listings of Sources for Further Help and Information

Gastrointestinal Diseases & Disorders Sourcebook, 2nd Edition

Basic Consumer Health Information about the Upper and Lower Gastrointestinal (GI) Tract, Including the Esophagus, Stomach, Intestines, Rectum, Liver, and Pancreas, with Facts about Gastroesophageal Reflux Disease, Gastritis, Hernias, Ulcers, Celiac Disease, Diverticulitis, Irritable Bowel Syndrome, Hemorrhoids, Gastrointestinal Cancers, and Other Diseases and Disorders Related to the Digestive Process

Along with Information about Commonly Used Diagnostic and Surgical Procedures, Statistics, Reports on Current Research Initiatives and Clinical Trials, a Glossary, and Resources for Additional Help and Information

Genetic Disorders Sourcebook, 3rd Edition

Basic Consumer Health Information about Hereditary Diseases and Disorders, Including Facts about the Human Genome, Genetic Inheritance Patterns, Disorders Associated with Specific Genes, Such as Sickle Cell Disease, Hemophilia, and Cystic Fibrosis, Chromosome Disorders, Such as Down Syndrome, Fragile X Syndrome, and Turner Syndrome, and Complex Diseases and Disorders Resulting from the Interaction of Environmental and Genetic Factors, Such as Allergies, Cancer, and Obesity

Along with Facts about Genetic Testing, Suggestions for Parents of Children with Special Needs, Reports on Current Research Initiatives, a Glossary of Genetic Terminology, and Resources for Additional Help and Information

Head Trauma Sourcebook

Basic Information for the Layperson about Open-Head and Closed-Head Injuries, Treatment Advances, Recovery, and Rehabilitation

Along with Reports on Current Research Initiatives

Edited by Karen Bellenir. 414 pages. 1997. 978-0-7808-0208-7.

Headache Sourcebook

Basic Consumer Health Information about Migraine, Tension, Cluster, Rebound and Other Types of Headaches, with Facts about the Cause and Prevention of Headaches, the Effects of Stress and the Environment, Headaches during Pregnancy and Menopause, and Childhood Headaches

Along with a Glossary and Other Resources for Additional Help and Information

Edited by Dawn D. Matthews. 362 pages. 2002. 978-0-7808-0337-4.

Healthy Aging Sourcebook

Basic Consumer Health Information about Maintaining Health through the Aging Process, Including Advice on Nutrition, Exercise, and Sleep, Help in Making Decisions about Midlife Issues and Retirement, and Guidance Concerning Practical and Informed Choices in Health Consumerism

Along with Data Concerning the Theories of Aging, Different Experiences in Aging by Minority Groups, and Facts about Aging Now and Aging in the Future; and Featuring a Glossary, a Guide to Consumer Help, Additional Suggested Reading, and Practical Resource Directory

Edited by Jenifer Swanson. 536 pages. 1999. 978-0-7808-0390-9.

SEE ALSO Physical & Mental Issues in Aging Sourcebook

Healthy Children Sourcebook

Basic Consumer Health Information about the Physical and Mental Development of Children between the Ages of 3 and 12, Including Routine Health Care, Preventative Health Services, Safety and First Aid,

Healthy Sleep, Dental Care, Nutrition, and Fitness, and Featuring Parenting Tips on Such Topics as Bedwetting, Choosing Day Care, Monitoring TV and Other Media, and Establishing a Foundation for Substance Abuse Prevention

Along with a Glossary of Commonly Used Pediatric Terms and Resources for Additional Help and Information.

Edited by Chad T. Kimball. 647 pages. 2003. 978-0-7808-0247-6.

SEE ALSO Childhood Diseases & Disorders Sourcebook

Healthy Heart Sourcebook for Women

Basic Consumer Health Information about Cardiac Issues Specific to Women, Including Facts about Major Risk Factors and Prevention, Treatment and Control Strategies, and Important Dietary Issues

Along with a Special Section Regarding the Pros and Cons of Hormone Replacement Therapy and Its Impact on Heart Health, and Additional Help, Including Recipes, a Glossary, and a Directory of Resources

Edited by Dawn D. Matthews. 336 pages. 2000. 978-0-7808-0329-9.

SEE ALSO Cardiovascular Diseases & Disorders Sourcebook, Women's Health Concerns Sourcebook

Hepatitis Sourcebook

Basic Consumer Health Information about Hepatitis A, Hepatitis B, Hepatitis C, and Other Forms of Hepatitis, Including Autoimmune Hepatitis, Alcoholic Hepatitis, Nonalcoholic Steatohepatitis, and Toxic Hepatitis, with

Facts about Risk Factors, Screening Methods, Diagnostic Tests, and Treatment Options

Along with Information on Liver Health, Tips for People Living with Chronic Hepatitis, Reports on Current Research Initiatives, a Glossary of Terms Related to Hepatitis, and a Directory of Sources for Further Help and Information

Edited by Sandra J. Judd. 597 pages. 2005. 978-0-7808-0749-5.

"Highly recommended."
— American Reference Books Annual, 2006

■

Household Safety Sourcebook

Basic Consumer Health Information about Household Safety, Including Information about Poisons, Chemicals, Fire, and Water Hazards in the Home

Along with Advice about the Safe Use of Home Maintenance Equipment, Choosing Toys and Nursery Furniture, Holiday and Recreation Safety, a Glossary, and Resources for Further Help and Information

Edited by Dawn D. Matthews. 606 pages. 2002. 978-0-7808-0338-1.

"This work will be useful in public libraries with large consumer health and wellness departments."
— American Reference Books Annual, 2003

"As a sourcebook on household safety this book meets its mark. It is encyclopedic in scope and covers a wide range of safety issues that are commonly seen in the home."
— E-Streams, Jul '02

■

Hypertension Sourcebook

Basic Consumer Health Information about the Causes, Diagnosis, and Treatment of High Blood Pressure, with Facts about Consequences, Complications, and Co-Occurring Disorders, Such as Coronary Heart Disease, Diabetes, Stroke, Kidney Disease, and Hypertensive Retinopathy, and Issues in Blood Pressure Control, Including Dietary Choices, Stress Management, and Medications

Along with Reports on Current Research Initiatives and Clinical Trials, a Glossary, and Resources for Additional Help and Information

Edited by Dawn D. Matthews and Karen Bellenir. 613 pages. 2004. 978-0-7808-0674-0.

"Academic, public, and medical libraries will want to add the *Hypertension Sourcebook* to their collections."
— E-Streams, Aug '05

"The strength of this source is the wide range of information given about hypertension."
— American Reference Books Annual, 2005

■

Immune System Disorders Sourcebook, 2nd Edition

Basic Consumer Health Information about Disorders of the Immune System, Including Immune System Function and Response, Diagnosis of Immune Disorders, Information about Inherited Immune Disease, Acquired Immune Disease, and Autoimmune Diseases, Including Primary Immune Deficiency, Acquired Immunodeficiency Syndrome (AIDS), Lupus, Multiple Sclerosis, Type 1 Diabetes, Rheumatoid Arthritis, and Graves' Disease

Along with Treatments, Tips for Coping with Immune Disorders, a Glossary, and a Directory of Additional Resources.

Edited by Joyce Brennfleck Shannon. 671 pages. 2005. 978-0-7808-0748-8.

"Highly recommended for academic and public libraries." — American Reference Books Annual, 2006

"The updated second edition is a 'must' for any consumer health library seeking a solid resource covering the treatments, symptoms, and options for immune disorder sufferers. . . . An excellent guide."
— MBR Bookwatch, Jan '06

■

Infant & Toddler Health Sourcebook

Basic Consumer Health Information about the Physical and Mental Development of Newborns, Infants, and Toddlers, Including Neonatal Concerns, Nutrition Recommendations, Immunization Schedules, Common Pediatric Disorders, Assessments and Milestones, Safety Tips, and Advice for Parents and Other Caregivers

Along with a Glossary of Terms and Resource Listings for Additional Help

Edited by Jenifer Swanson. 585 pages. 2000. 978-0-7808-0246-9.

"As a reference for the general public, this would be useful in any library." — E-Streams, May '01

"Recommended reference source."
— Booklist, American Library Association, Feb '01

"This is a good source for general use."
— American Reference Books Annual, 2001

■

Infectious Diseases Sourcebook

Basic Consumer Health Information about Non-Contagious Bacterial, Viral, Prion, Fungal, and Parasitic Diseases Spread by Food and Water, Insects and Animals, or Environmental Contact, Including Botulism, E. Coli, Encephalitis, Legionnaires' Disease, Lyme Disease, Malaria, Plague, Rabies, Salmonella, Tetanus, and Others, and Facts about Newly Emerging Diseases, Such as Hantavirus, Mad Cow Disease, Monkeypox, and West Nile Virus

Along with Information about Preventing Disease Transmission, the Threat of Bioterrorism, and Current Research Initiatives, with a Glossary and Directory of Resources for More Information

Edited by Karen Bellenir. 634 pages. 2004. 978-0-7808-0675-7.

Injury & Trauma Sourcebook

Basic Consumer Health Information about the Impact of Injury, the Diagnosis and Treatment of Common and Traumatic Injuries, Emergency Care, and Specific Injuries Related to Home, Community, Workplace, Transportation, and Recreation

Along with Guidelines for Injury Prevention, a Glossary, and a Directory of Additional Resources

Edited by Joyce Brennfleck Shannon. 696 pages. 2002. 978-0-7808-0421-0.

Kidney & Urinary Tract Diseases & Disorders Sourcebook

SEE *Urinary Tract & Kidney Diseases & Disorders Sourcebook*

Learning Disabilities Sourcebook, 2nd Edition

Basic Consumer Health Information about Learning Disabilities, Including Dyslexia, Developmental Speech and Language Disabilities, Non-Verbal Learning Disorders, Developmental Arithmetic Disorder, Developmental Writing Disorder, and Other Conditions That Impede Learning Such as Attention Deficit/Hyperactivity Disorder, Brain Injury, Hearing Impairment, Klinefelter Syndrome, Dyspraxia, and Tourette's Syndrome

Along with Facts about Educational Issues and Assistive Technology, Coping Strategies, a Glossary of Related Terms, and Resources for Further Help and Information

Edited by Dawn D. Matthews. 621 pages. 2003. 978-0-7808-0626-9.

Leukemia Sourcebook

Basic Consumer Health Information about Adult and Childhood Leukemias, Including Acute Lymphocytic Leukemia (ALL), Chronic Lymphocytic Leukemia (CLL), Acute Myelogenous Leukemia (AML), Chronic Myelogenous Leukemia (CML), and Hairy Cell Leukemia, and Treatments Such as Chemotherapy, Radiation Therapy, Peripheral Blood Stem Cell and Marrow Transplantation, and Immunotherapy

Along with Tips for Life During and After Treatment, a Glossary, and Directories of Additional Resources

Edited by Joyce Brennfleck Shannon. 587 pages. 2003. 978-0-7808-0627-6.

Liver Disorders Sourcebook

Basic Consumer Health Information about the Liver and How It Works; Liver Diseases, Including Cancer, Cirrhosis, Hepatitis, and Toxic and Drug Related Diseases; Tips for Maintaining a Healthy Liver; Laboratory Tests, Radiology Tests, and Facts about Liver Transplantation

Along with a Section on Support Groups, a Glossary, and Resource Listings

Edited by Joyce Brennfleck Shannon. 591 pages. 2000. 978-0-7808-0383-1.

"A valuable resource."
—*American Reference Books Annual, 2001*

"This title is recommended for health sciences and public libraries with consumer health collections."
—*E-Streams, Oct '00*

"Recommended reference source."
—*Booklist, American Library Association, Jun '00*

■

Lung Disorders Sourcebook

Basic Consumer Health Information about Emphysema, Pneumonia, Tuberculosis, Asthma, Cystic Fibrosis, and Other Lung Disorders, Including Facts about Diagnostic Procedures, Treatment Strategies, Disease Prevention Efforts, and Such Risk Factors as Smoking, Air Pollution, and Exposure to Asbestos, Radon, and Other Agents

Along with a Glossary and Resources for Additional Help and Information

Edited by Dawn D. Matthews. 678 pages. 2002. 978-0-7808-0339-8.

"This title is a great addition for public and school libraries because it provides concise health information on the lungs."
—*American Reference Books Annual, 2003*

"Highly recommended for academic and medical reference collections." —*Library Bookwatch, Sep '02*

SEE ALSO Respiratory Diseases & Disorders Sourcebook

■

Medical Tests Sourcebook, 2nd Edition

Basic Consumer Health Information about Medical Tests, Including Age-Specific Health Tests, Important Health Screenings and Exams, Home-Use Tests, Blood and Specimen Tests, Electrical Tests, Scope Tests, Genetic Testing, and Imaging Tests, Such as X-Rays, Ultrasound, Computed Tomography, Magnetic Resonance Imaging, Angiography, and Nuclear Medicine

Along with a Glossary and Directory of Additional Resources

Edited by Joyce Brennfleck Shannon. 654 pages. 2004. 978-0-7808-0670-2.

"Recommended for hospital and health sciences libraries with consumer health collections."
—*E-Streams, Mar '00*

"This is an overall excellent reference with a wealth of general knowledge that may aid those who are reluctant to get vital tests performed."
—*Today's Librarian, Jan '00*

"A valuable reference guide."
—*American Reference Books Annual, 2000*

■

Men's Health Concerns Sourcebook, 2nd Edition

Basic Consumer Health Information about the Medical and Mental Concerns of Men, Including Theories about the Shorter Male Lifespan, the Leading Causes of Death and Disability, Physical Concerns of Special Significance to Men, Reproductive and Sexual Concerns, Sexually Transmitted Diseases, Men's Mental and Emotional Health, and Lifestyle Choices That Affect Wellness, Such as Nutrition, Fitness, and Substance Use

Along with a Glossary of Related Terms and a Directory of Organizational Resources in Men's Health

Edited by Robert Aquinas McNally. 644 pages. 2004. 978-0-7808-0671-9.

"A very accessible reference for non-specialist general readers and consumers." —*The Bookwatch, Jun '04*

"This comprehensive resource and the series are highly recommended."
—*American Reference Books Annual, 2000*

"Recommended reference source."
—*Booklist, American Library Association, Dec '98*

■

Mental Health Disorders Sourcebook, 3rd Edition

Basic Consumer Health Information about Mental and Emotional Health and Mental Illness, Including Facts about Depression, Bipolar Disorder, and Other Mood Disorders, Phobias, Post-Traumatic Stress Disorder (PTSD), Obsessive-Compulsive Disorder, and Other Anxiety Disorders, Impulse Control Disorders, Eating Disorders, Personality Disorders, and Psychotic Disorders, Including Schizophrenia and Dissociative Disorders

Along with Statistical Information, a Special Section Concerning Mental Health Issues in Children and Adolescents, a Glossary, and Directories of Resources for Additional Help and Information

Edited by Karen Bellenir. 661 pages. 2005. 978-0-7808-0747-1.

"Recommended for public libraries and academic libraries with an undergraduate program in psychology."
—*American Reference Books Annual, 2006*

"Recommended reference source."
—*Booklist, American Library Association, Jun '00*

Mental Retardation Sourcebook

Basic Consumer Health Information about Mental Retardation and Its Causes, Including Down Syndrome, Fetal Alcohol Syndrome, Fragile X Syndrome, Genetic Conditions, Injury, and Environmental Sources Along with Preventive Strategies, Parenting Issues, Educational Implications, Health Care Needs, Employment and Economic Matters, Legal Issues, a Glossary, and a Resource Listing for Additional Help and Information

Edited by Joyce Brennfleck Shannon. 642 pages. 2000. 978-0-7808-0377-0.

"Public libraries will find the book useful for reference and as a beginning research point for students, parents, and caregivers."
— *American Reference Books Annual, 2001*

"The strength of this work is that it compiles many basic fact sheets and addresses for further information in one volume. It is intended and suitable for the general public. This sourcebook is relevant to any collection providing health information to the general public."
— *E-Streams, Nov '00*

"From preventing retardation to parenting and family challenges, this covers health, social and legal issues and will prove an invaluable overview."
— *Reviewer's Bookwatch, Jul '00*

∎

Movement Disorders Sourcebook

Basic Consumer Health Information about Neurological Movement Disorders, Including Essential Tremor, Parkinson's Disease, Dystonia, Cerebral Palsy, Huntington's Disease, Myasthenia Gravis, Multiple Sclerosis, and Other Early-Onset and Adult-Onset Movement Disorders, Their Symptoms and Causes, Diagnostic Tests, and Treatments Along with Mobility and Assistive Technology Information, a Glossary, and a Directory of Additional Resources

Edited by Joyce Brennfleck Shannon. 655 pages. 2003. 978-0-7808-0628-3.

". . . a good resource for consumers and recommended for public, community college and undergraduate libraries." — *American Reference Books Annual, 2004*

∎

Muscular Dystrophy Sourcebook

Basic Consumer Health Information about Congenital, Childhood-Onset, and Adult-Onset Forms of Muscular Dystrophy, Such as Duchenne, Becker, Emery-Dreifuss, Distal, Limb-Girdle, Facioscapulohumeral (FSHD), Myotonic, and Ophthalmoplegic Muscular Dystrophies, Including Facts about Diagnostic Tests, Medical and Physical Therapies, Management of Co-Occurring Conditions, and Parenting Guidelines Along with Practical Tips for Home Care, a Glossary, and Directories of Additional Resources

Edited by Joyce Brennfleck Shannon. 577 pages. 2004. 978-0-7808-0676-4.

"This book is highly recommended for public and academic libraries as well as health care offices that support the information needs of patients and their families."
— *E-Streams, Apr '05*

"Excellent reference." — *The Bookwatch, Jan '05*

∎

Obesity Sourcebook

Basic Consumer Health Information about Diseases and Other Problems Associated with Obesity, and Including Facts about Risk Factors, Prevention Issues, and Management Approaches Along with Statistical and Demographic Data, Information about Special Populations, Research Updates, a Glossary, and Source Listings for Further Help and Information

Edited by Wilma Caldwell and Chad T. Kimball. 376 pages. 2001. 978-0-7808-0333-6.

"The book synthesizes the reliable medical literature on obesity into one easy-to-read and useful resource for the general public."
— *American Reference Books Annual, 2002*

"This is a very useful resource book for the lay public."
— *Doody's Review Service, Nov '01*

"Well suited for the health reference collection of a public library or an academic health science library that serves the general population." — *E-Streams, Sep '01*

"Recommended reference source."
— *Booklist, American Library Association, Apr '01*

"Recommended pick both for specialty health library collections and any general consumer health reference collection." — *The Bookwatch, Apr '01*

∎

Oral Health Sourcebook

SEE *Dental Care & Oral Health Sourcebook*

∎

Osteoporosis Sourcebook

Basic Consumer Health Information about Primary and Secondary Osteoporosis and Juvenile Osteoporosis and Related Conditions, Including Fibrous Dysplasia, Gaucher Disease, Hyperthyroidism, Hypophosphatasia, Myeloma, Osteopetrosis, Osteogenesis Imperfecta, and Paget's Disease Along with Information about Risk Factors, Treatments, Traditional and Non-Traditional Pain Management, a Glossary of Related Terms, and a Directory of Resources

Edited by Allan R. Cook. 584 pages. 2001. 978-0-7808-0239-1.

"This would be a book to be kept in a staff or patient library. The targeted audience is the layperson, but the therapist who needs a quick bit of information on a particular topic will also find the book useful."
— *Physical Therapy, Jan '02*

Pain Sourcebook, 2nd Edition

Basic Consumer Health Information about Specific Forms of Acute and Chronic Pain, Including Muscle and Skeletal Pain, Nerve Pain, Cancer Pain, and Disorders Characterized by Pain, Such as Fibromyalgia, Shingles, Angina, Arthritis, and Headaches

Along with Information about Pain Medications and Management Techniques, Complementary and Alternative Pain Relief Options, Tips for People Living with Chronic Pain, a Glossary, and a Directory of Sources for Further Information

Edited by Karen Bellenir. 670 pages. 2002. 978-0-7808-0612-2.

Pediatric Cancer Sourcebook

Basic Consumer Health Information about Leukemias, Brain Tumors, Sarcomas, Lymphomas, and Other Cancers in Infants, Children, and Adolescents, Including Descriptions of Cancers, Treatments, and Coping Strategies

Along with Suggestions for Parents, Caregivers, and Concerned Relatives, a Glossary of Cancer Terms, and Resource Listings

Edited by Edward J. Prucha. 587 pages. 1999. 978-0-7808-0245-2.

Physical & Mental Issues in Aging Sourcebook

Basic Consumer Health Information on Physical and Mental Disorders Associated with the Aging Process, Including Concerns about Cardiovascular Disease, Pulmonary Disease, Oral Health, Digestive Disorders, Musculoskeletal and Skin Disorders, Metabolic Changes, Sexual and Reproductive Issues, and Changes in Vision, Hearing, and Other Senses

Along with Data about Longevity and Causes of Death, Information on Acute and Chronic Pain, Descriptions of Mental Concerns, a Glossary of Terms, and Resource Listings for Additional Help

Edited by Jenifer Swanson. 660 pages. 1999. 978-0-7808-0233-9.

Podiatry Sourcebook, 2nd Edition

Basic Consumer Health Information about Disorders, Diseases, Deformities, and Injuries that Affect the Foot and Ankle, Including Sprains, Corns, Calluses, Bunions, Plantar Warts, Plantar Fasciitis, Neuromas, Clubfoot, Flat Feet, Achilles Tendonitis, and Much More

Along with Information about Selecting a Foot Care Specialist, Foot Fitness, Shoes and Socks, Diagnostic Tests and Corrective Procedures, Financial Assistance for Corrective Devices, a Glossary of Related Terms, and a Directory of Resources for Additional Help and Information

Edited by Ivy L. Alexander. 543 pages. 2007. 978-0-7808-0944-4.

"Recommended reference source."
— Booklist, American Library Association, Feb '02

"There is a lot of information presented here on a topic that is usually only covered sparingly in most larger comprehensive medical encyclopedias."
— American Reference Books Annual, 2002

∎

Pregnancy & Birth Sourcebook, 2nd Edition

Basic Consumer Health Information about Conception and Pregnancy, Including Facts about Fertility, Infertility, Pregnancy Symptoms and Complications, Fetal Growth and Development, Labor, Delivery, and the Postpartum Period, as Well as Information about Maintaining Health and Wellness during Pregnancy and Caring for a Newborn

Along with Information about Public Health Assistance for Low-Income Pregnant Women, a Glossary, and Directories of Agencies and Organizations Providing Help and Support

Edited by Amy L. Sutton. 626 pages. 2004. 978-0-7808-0672-6.

"Will appeal to public and school reference collections strong in medicine and women's health. . . . Deserves a spot on any medical reference shelf."
— The Bookwatch, Jul '04

"A well-organized handbook. Recommended."
— Choice, Association of College & Research Libraries, Apr '98

"Recommended reference source."
— Booklist, American Library Association, Mar '98

"Recommended for public libraries."
— American Reference Books Annual, 1998

SEE ALSO Breastfeeding Sourcebook, Congenital Disorders Sourcebook, Family Planning Sourcebook

∎

Prostate & Urological Disorders Sourcebook

Basic Consumer Health Information about Urogenital and Sexual Disorders in Men, Including Prostate and Other Andrological Cancers, Prostatitis, Benign Prostatic Hyperplasia, Testicular and Penile Trauma, Cryptorchidism, Peyronie Disease, Erectile Dysfunction, and Male Factor Infertility, and Facts about Commonly Used Tests and Procedures, Such as Prostatectomy, Vasectomy, Vasectomy Reversal, Penile Implants, and Semen Analysis

Along with a Glossary of Andrological Terms and a Directory of Resources for Additional Information

Edited by Karen Bellenir. 631 pages. 2005. 978-0-7808-0797-6.

Prostate Cancer Sourcebook

Basic Consumer Health Information about Prostate Cancer, Including Information about the Associated Risk Factors, Detection, Diagnosis, and Treatment of Prostate Cancer

Along with Information on Non-Malignant Prostate Conditions, and Featuring a Section Listing Support and Treatment Centers and a Glossary of Related Terms

Edited by Dawn D. Matthews. 358 pages. 2001. 978-0-7808-0324-4.

"Recommended reference source."
— Booklist, American Library Association, Jan '02

"A valuable resource for health care consumers seeking information on the subject. . . . All text is written in a clear, easy-to-understand language that avoids technical jargon. Any library that collects consumer health resources would strengthen their collection with the addition of the Prostate Cancer Sourcebook."
— American Reference Books Annual, 2002

SEE ALSO Men's Health Concerns Sourcebook

∎

Reconstructive & Cosmetic Surgery Sourcebook

Basic Consumer Health Information on Cosmetic and Reconstructive Plastic Surgery, Including Statistical Information about Different Surgical Procedures, Things to Consider Prior to Surgery, Plastic Surgery Techniques and Tools, Emotional and Psychological Considerations, and Procedure-Specific Information

Along with a Glossary of Terms and a Listing of Resources for Additional Help and Information

Edited by M. Lisa Weatherford. 374 pages. 2001. 978-0-7808-0214-8.

"An excellent reference that addresses cosmetic and medically necessary reconstructive surgeries. . . . The style of the prose is calm and reassuring, discussing the many positive outcomes now available due to advances in surgical techniques."
— American Reference Books Annual, 2002

"Recommended for health science libraries that are open to the public, as well as hospital libraries that are open to the patients. This book is a good resource for the consumer interested in plastic surgery."
— E-Streams, Dec '01

"Recommended reference source."
— Booklist, American Library Association, Jul '01

∎

Rehabilitation Sourcebook

Basic Consumer Health Information about Rehabilitation for People Recovering from Heart Surgery, Spinal Cord Injury, Stroke, Orthopedic Impairments, Amputation, Pulmonary Impairments, Traumatic Injury, and More, Including Physical Therapy, Occupational Therapy, Speech/Language Therapy, Massage Therapy, Dance Therapy, Art Therapy, and Recreational Therapy

Along with Information on Assistive and Adaptive Devices, a Glossary, and Resources for Additional Help and Information

Edited by Dawn D. Matthews. 531 pages. 1999. 978-0-7808-0236-0.

"This is an excellent resource for public library reference and health collections."
— American Reference Books Annual, 2001

"Recommended reference source."
— Booklist, American Library Association, May '00

■

Respiratory Diseases & Disorders Sourcebook

Basic Information about Respiratory Diseases and Disorders, Including Asthma, Cystic Fibrosis, Pneumonia, the Common Cold, Influenza, and Others, Featuring Facts about the Respiratory System, Statistical and Demographic Data, Treatments, Self-Help Management Suggestions, and Current Research Initiatives

Edited by Allan R. Cook and Peter D. Dresser. 771 pages. 1995. 978-0-7808-0037-3.

"Designed for the layperson and for patients and their families coping with respiratory illness. . . . an extensive array of information on diagnosis, treatment, management, and prevention of respiratory illnesses for the general reader." — Choice, Association of College & Research Libraries, Jun '96

"A highly recommended text for all collections. It is a comforting reminder of the power of knowledge that good books carry between their covers."
— Academic Library Book Review, Spring '96

"A comprehensive collection of authoritative information presented in a nontechnical, humanitarian style for patients, families, and caregivers."
— Association of Operating Room Nurses, Sep/Oct '95

SEE ALSO Lung Disorders Sourcebook

■

Sexually Transmitted Diseases Sourcebook, 3rd Edition

Basic Consumer Health Information about Chlamydial Infections, Gonorrhea, Hepatitis, Herpes, HIV/AIDS, Human Papillomavirus, Pubic Lice, Scabies, Syphilis, Trichomoniasis, Vaginal Infections, and Other Sexually Transmitted Diseases, Including Facts about Risk Factors, Symptoms, Diagnosis, Treatment, and the Prevention of Sexually Transmitted Infections

Along with Updates on Current Research Initiatives, a Glossary of Related Terms, and Resources for Additional Help and Information

Edited by Amy L. Sutton. 629 pages. 2006. 978-0-7808-0824-9.

"Recommended for consumer health collections in public libraries, and secondary school and community college libraries."
— American Reference Books Annual, 2002

"Every school and public library should have a copy of this comprehensive and user-friendly reference book."
— Choice, Association of College & Research Libraries, Sep '01

"This is a highly recommended book. This is an especially important book for all school and public libraries."
— AIDS Book Review Journal, Jul-Aug '01

"Recommended reference source."
— Booklist, American Library Association, Apr '01

■

Sleep Disorders Sourcebook, 2nd Edition

Basic Consumer Health Information about Sleep and Sleep Disorders, Including Insomnia, Sleep Apnea, Restless Legs Syndrome, Narcolepsy, Parasomnias, and Other Health Problems That Affect Sleep, Plus Facts about Diagnostic Procedures, Treatment Strategies, Sleep Medications, and Tips for Improving Sleep Quality

Along with a Glossary of Related Terms and Resources for Additional Help and Information

Edited by Amy L. Sutton. 567 pages. 2005. 978-0-7808-0743-3.

"This book will be useful for just about everybody, especially the 40 million Americans with sleep disorders."
— American Reference Books Annual, 2006

"Recommended for public libraries and libraries supporting health care professionals." — E-Streams, Sep '05

". . . key medical library acquisition."
— The Bookwatch, Jun '05

■

Smoking Concerns Sourcebook

Basic Consumer Health Information about Nicotine Addiction and Smoking Cessation, Featuring Facts about the Health Effects of Tobacco Use, Including Lung and Other Cancers, Heart Disease, Stroke, and Respiratory Disorders, Such as Emphysema and Chronic Bronchitis

Along with Information about Smoking Prevention Programs, Suggestions for Achieving and Maintaining a Smoke-Free Lifestyle, Statistics about Tobacco Use, Reports on Current Research Initiatives, a Glossary of Related Terms, and Directories of Resources for Additional Help and Information

Edited by Karen Bellenir. 621 pages. 2004. 978-0-7808-0323-7.

"Provides everything needed for the student or general reader seeking practical details on the effects of tobacco use." — The Bookwatch, Mar '05

"Public libraries and consumer health care libraries will find this work useful."
— American Reference Books Annual, 2005

Sports Injuries Sourcebook, 3rd Edition

Basic Consumer Health Information about Sprains and Strains, Fractures, Growth Plate Injuries, Overtraining Injuries, and Injuries to the Head, Face, Shoulders, Elbows, Hands, Spinal Column, Knees, Ankles, and Feet, and with Facts about Heat-Related Illness, Steroids and Sport Supplements, Protective Equipment, Diagnostic Procedures, Treatment Options, and Rehabilitation

Along with a Glossary of Related Terms and a Directory of Resources for Additional Help and Information

Edited by Sandra J. Judd. 651 pages. 2007. 978-0-7808-0949-9.

"This is an excellent reference for consumers and it is recommended for public, community college, and undergraduate libraries."
— American Reference Books Annual, 2003

"Recommended reference source."
— Booklist, American Library Association, Feb '03

Stress-Related Disorders Sourcebook

Basic Consumer Health Information about Stress and Stress-Related Disorders, Including Stress Origins and Signals, Environmental Stress at Work and Home, Mental and Emotional Stress Associated with Depression, Post-Traumatic Stress Disorder, Panic Disorder, Suicide, and the Physical Effects of Stress on the Cardiovascular, Immune, and Nervous Systems

Along with Stress Management Techniques, a Glossary, and a Listing of Additional Resources

Edited by Joyce Brennfleck Shannon. 610 pages. 2002. 978-0-7808-0560-6.

"Well written for a general readership, the Stress-Related Disorders Sourcebook is a useful addition to the health reference literature."
— American Reference Books Annual, 2003

"I am impressed by the amount of information. It offers a thorough overview of the causes and consequences of stress for the layperson. . . . A well-done and thorough reference guide for professionals and nonprofessionals alike." — Doody's Review Service, Dec '02

Stroke Sourcebook

Basic Consumer Health Information about Stroke, Including Ischemic, Hemorrhagic, Transient Ischemic Attack (TIA), and Pediatric Stroke, Stroke Triggers and Risks, Diagnostic Tests, Treatments, and Rehabilitation Information

Along with Stroke Prevention Guidelines, Legal and Financial Information, a Glossary, and a Directory of Additional Resources

Edited by Joyce Brennfleck Shannon. 606 pages. 2003. 978-0-7808-0630-6.

"This volume is highly recommended and should be in every medical, hospital, and public library."
— American Reference Books Annual, 2004

"Highly recommended for the amount and variety of topics and information covered." — Choice, Nov '03

Surgery Sourcebook

Basic Consumer Health Information about Inpatient and Outpatient Surgeries, Including Cardiac, Vascular, Orthopedic, Ocular, Reconstructive, Cosmetic, Gynecologic, and Ear, Nose, and Throat Procedures and More

Along with Information about Operating Room Policies and Instruments, Laser Surgery Techniques, Hospital Errors, Statistical Data, a Glossary, and Listings of Sources for Further Help and Information

Edited by Annemarie S. Muth and Karen Bellenir. 596 pages. 2002. 978-0-7808-0380-0.

"Large public libraries and medical libraries would benefit from this material in their reference collections."
— American Reference Books Annual, 2004

"Invaluable reference for public and school library collections alike." — Library Bookwatch, Apr '03

Thyroid Disorders Sourcebook

Basic Consumer Health Information about Disorders of the Thyroid and Parathyroid Glands, Including Hypothyroidism, Hyperthyroidism, Graves Disease, Hashimoto Thyroiditis, Thyroid Cancer, and Parathyroid Disorders, Featuring Facts about Symptoms, Risk Factors, Tests, and Treatments

Along with Information about the Effects of Thyroid Imbalance on Other Body Systems, Environmental Factors That Affect the Thyroid Gland, a Glossary, and a Directory of Additional Resources

Edited by Joyce Brennfleck Shannon. 599 pages. 2005. 978-0-7808-0745-7.

"Recommended for consumer health collections."
— American Reference Books Annual, 2006

"Highly recommended pick for basic consumer health reference holdings at all levels."
— The Bookwatch, Aug '05

Transplantation Sourcebook

Basic Consumer Health Information about Organ and Tissue Transplantation, Including Physical and Financial Preparations, Procedures and Issues Relating to Specific Solid Organ and Tissue Transplants, Rehabilitation, Pediatric Transplant Information, the Future of Transplantation, and Organ and Tissue Donation

Along with a Glossary and Listings of Additional Resources

Edited by Joyce Brennfleck Shannon. 628 pages. 2002. 978-0-7808-0322-0.

"Along with these advances [in transplantation technology] have come a number of daunting questions for potential transplant patients, their families, and their health care providers. This reference text is the best single tool to address many of these questions. . . . It will be a much-needed addition to the reference collections in health care, academic, and large public libraries."
— American Reference Books Annual, 2003

"Recommended for libraries with an interest in offering consumer health information."   — E-Streams, Jul '02

"This is a unique and valuable resource for patients facing transplantation and their families."
— Doody's Review Service, Jun '02

Traveler's Health Sourcebook

Basic Consumer Health Information for Travelers, Including Physical and Medical Preparations, Transportation Health and Safety, Essential Information about Food and Water, Sun Exposure, Insect and Snake Bites, Camping and Wilderness Medicine, and Travel with Physical or Medical Disabilities

Along with International Travel Tips, Vaccination Recommendations, Geographical Health Issues, Disease Risks, a Glossary, and a Listing of Additional Resources

Edited by Joyce Brennfleck Shannon. 613 pages. 2000. 978-0-7808-0384-8.

"Recommended reference source."
— Booklist, American Library Association, Feb '01

"This book is recommended for any public library, any travel collection, and especially any collection for the physically disabled."
— American Reference Books Annual, 2001

SEE ALSO Worldwide Health Sourcebook

Urinary Tract & Kidney Diseases & Disorders Sourcebook, 2nd Edition

Basic Consumer Health Information about the Urinary System, Including the Bladder, Urethra, Ureters, and Kidneys, with Facts about Urinary Tract Infections, Incontinence, Congenital Disorders, Kidney Stones, Cancers of the Urinary Tract and Kidneys, Kidney Failure, Dialysis, and Kidney Transplantation

Along with Statistical and Demographic Information, Reports on Current Research in Kidney and Urologic Health, a Summary of Commonly Used Diagnostic Tests, a Glossary of Related Terms, and a Directory of Resources for Additional Help and Information

Edited by Ivy L. Alexander. 649 pages. 2005. 978-0-7808-0750-1.

"A good choice for a consumer health information library or for a medical library needing information to refer to their patients."
— American Reference Books Annual, 2006

Vegetarian Sourcebook

Basic Consumer Health Information about Vegetarian Diets, Lifestyle, and Philosophy, Including Definitions of Vegetarianism and Veganism, Tips about Adopting Vegetarianism, Creating a Vegetarian Pantry, and Meeting Nutritional Needs of Vegetarians, with Facts Regarding Vegetarianism's Effect on Pregnant and Lactating Women, Children, Athletes, and Senior Citizens

Along with a Glossary of Commonly Used Vegetarian Terms and Resources for Additional Help and Information

Edited by Chad T. Kimball. 360 pages. 2002. 978-0-7808-0439-5.

"Organizes into one concise volume the answers to the most common questions concerning vegetarian diets and lifestyles. This title is recommended for public and secondary school libraries."   — E-Streams, Apr '03

"Invaluable reference for public and school library collections alike."   — Library Bookwatch, Apr '03

"The articles in this volume are easy to read and come from authoritative sources. The book does not necessarily support the vegetarian diet but instead provides the pros and cons of this important decision. The Vegetarian Sourcebook is recommended for public libraries and consumer health libraries."
— American Reference Books Annual, 2003

SEE ALSO Diet & Nutrition Sourcebook

Women's Health Concerns Sourcebook, 2nd Edition

Basic Consumer Health Information about the Medical and Mental Concerns of Women, Including Maintaining Health and Wellness, Gynecological Concerns, Breast Health, Sexuality and Reproductive Issues, Menopause, Cancer in Women, Leading Causes of Death and Disability among Women, Physical Concerns of Special Significance to Women, and Women's Mental and Emotional Health

Along with a Glossary of Related Terms and Directories of Resources for Additional Help and Information

Edited by Amy L. Sutton. 746 pages. 2004. 978-0-7808-0673-3.

"This is a useful reference book, which makes the reader knowledgeable about several issues that concern women's health. It is recommended for public libraries and home library collections."   — E-Streams, May '05

"A useful addition to public and consumer health library collections."
— American Reference Books Annual, 2005

"A highly recommended title."
— The Bookwatch, May '04

"Handy compilation. There is an impressive range of diseases, devices, disorders, procedures, and other physical and emotional issues covered . . . well organized, illustrated, and indexed."   — Choice, Association of College & Research Libraries, Jan '98

SEE ALSO Breast Cancer Sourcebook, Cancer Sourcebook for Women, Healthy Heart Sourcebook for Women, Osteoporosis Sourcebook

Workplace Health & Safety Sourcebook

Basic Consumer Health Information about Workplace Health and Safety, Including the Effect of Workplace Hazards on the Lungs, Skin, Heart, Ears, Eyes, Brain, Reproductive Organs, Musculoskeletal System, and Other Organs and Body Parts

Along with Information about Occupational Cancer, Personal Protective Equipment, Toxic and Hazardous Chemicals, Child Labor, Stress, and Workplace Violence

Edited by Chad T. Kimball. 626 pages. 2000. 978-0-7808-0231-5.

"As a reference for the general public, this would be useful in any library." — *E-Streams, Jun '01*

"Provides helpful information for primary care physicians and other caregivers interested in occupational medicine. . . . General readers; professionals."
— *Choice, Association of College & Research Libraries, May '01*

"Recommended reference source."
— *Booklist, American Library Association, Feb '01*

"Highly recommended." — *The Bookwatch, Jan '01*

Worldwide Health Sourcebook

Basic Information about Global Health Issues, Including Malnutrition, Reproductive Health, Disease Dispersion and Prevention, Emerging Diseases, Risky Health Behaviors, and the Leading Causes of Death

Along with Global Health Concerns for Children, Women, and the Elderly, Mental Health Issues, Research and Technology Advancements, and Economic, Environmental, and Political Health Implications, a Glossary, and a Resource Listing for Additional Help and Information

Edited by Joyce Brennfleck Shannon. 614 pages. 2001. 978-0-7808-0330-5.

"Named an Outstanding Academic Title."
— *Choice, Association of College & Research Libraries, Jan '02*

"Yet another handy but also unique compilation in the extensive *Health Reference Series*, this is a useful work because many of the international publications reprinted or excerpted are not readily available. Highly recommended." — *Choice, Association of College & Research Libraries, Nov '01*

"Recommended reference source."
— *Booklist, American Library Association, Oct '01*

SEE ALSO Traveler's Health Sourcebook

Teen Health Series
Helping Young Adults Understand, Manage, and Avoid Serious Illness

List price $65 per volume. **School and library price $58 per volume.**

Alcohol Information for Teens
Health Tips about Alcohol and Alcoholism
Including Facts about Underage Drinking, Preventing Teen Alcohol Use, Alcohol's Effects on the Brain and the Body, Alcohol Abuse Treatment, Help for Children of Alcoholics, and More

Edited by Joyce Brennfleck Shannon. 370 pages. 2005. 978-0-7808-0741-9.

"Boxed facts and tips add visual interest to the well-researched and clearly written text."
— *Curriculum Connection, Apr '06*

Allergy Information for Teens
Health Tips about Allergic Reactions Such as Anaphylaxis, Respiratory Problems, and Rashes
Including Facts about Identifying and Managing Allergies to Food, Pollen, Mold, Animals, Chemicals, Drugs, and Other Substances

Edited by Karen Bellenir. 410 pages. 2006. 978-0-7808-0799-0.

Asthma Information for Teens
Health Tips about Managing Asthma and Related Concerns
Including Facts about Asthma Causes, Triggers, Symptoms, Diagnosis, and Treatment

Edited by Karen Bellenir. 386 pages. 2005. 978-0-7808-0770-9.

"Highly recommended for medical libraries, public school libraries, and public libraries."
— *American Reference Books Annual, 2006*

"It is so clearly written and well organized that even hesitant readers will be able to find the facts they need, whether for reports or personal information. . . . A succinct but complete resource."
— *School Library Journal, Sep '05*

Body Information for Teens
Health Tips about Maintaining Well-Being for a Lifetime
Including Facts about the Development and Functioning of the Body's Systems, Organs, and Structures and the Health Impact of Lifestyle Choices

Edited by Sandra Augustyn Lawton. 458 pages. 2007. 978-0-7808-0443-2.

Cancer Information for Teens
Health Tips about Cancer Awareness, Prevention, Diagnosis, and Treatment
Including Facts about Frequently Occurring Cancers, Cancer Risk Factors, and Coping Strategies for Teens Fighting Cancer or Dealing with Cancer in Friends or Family Members

Edited by Wilma R. Caldwell. 428 pages. 2004. 978-0-7808-0678-8.

"Recommended for school libraries, or consumer libraries that see a lot of use by teens."
— *E-Streams, May '05*

"A valuable educational tool."
— *American Reference Books Annual, 2005*

"Young adults and their parents alike will find this new addition to the *Teen Health Series* an important reference to cancer in teens."
— *Children's Bookwatch, Feb '05*

Complementary and Alternative Medicine Information for Teens
Health Tips about Non-Traditional and Non-Western Medical Practices
Including Information about Acupuncture, Chiropractic Medicine, Dietary and Herbal Supplements, Hypnosis, Massage Therapy, Prayer and Spirituality, Reflexology, Yoga, and More

Edited by Sandra Augustyn Lawton. 405 pages. 2006. 978-0-7808-0966-6.

Diabetes Information for Teens
Health Tips about Managing Diabetes and Preventing Related Complications
Including Information about Insulin, Glucose Control, Healthy Eating, Physical Activity, and Learning to Live with Diabetes

Edited by Sandra Augustyn Lawton. 410 pages. 2006. 978-0-7808-0811-9.

645

Diet Information for Teens, 2nd Edition

Health Tips about Diet and Nutrition

Including Facts about Dietary Guidelines, Food Groups, Nutrients, Healthy Meals, Snacks, Weight Control, Medical Concerns Related to Diet, and More

Edited by Karen Bellenir. 432 pages. 2006. 978-0-7808-0820-1.

"Full of helpful insights and facts throughout the book. . . . An excellent resource to be placed in public libraries or even in personal collections."
— American Reference Books Annual, 2002

"Recommended for middle and high school libraries and media centers as well as academic libraries that educate future teachers of teenagers. It is also a suitable addition to health science libraries that serve patrons who are interested in teen health promotion and education." — E-Streams, Oct '01

"This comprehensive book would be beneficial to collections that need information about nutrition, dietary guidelines, meal planning, and weight control. . . . This reference is so easy to use that its purchase is recommended." — The Book Report, Sep-Oct '01

"This book is written in an easy to understand format describing issues that many teens face every day, and then provides thoughtful explanations so that teens can make informed decisions. This is an interesting book that provides important facts and information for today's teens." — Doody's Health Sciences Book Review Journal, Jul-Aug '01

"A comprehensive compendium of diet and nutrition. The information is presented in a straightforward, plain-spoken manner. This title will be useful to those working on reports on a variety of topics, as well as to general readers concerned about their dietary health." — School Library Journal, Jun '01

Drug Information for Teens, 2nd Edition

Health Tips about the Physical and Mental Effects of Substance Abuse

Including Information about Marijuana, Inhalants, Club Drugs, Stimulants, Hallucinogens, Opiates, Prescription and Over-the-Counter Drugs, Herbal Products, Tobacco, Alcohol, and More

Edited by Sandra Augustyn Lawton. 468 pages. 2006. 978-0-7808-0862-1.

"A clearly written resource for general readers and researchers alike." — School Library Journal

"This book is well-balanced. . . . a must for public and school libraries."
— VOYA: Voice of Youth Advocates, Dec '03

"The chapters are quick to make a connection to their teenage reading audience. The prose is straightforward and the book lends itself to spot reading. It should be useful both for practical information and for research, and it is suitable for public and school libraries." — American Reference Books Annual, 2003

"Recommended reference source."
— Booklist, American Library Association, Feb '03

"This is an excellent resource for teens and their parents. Education about drugs and substances is key to discouraging teen drug abuse and this book provides this much needed information in a way that is interesting and factual." — Doody's Review Service, Dec '02

Eating Disorders Information for Teens

Health Tips about Anorexia, Bulimia, Binge Eating, and Other Eating Disorders

Including Information on the Causes, Prevention, and Treatment of Eating Disorders, and Such Other Issues as Maintaining Healthy Eating and Exercise Habits

Edited by Sandra Augustyn Lawton. 337 pages. 2005. 978-0-7808-0783-9.

"An excellent resource for teens and those who work with them."
— VOYA: Voice of Youth Advocates, Apr '06

"A welcome addition to high school and undergraduate libraries." — American Reference Books Annual, 2006

"This book covers the topic in a lucid manner but delves deeper into every aspect of an eating disorder. A solid addition for any nonfiction or reference collection." — School Library Journal, Dec '05

Fitness Information for Teens

Health Tips about Exercise, Physical Well-Being, and Health Maintenance

Including Facts about Aerobic and Anaerobic Conditioning, Stretching, Body Shape and Body Image, Sports Training, Nutrition, and Activities for Non-Athletes

Edited by Karen Bellenir. 425 pages. 2004. 978-0-7808-0679-5.

"Another excellent offering from Omnigraphics in their Teen Health Series. . . . This book will be a great addition to any public, junior high, senior high, or secondary school library."
— American Reference Books Annual, 2005

Learning Disabilities Information for Teens

Health Tips about Academic Skills Disorders and Other Disabilities That Affect Learning

Including Information about Common Signs of Learning Disabilities, School Issues, Learning to Live with a Learning Disability, and Other Related Issues

Edited by Sandra Augustyn Lawton. 337 pages. 2005. 978-0-7808-0796-9.

"This book provides a wealth of information for any reader interested in the signs, causes, and consequences

of learning disabilities, as well as related legal rights and educational interventions. . . . Public and academic libraries should want this title for both students and general readers."
— *American Reference Books Annual, 2006*

■

Mental Health Information for Teens, 2nd Edition

Health Tips about Mental Wellness and Mental Illness

Including Facts about Mental and Emotional Health, Depression and Other Mood Disorders, Anxiety Disorders, Behavior Disorders, Self-Injury, Psychosis, Schizophrenia, and More

Edited by Karen Bellenir. 400 pages. 2006. 978-0-7808-0863-8.

"In both language and approach, this user-friendly entry in the *Teen Health Series* is on target for teens needing information on mental health concerns."
— *Booklist, American Library Association, Jan '02*

"Readers will find the material accessible and informative, with the shaded notes, facts, and embedded glossary insets adding appropriately to the already interesting and succinct presentation."
— *School Library Journal, Jan '02*

"This title is highly recommended for any library that serves adolescents and parents/caregivers of adolescents."
— *E-Streams, Jan '02*

"Recommended for high school libraries and young adult collections in public libraries. Both health professionals and teenagers will find this book useful."
— *American Reference Books Annual, 2002*

"This is a nice book written to enlighten the society, primarily teenagers, about common teen mental health issues. It is highly recommended to teachers and parents as well as adolescents."
— *Doody's Review Service, Dec '01*

■

Sexual Health Information for Teens

Health Tips about Sexual Development, Human Reproduction, and Sexually Transmitted Diseases

Including Facts about Puberty, Reproductive Health, Chlamydia, Human Papillomavirus, Pelvic Inflammatory Disease, Herpes, AIDS, Contraception, Pregnancy, and More

Edited by Deborah A. Stanley. 391 pages. 2003. 978-0-7808-0445-6.

"This work should be included in all high school libraries and many larger public libraries. . . . highly recommended."
— *American Reference Books Annual, 2004*

"*Sexual Health* approaches its subject with appropriate seriousness and offers easily accessible advice and information."
— *School Library Journal, Feb '04*

Skin Health Information for Teens

Health Tips about Dermatological Concerns and Skin Cancer Risks

Including Facts about Acne, Warts, Hives, and Other Conditions and Lifestyle Choices, Such as Tanning, Tattooing, and Piercing, That Affect the Skin, Nails, Scalp, and Hair

Edited by Robert Aquinas McNally. 429 pages. 2003. 978-0-7808-0446-3.

"This volume, as with others in the series, will be a useful addition to school and public library collections."
— *American Reference Books Annual, 2004*

"There is no doubt that this reference tool is valuable."
— *VOYA: Voice of Youth Advocates, Feb '04*

"This volume serves as a one-stop source and should be a necessity for any health collection."
— *Library Media Connection*

■

Sports Injuries Information for Teens

Health Tips about Sports Injuries and Injury Protection

Including Facts about Specific Injuries, Emergency Treatment, Rehabilitation, Sports Safety, Competition Stress, Fitness, Sports Nutrition, Steroid Risks, and More

Edited by Joyce Brennfleck Shannon. 405 pages. 2003. 978-0-7808-0447-0.

"This work will be useful in the young adult collections of public libraries as well as high school libraries."
— *American Reference Books Annual, 2004*

■

Suicide Information for Teens

Health Tips about Suicide Causes and Prevention

Including Facts about Depression, Risk Factors, Getting Help, Survivor Support, and More

Edited by Joyce Brennfleck Shannon. 368 pages. 2005. 978-0-7808-0737-2.

■

Tobacco Information for Teens

Health Tips about the Hazards of Using Cigarettes, Smokeless Tobacco, and Other Nicotine Products

Including Facts about Nicotine Addiction, Immediate and Long-Term Health Effects of Tobacco Use, Related Cancers, Smoking Cessation, Tobacco Use Prevention, and Tobacco Use Statistics

Edited by Karen Bellenir. 440 pages. 2007. 978-0-7808-0976-5.

Health Reference Series

Adolescent Health Sourcebook, 2nd Edition

Adult Health Concerns Sourcebook

AIDS Sourcebook, 4th Edition

Alcoholism Sourcebook, 2nd Edition

Allergies Sourcebook, 3rd Edition

Alzheimer Disease Sourcebook, 4th Edition

Arthritis Sourcebook, 2nd Edition

Asthma Sourcebook, 2nd Edition

Attention Deficit Disorder Sourcebook

Autism & Pervasive Developmental Disorders Sourcebook

Back & Neck Sourcebook, 2nd Edition

Blood & Circulatory Disorders Sourcebook, 2nd Edition

Brain Disorders Sourcebook, 2nd Edition

Breast Cancer Sourcebook, 2nd Edition

Breastfeeding Sourcebook

Burns Sourcebook

Cancer Sourcebook, 5th Edition

Cancer Sourcebook for Women, 3rd Edition

Cancer Survivorship Sourcebook

Cardiovascular Diseases & Disorders Sourcebook, 3rd Edition

Caregiving Sourcebook

Child Abuse Sourcebook

Childhood Diseases & Disorders Sourcebook

Colds, Flu & Other Common Ailments Sourcebook

Communication Disorders Sourcebook

Complementary & Alternative Medicine Sourcebook, 3rd Edition

Congenital Disorders Sourcebook, 2nd Edition

Contagious Diseases Sourcebook

Cosmetic & Reconstructive Surgery Sourcebook, 2nd Edition

Death & Dying Sourcebook, 2nd Edition

Dental Care and Oral Health Sourcebook, 3rd Edition

Depression Sourcebook, 2nd Edition

Dermatological Disorders Sourcebook, 2nd Edition

Diabetes Sourcebook, 4th Edition

Diet & Nutrition Sourcebook, 3rd Edition

Digestive Diseases & Disorder Sourcebook

Disabilities Sourcebook

Disease Management Sourcebook

Domestic Violence Sourcebook, 2nd Edition

Drug Abuse Sourcebook, 2nd Edition

Ear, Nose & Throat Disorders Sourcebook, 2nd Edition

Eating Disorders Sourcebook, 2nd Edition

Emergency Medical Services Sourcebook

Endocrine & Metabolic Disorders Sourcebook, 2nd Edition

EnvironmentalHealth Sourcebook, 2nd Edition

Ethnic Diseases Sourcebook

Eye Care Sourcebook, 3rd Edition

Family Planning Sourcebook

Fitness & Exercise Sourcebook, 3rd Edition

Food Safety Sourcebook

Forensic Medicine Sourcebook

Gastrointestinal Diseases & Disorders Sourcebook, 2nd Edition

Genetic Disorders Sourcebook, 3rd Edition

Head Trauma Sourcebook

Headache Sourcebook

Health Insurance Sourcebook

Healthy Aging Sourcebook

Healthy Children Sourcebook

Healthy Heart Sourcebook for Women

Hepatitis Sourcebook

Household Safety Sourcebook

Hypertension Sourcebook

Immune System Disorders Sourcebook, 2nd Edition

Infant & Toddler Health Sourcebook

Infectious Diseases Sourcebook

90 HORSENECK ROAD
MONTVILLE, N.J. 07045